Surgical Patient Care for Veterinary Technicians and Nurses

Surgical Patient Care for Veterinary Technicians and Nurses

Second Edition

Edited by

Gerianne Holzman
University of Wisconsin,
School of Veterinary Medicine Veterinary Technician
Emerita
Madison, WI

Teri Raffel Kleist
Madison College Veterinary Technician Program (Retired)
Madison, WI

WILEY Blackwell

Published by John Wiley & Sons, Inc., Hoboken, New Jersey.
Published simultaneously in Canada.

Edition History
First Edition © 2015 by John Wiley & Sons, Inc.

Library of Congress Cataloging-in-Publication Data

Names: Holzman, Gerianne, editor. | Kleist, Teri Raffel, 1961– editor. | Holzman, Gerianne. Surgical patient care for veterinary technicians and nurses.
Title: Surgical patient care for veterinary technicians and nurses / edited by Gerianne Holzman, Teri Raffel Kleist.
Description: Second edition. | Hoboken New Jersey : Wiley-Blackwell, [2024] | Includes index.
Identifiers: LCCN 2023035265 (print) | LCCN 2023035266 (ebook) | ISBN 9781119760092 (paperback) | ISBN 9781119760306 (Adobe PDF) | ISBN 9781119760290 (epub)
Subjects: MESH: Surgical Procedures, Operative–veterinary | Surgery, Veterinary–methods | Animal Technicians
Classification: LCC SF911 (print) | LCC SF911 (ebook) | NLM SF 911 | DDC 636.089/7–dc23/eng/20231004
LC record available at https://lccn.loc.gov/2023035265
LC ebook record available at https://lccn.loc.gov/2023035266

Cover Design: Wiley
Cover Image: Courtesy of Teri Kleist; Gerianne Holzman

Set in 9.5/12.5pt STIXTwoText by Straive, Pondicherry, India

SKY10060478_112323

Contents

Foreword to the First Edition *xv*
Preface *xvii*
Acknowledgments *xix*
Author Biographies *xxi*
List of Contributors *xxv*
About the Companion Website *xxvii*

1 **History and Physical Examination** *1*
Gerianne Holzman and Lana Bishop
History *1*
Vaccinations *2*
Parasites *2*
Diet *2*
Allergies *3*
Current Medication *3*
Patient's Lifestyle *3*
Medical History *3*
Client Expectation *4*
Physical Exam *5*
Temperature, Pulse, Respiration, and Weight *5*
Body Condition Score *5*
General Appearance *7*
Attitude *7*
Locomotion *8*
Head and Face *9*
Oral Pharynx *10*
Lymph Nodes *10*
Integument *10*
Musculoskeletal *10*
Perineum *13*
Abdominal Cavity *14*
Respiratory System *14*
Cardiovascular System *14*
Nervous System *15*
References *16*

2 **Preoperative Planning** *17*
Gerianne Holzman and Lana Bishop
Laboratory Tests *17*
Complete Blood Count *18*
Serum Chemistry Panel *18*
Coagulation Tests *21*
Blood Collection Tubes *21*
Urinalysis *21*
Other Diagnostic Tests *24*
Abdominocentesis *25*
Arthrocentesis *25*
Fine Needle Aspirate *27*
Imaging *28*
Personal Protection *29*
Radiographs *30*
Computed Tomography Scan and Magnetic Resonance Imaging *31*
Ultrasound *33*
Contrast Studies *36*
Cystogram *36*
Esophagram *36*
Arthrogram *37*
Enterogram *37*
Medications *37*
Antibiotics *37*
Analgesics *38*
Pathophysiology of Pain *38*
Where to Control Pain *38*
When to Control Pain *38*
Non-steroidal Anti-inflammatory Drugs (NSAIDs) *41*
Opioids *41*
References *43*

3 **Asepsis and Infection Control** *45*
Teri Raffel Kleist and Cassandra Simmons
Surgical Suite Preparation *45*
Theater Design *45*
Air Exchanges *45*
Surgical Attire *46*
Traffic *47*
Cleaning *48*
Before the First Case of the Day *48*
In Between Cases *48*
Terminal Cleaning – End of Day *49*
Solutions to Use for Cleaning *49*

Sodium Hypochlorite *49*
Potassium Peroxymonosulfate *50*
Quaternary Ammoniums *50*
Accelerated Hydrogen Peroxide *50*
Patient Preparation *50*
Clipping *51*
Abdominal *52*
Thoracic *52*
Orthopedic *54*
Neurologic *55*
Miscellaneous Sites *56*
Ophthalmic *56*
Aural *57*
Head and Mouth *57*
Perineal *57*
Open Wound Clipping *58*
Clipper Care *59*
Patient Skin Preparation *59*
Surgical Scrub Products *59*
Chlorhexidine *59*
Povidone-Iodine *59*
Rinsing Agents *60*
Final Paint Solutions *60*
Patient Prep Patterns *62*
Target Pattern *62*
Orthopedic Prep *63*
Perineal *65*
Patient Positioning *66*
Patient Warming *69*
Heated Surgery Tables *69*
Circulating Water Blankets *69*
Convection Warming Systems *70*
Solid Warming Pads *70*
Alternative Methods *70*
Patient Sterile Prep *71*
Personnel Preparation *73*
Attire *73*
Surgeons Hand Scrub *74*
Surgical Hand Rub *78*
Drying the Hands and Arms *78*
Gowning *80*
Gloving *83*
Closed Gloving *83*
Open Gloving *86*
Assisted Gloving *89*

Removing a Contaminate Glove 90
Double Gloving 90
Stress Mats 91
Instrumentation 92
Instrument Manufacturing 92
General Surgery Instruments 94
Scissors 94
Towel Clamps 97
Scalpel Handles and Scalpel Blades 97
Hemostatic Forceps 98
Thumb Tissue Forceps 99
Needle Holders 101
Hand-Held Retractors 102
Miscellaneous Instruments 104
Snook Spay Hook 104
Dowling Spay Retractor 104
Grooved Director 104
Alligator Forceps 104
Allis Tissue Forceps 105
Needle Rack 105
Abdominal Instrumentation 105
Retractors 105
Abdominal Intestinal Forceps 106
Thoracic Instruments 106
Retractors 106
Thoracic Scissors 106
Thumb Tissue Forceps 107
Vascular Clamps 107
Satinsky/Cooley 107
Orthopedic Instruments 108
Retractors 108
Ronguers 110
Periosteal Elevators 110
Osteotomes 111
Chisels 111
Mallet 111
Bone Holding/Reduction Forceps 111
Bone Cutters 113
Jacob's Chuck 113
Power Equipment 113
Internal Fixation Implants 114
Intramedullary Pins 114
Orthopedic Wire 115
Wire Twisters 115
Pin/Bolt Cutters 116
Interlocking Nails 117

Bone Plates 117
Bone Screws 118
Arthroscopic Instrumentation 120
Laparoscopic Instruments 122
Neurologic Instrumentation 123
Ophthalmic Instrumentation 124
Instrument Cleaning and Care 126
Manual Cleaning 127
Ultrasonic Cleaning 127
Instrument Lubrication 129
Instrument Maintenance 130
Pack Preparation 131
Pack Wrapping and Instrument Packaging 136
Methods of Wrapping Packs 138
Sterilization 141
Chemical 142
Steam 143
Loading the Autoclave 145
Autoclave Maintenance 146
Ethylene Oxide Sterilization (ETO, EtO, or EO) 147
Plasma Sterilization 147
Monitoring the Sterilization Process 148
Physical Monitors 148
Chemical Indicators 148
Biological Indicators 149
Shelf Life 150
Reference 151
Webliography 151

4 Intraoperative Surgical Assistant and Circulating Nurse *153*
Teri Raffel Kleist and Cassandra Simmons
Patient Positioning 154
Sterile Patient Prep 157
Patient Draping 158
Non-orthopedic Draping (Soft Tissue, Neuro, etc.) 159
Orthopedic Draping 162
Other Responsibilities 163
Setting Up the Instrument Table 164
Passing Surgical Instruments 164
Scalpel Handle and Blade 164
Ring-Handled Instruments 164
Thumb Tissue Forceps 165
Lavaging 165
Hemostasis 167
Suction 169

Retraction 170
Instrument Maintenance 170
Scalpel Blade/Handle Assembly 171
Sponge/Instrument Count 171
Procedure Specific Duties 173
Suture Materials and Suture Patterns 174
Characteristics 174
Sizing 176
Classification 176
Absorbable vs. Non-absorbable 176
Monofilament vs. Multifilament 177
Natural/Organic vs. Synthetic 178
Suture Material 178
Absorbable Sutures – Monofilament 178
Absorbable – Multifilament 179
Non-absorbable Suture – Monofilament 179
Non-absorbable – Multifilament 179
Suture Patterns 180
Continuous Patterns 180
Simple Continuous 180
Ford Interlocking 181
Lembert, Cushing, and Connell Patterns 182
Interrupted Patterns 182
Simple Interrupted 182
Horizontal Mattress 182
Cruciate Pattern 183
Vertical Mattress 183
Cutting Suture 184
Internal Sutures 184
External Sutures 185
Staples 185
External (Skin) Staples 185
Internal Staples 186
Circulating Nurse 187
Setting Up the Room 187
Opening Packs 188
Monitoring Aseptic Technique 193
Monitoring the Room During the Surgery 193
References 195
Additional Resources 195
Further Reading 195

5 **Surgical Procedures** 196
Teri Raffel Kleist, JoAnne Mead, and Gerianne Holzman
Abdominal 196
Digestive 196
GDV Gastric Dilatation Volvulus (Bloat) 196

Gastric Foreign Body *197*
Intestinal Foreign Body *198*
Exploratory Laparotomy *199*
Gallbladder *200*
Cholecystectomy *200*
Liver *201*
Liver Lobectomy *201*
Portosystemic Shunt (PSS) *203*
Reproductive *203*
Cesarean Section *203*
Orchiectomy (Neuter/Castration) *204*
Ovariohysterectomy (OHE/Neuter/Spay) *206*
Spleen *207*
Splenectomy *207*
Urinary *208*
Cystotomy *208*
Nephrectomy *210*
Perineal Urethrostomy – Male Cats *211*
Subcutaneous Ureteral Bypass (SUB) *212*
Head and Neck *212*
Auditory *212*
External Ear Canal and Pinna *212*
Otitis Media and Otitis Interna *214*
Ophthalmic *215*
Distichiasis *215*
Entropion *215*
Enucleation *216*
Neoplasia of the Eye *217*
Thyroidectomy *217*
Upper Respiratory System *218*
Elongated Soft Palate *218*
Laryngeal Paralysis *220*
Stenotic Nares *221*
Minimally Invasive *222*
Arthroscopy *222*
Laparoscopy *223*
Thoracoscopy *224*
Neurosurgery *227*
Spine *227*
Cervical *227*
Thoracolumbar *227*
Orthopedic *228*
Fractures *228*
Forelimb *232*
Shoulder *232*
Elbow *233*
Radius/Ulna *237*

Carpus *239*
Digits *240*
Hindlimb *243*
Pelvis *243*
Hip Dysplasia *243*
Stifle *249*
Cranial Cruciate Ligament (CCL) Rupture *249*
Patella Luxation *253*
Tarsus *253*
Tarsus – Achilles Tendon Repair *253*
Arthrodesis *255*
Thoracic *256*
Cardiovascular *256*
Thoracotomy / Patent Ductus Arteriosus (PDA) *256*
Persistent Right Aortic Arch (PRAA) *257*
Respiratory *258*
Lung Lobectomy *258*
Tracheal Collapse *259*
Other Surgery *262*
Anal Sacculectomy *262*
Perineal Hernia *263*
Mastectomy *264*
References *266*
Additional Resources *267*
References *267*
Webliography *268*

6 Wound Management *269*
Gerianne Holzman and JoAnne Mead
Types of Wounds *269*
Phases of Wound Healing *270*
Delays in Wound Healing *272*
General Wound Care *274*
Negative Pressure Wound Therapy *280*
Burns *282*
Thermal Burns *282*
Thermal Burn Treatment *283*
Frostbite *286*
Frostbite Treatment *286*
Chemical Burns *287*
Chemical Burn Treatment *287*
Electrical Burns *287*
References *287*

7 Postoperative Care *289*
Gerianne Holzman and Sandra Engelmeyer
Anesthesia Recovery *289*

Self-Trauma *290*
Housing *291*
Bedding *291*
Pads *291*
Perforated Mats *291*
Other Mats *292*
Other Bedding *292*
Cage Lining *293*
Boxes/Hiding Spots *293*
Cage Height *293*
Pheromones *294*
Nutritional Support *294*
Urinary Bladder Care *294*
Bandages *295*
External Coaptation Concepts *295*
Types of Support *296*
Temporary Support *296*
Supplemental Support *296*
Primary Support *297*
Considerations *297*
Anatomy of a Bandage *298*
Soft Padded *299*
Application of a Limb Bandage *299*
Robert Jones *303*
Splints *305*
Purposes *305*
Splint Materials *305*
Splint Application *306*
Spica Splints *307*
Casts *310*
Cast Application *310*
External Coaptation Complications and Care *312*
External Skeletal Fixation (ESF) Devices *314*
Slings *315*
References *317*

8 **Aftercare and Home Care** *319*
Gerianne Holzman and Sandra Engelmeyer
Client Instructions *319*
Written Instructions *319*
Hands-on Demonstrations *321*
Feeding Instructions *322*
Elimination *324*
Exercise *325*
Support Devices *325*
Physical Rehabilitation *326*
Cryotherapy *329*

Heat *329*
Massage *329*
Passive Range of Motion *329*
Therapeutic Exercises *331*
Follow-Up *332*
References *334*

Glossary *335*
Index *341*

Foreword to the First Edition

It is a privilege to write the Foreword to *Veterinary Surgical Patient Care* by Gerianne Holzman and Teresa (Teri) Raffel. The objective of the authors was to create a comprehensive text targeted to the veterinary technician interested or involved with all aspects of veterinary surgical practice. This text follows a logical progression beginning with deciphering clinical information by history taking and physical examination; then onto preoperative planning, asepsis, infection control, a description of common surgical procedures, and a description of common surgical instruments; and finishing with postoperative patient care. The authors support each chapter with eloquent details and illustrations derived from their clinical experience, highlighting the crucial role played by the veterinary technician at each step. This text offers a unique perspective for veterinary technicians by two very capable veterinary technicians and educators.

The authors, Gerianne Holzman and Teresa Raffel, bring a wealth of clinical experience to this book. Both graduates of Madison Area Technical College, they quickly brought their combined talents to the academic environment of the newly created School of Veterinary Medicine in Madison, Wisconsin, in the mid-1980s. When I was recruited at University of Wisconsin in 1984, I was a young and relatively naïve veterinary surgeon specializing in orthopedic surgery. Geri and Teri were instrumental in the refinement and development of my skills, both inside and outside of the operating room. Over the ensuing years, the authors have continued to educate and groom thousands of veterinary surgeons, veterinary students, and veterinary technicians. This book will stand as a legacy to their perseverance and endurance and will serve as a primer for all those interested in the practice of veterinary surgery.

Paul Manley, DVM, MSc, DACVS
Professor Emeritus
School of Veterinary Medicine
University of Wisconsin, Madison

Preface

Welcome to the second edition of *Surgical Patient Care for Veterinary Technicians and Nurses*. The authors and editors updated and revised the book to address the needs of veterinary professionals in their daily patient care.

Veterinary technicians play an integral role in veterinary surgical patient care; however, this care begins before the patient enters the surgical suite and does not end when the patient goes home. A patient's history and physical exam impact preoperative care and surgical planning. While communicating with clients and performing physical exams, the veterinary technician aids in accumulating information to complete a patient's record.

Preoperative care of patients includes obtaining laboratory samples, radiographs, and medications. Additional needs vary to provide for the maximum physical and mental comfort of patients. Keeping patients calm and quiet during the entire perioperative period aids in healing and may lessen pain medication needs. A veterinary technician well versed in preoperative coordination contributes to the anesthetic and surgical plan.

Veterinary technicians not only prepare a patient for a surgical procedure by shaving hair and cleaning a surgical site; they employ their extensive knowledge of appropriate prepping techniques and materials for the specific situation. Technicians play an integral role in monitoring the surgical team and maintaining the surgical suite, instruments, and equipment in a sterile environment. Veterinary technicians assist in surgical procedures. Knowledge of a variety of common surgeries provides a capable assistant to the veterinary surgeon.

Veterinary technicians are essential in providing postoperative patient care while monitoring for pain control, surgical complications, and comfort. A well-trained veterinary technician recognizes and tends to patients' needs. This may include immediate action and communication with a veterinarian. A veterinary technician experienced in bandage techniques and wound care frees up a veterinarian's time and provides more efficient patient care.

Communicating with clients after discharge is a great vehicle to increase client compliance, improve patient care, and promote a veterinary practice.

October 2023 *Gerianne and Teri*

Acknowledgments

Surgical Patient Care for Veterinary Technicians and Nurses came together to address the needs of veterinary professionals as they pursued their interests in veterinary surgery. We are proud to introduce the Second Edition of our book, written exclusively by veterinary technicians. This book has been a dream for both of us. While writing and editing both editions, we each experienced extreme personal challenges causing several delays in publication. However, the strong desire to provide a great resource for technicians, and a very understanding literary staff, helped us to persevere and finish the long journey to completion. Our combined experience, of over 80 years plus those of our co-authors, shows in the personal knowledge conveyed in these pages. However, we could not have completed this book without the help of many individuals. We thank our co-authors – Lana Bishop, Sandra Engelmeyer, JoAnne Mead, and Cassandra Simmons.

We particularly thank and recognize the following people for their inspiration, assistance, guidance, time, patience, and knowledge: Paul Manley, Susan Schaefer, Peter Muir, Jason Bleedorn, Robert Hardie, Dale Bjorling, Jonathan McAnulty, C.C. Sheldon, Krystal Telfer, the staff of Wiley-Blackwell, and the many surgeons, residents, and technicians we have had the pleasure of working with through our careers. The thousands of veterinary medical and technician students, who taught us many lessons as we shared our knowledge with them, were instrumental in our growth as veterinary technicians. Finally, we thank our families for their support and encouragement: Rob Zimmerman, Sherry Freiberg, Penny Lamb, Bob J. Holzman, Tony Raffel, Patrick Raffel, Peter Raffel, Gerry Stoeberl, Carol Sliwka, and Peggy Marvin. We acknowledge those who inspired us and are no longer present to receive our thanks: Eb Rosin, Carole Vick, Ann and Bob F. Holzman, Tom Stoeberl, and Mary Ann and George Stoeberl.

We encourage all veterinary technicians and veterinary professionals to pursue their dreams, advance their careers, explore new challenges, but most of all, have fun while enjoying one of the best jobs in the world!

March 2023 *Gerianne and Teri*

Author Biographies

Gerianne Holzman, CVT, VTS (Dentistry) (Retired)
After practicing for 40 years, Gerianne retired from veterinary practice in 2018. She began her career in a private small animal practice before entering the world of academia. Gerianne was one of the original veterinary technicians hired, in 1983, at the brand-new University of Wisconsin School of Veterinary Medicine (UW-SVM). She worked with all the surgical services performing preoperative and postoperative care. Her lifelong friendship with Teri began with their interactions while caring for surgical patients. This carried into professional organizations (including both serving as president of the Wisconsin Veterinary Technician Association), presentations, and their personal lives. Gerianne helped to create the UW Veterinary Care's dentistry service while becoming a charter member of the Academy of Veterinary Dental Technicians. She worked with and taught thousands of veterinary medical students and hundreds of surgery and dentistry residents. Over time, Gerianne's horizons expanded beyond the surgical ward and she originated the positions of feline renal transplant coordinator and orthopedic coordinator. While taking her away from her love of teaching, these positions provided her with more autonomy and client interaction. Over the years, peers and graduating veterinary medical students recognized her, many times, as an outstanding teacher. Gerianne retired from practice as a veterinary technician, emerita in 2015. She continued to work at the UW-SVM as the first clinical studies coordinator before finally leaving veterinary medicine for good. Gerianne now fills her days volunteering, traveling, and spending time with her husband and pets.

Teri Raffel Kleist, CVT, VTS (Surgery)
Having over 40 years of experience as a certified veterinary technician, Teri started her career in a mixed animal practice in Wisconsin after graduating from Madison Area Technical College's Veterinary Technician program. She then traveled to Purdue University where she began to discover her love of surgery while being employed as a surgical technician in the small animal surgery department. A new veterinary medical school opened in Wisconsin, and Teri applied for a position to bring her back to her home state. Teri and Gerianne's paths crossed when Teri traveled back to Wisconsin to join the original surgical staff at the University of Wisconsin. Teri obtained the position of a lead surgery tech serving both small animal and large animal patients. Teri enjoyed teaching hands-on skills to fourth-year veterinary students while instructing these future veterinarians on the need for great technical assistance. Teri eventually moved on to teaching these same skills to veterinary technician students in the veterinary technician program at Madison College. After 30 years at Madison College, Teri retired in 2021. She is a charter member of the Academy of Veterinary Surgery Technicians, earning her VTS in 2013, and remains busy with the credentialing exam that this organization offers. Teri has been involved with organized veterinary

medicine on the local and national level for many years, holding many board positions for National Association of Veterinary Technicians (NAVTA), American Association of Veterinary State Boards (AAVSB), and Wisconsin Veterinary Technician Association (WVTA). Teri has contributed to multiple veterinary technician textbooks, in addition to co-authoring the first edition of this book. She has published several articles in veterinary journals as well. In her retirement, she continues that involvement and is currently the Surgery Summit laboratory technician and the Veterinary Technician Seminar Chair on the Continuing Education committee for American College of Veterinary Surgeons (ACVS). In 2022 she went back to her early career roots and love of all things surgical and now works part-time in a surgical referral practice in Madison, WI.

Lana Bishop, RVT, VTS (Surgery)
Lana is a technician training coordinator at BluePearl Pet Hospital in Iowa. She graduated from Des Moines Area Community College in 2011 with an AAS degree in Veterinary Technology and became a registered veterinary technician (RVT) that same year after passing the national and state exams. After spending her first few years as an RVT in general practice, Lana decided to pursue her interest in surgery, and she started her career at Iowa Veterinary Referral Center (now BluePearl Pet Hospital) in 2014 as a technician in the surgical department. At BluePearl her interest grew into her passion as more opportunities became available to technicians. She continued to grow her knowledge through collaboration with veterinarians/technicians at the hospital, continuing education and independent study. She concentrated on learning advanced analgesia techniques, surgical techniques, and surgical instrument/suite management. In 2018, she became the surgery technician supervisor, leading a team of RVTs and assistants in the four-surgeon department. Lana proudly earned her VTS as a member of the Academy of Veterinary Surgical Technicians (AVST) in 2019. In 2022 she became a technician training coordinator.

Sandra Engelmeyer, BS, CVT, RVT, VTS (Surgery)
Sandra graduated from Iowa State University with a BS in Animal Science in 2009 and has been a licensed veterinary technician since 2010. She has been in specialty surgery since 2014 and has a VTS in Surgery. Sandra has spoken at conferences on surgical topics and serves on the executive board of the Academy of Veterinary Surgical Technicians (AVST). She works with Blue Pearl Veterinary Partners in Minnesota as a surgery technician.

JoAnne Mead, AAS, RVT, VTS (Surgery)
JoAnne has worked at the North Carolina State University-College of Veterinary Medicine for over 26 years. She started in the large animal hospital, anesthesia, small animal ICU, and research. She then discovered her true passion in the surgery department. JoAnne earned her VTS in Surgery from the Academy of Veterinary Surgical Technicians in 2017. She has been active in the academy, most recently as a member of the Exam committee. Her contribution to the second edition is her inaugural work in her writing career.

Cassandra Simmons, RVT, LAT, VTS (Surgery)
Cassandra graduated from Purdue University's Veterinary Technology Program in 1990. The following year she started her surgical nursing career as an RVT in the Hillenbrand Biomedical Engineering Research Center at Purdue University. In 1991 she obtained her Laboratory Animal Technician (LAT) certification. From 2008 to 2011, she worked as a bio-technician supervisor at ACELL, Inc., in Lafayette, IN. She then became an instructional surgical nurse in the Department of Small Animal Surgery at Purdue University's Veterinary Teaching Hospital. While in this

position, Cassandra served as the veterinary technician student rotation supervisor for four years. She is currently the lecturer for the Purdue College of Veterinary Medicine Veterinary Technology Program Operating Room and Surgical Nursing Protocol course. She is the coordinating technician for the Junior DVM Surgery courses and Junior Surgery Facility Manager. Cassandra obtained her VTS in surgery, through the Academy of Veterinary Surgical Technicians, in 2017. She is also a member of the Indiana Veterinary Technology Association (IVTA) and NAVTA.

List of Contributors

Editor and Author

Gerianne Holzman, CVT, VTS (Dentistry) (Retired)
University of Wisconsin
School of Veterinary Medicine
Middleton, WI, USA

Editor and Author

Teri Raffel Kleist, CVT, VTS (Surgery) (Retired)
Madison College
Madison, WI, USA

Author

Lana Bishop, RVT, VTS (Surgery)
Blue Pearl Pet Hospital
Des Moines, IA, USA

Author

Sandra Engelmeyer, BS, CVT, RVT, VTS (Surgery)
Blue Pearl Veterinary Partners
Golden Valley, MN, USA

Author

JoAnne Mead, AAS, RVT, VTS (Surgery)
North Carolina State University
College of Veteirnary Medicine
Surgery Department
Raleigh, NC, USA

Author

Cassandra Simmons, RVT, LAT, VTS (Surgery)
College of Veterinary Medicine
Purdue University
Veterinary Technology Program
West Lafayette, IN, USA

About the Companion Website

This book is accompanied by a companion website:

www.wiley.com/go/holzman/patient

This website includes:

i) MCQs
ii) Videos

1

History and Physical Examination

Gerianne Holzman[1] and Lana Bishop[2]

[1] *University of Wisconsin, School of Veterinary Medicine, Emerita, Madison, WI, USA*
[2] *Blue Pearl Pet Hospital, Des Moines, IA, USA*

The history and physical exam provide the basis for all patient care. Without this information, the veterinarian cannot formulate a correct diagnosis and treatment plan. Veterinary technicians provide an invaluable service in deciphering a client's perception of the problem while determining their true concerns. These may not be the same as the patient's actual medical condition. For example, a client brings a pet in for behavioral problems of urinating in the house. The client thinks the cat is "mad" because it is left alone for many hours. The client's concern is for the cat to stop urinating in the house. Questions are asked about litter pan behavior, urine color, and the cat's attitude. The patient shows pain on abdominal palpation and distended bladder. After consultation with the surgeon, it is decided to perform abdominal radiographs on this patient. Radiographs show the cat has cystic calculi (Figure 1.1). After discussing medical versus surgical options with the client, it is decided to surgically remove the bladder stones.

History

Surgical patients may present with many or no other medical conditions other than the original complaint. A careful medical history contributes to the patient's diagnosis, prognosis, and treatment plan. A complete history includes:

- Vaccinations
- Heartworm testing/preventative
- Diet
- Allergies
- Current medication
- Patient's lifestyle
- Medical and surgical history
- Client expectations

Surgical Patient Care for Veterinary Technicians and Nurses, Second Edition.
Edited by Gerianne Holzman and Teri Raffel Kleist.

Companion website: www.wiley.com/go/holzman/patient

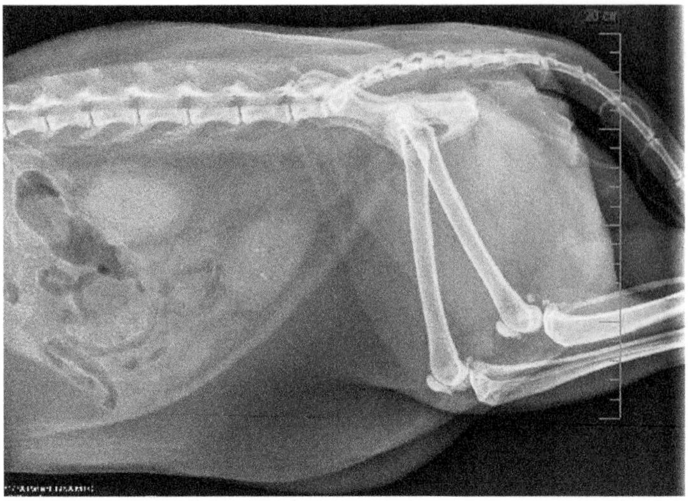

Figure 1.1 Lateral radiograph of a cat with cystic calculi. *Source:* Courtesy of Amy Lang.

Vaccinations

Hospitalized patients may be exposed to many communicable diseases. Suggested canine vaccinations include distemper, adenovirus, parainfluenza, parvovirus, leptospirosis, rabies, and possibly Bordetella and influenza. Feline vaccinations include viral rhinotracheitis, calicivirus, rabies, and panleukopenia. Care is taken to protect unvaccinated emergency patients with minimal inter-patient contact. Hospital policy and local regulations dictate vaccination requirements. In an emergency setting, the vaccination records may not be attainable at intake and treatment will still be initiated carefully.

Parasites

Every state reports cases of heartworm disease. Preventative treatment promotes patients' good health. Patients with active or prior heartworm disease pose an anesthetic risk. The client is quizzed to determine the status of heartworm testing and preventative. Flea infestation is avoided in the veterinary hospital with appropriate prevention, therefore determining a client's use of flea and tick preventative is imperative. Many intestinal parasites can also be prevented with these medications. Some intestinal parasites can be zoonotic such as giardia.

Diet

Diet affects all aspects of a patient's health. Knowledge of a patient's dietary habits aids treatment plans. For example, young puppies fed a high-calcium diet can succumb to developmental orthopedic conditions. Obesity causes stress to most body systems including heart, lungs, and joints. Determining if a patient's feeding schedule is free choice or meal feeding aids in formulating weight management plans. Between-meal snacks contribute to obesity. Maintaining a patient's current diet while hospitalized avoids gastrointestinal upset from food change. However, clients providing raw food diets might create an in-hospital storage problem and hazard for hospital personnel. Patients undergoing oral or facial surgery may need a softened diet postoperatively. Crushing a normal diet of dry kibble and soaking for a short time in water maintains the animal's normal diet. There are also many non-traditional diets such as grain free, raw, and home cooked. Nutritional balance may not be obtained with these diets and other health issues can arise from them. Dilated cardiomyopathy (DCM) can be the result of grain-free diets according to the FDA and a study by the University of California, Davis [1].

Allergies

Food allergies are prevalent in the veterinary patient population. Determining a patient's food allergies avoids gastrointestinal problems while hospitalized. Unidentified medication allergies can cause very serious complications during hospitalization, surgery, and recovery. Obtaining information on past sedation and anesthetic episodes provides guidelines for future needs. Patients with a history of a poor response to anesthesia must be more closely monitored during any surgical procedure and recovery. Anesthetic complications include vomiting, diarrhea, cardiac arrhythmias, breathing difficulties, blood pressure changes, and slow recovery. Other previous or ongoing allergic reactions to medications or environmental conditions must also be noted.

Current Medication

A patient's current and prior medication and supplement history influences future treatment plans. For example, patients receiving anti-inflammatory medications need a "wash-out" period (three to seven days) prior to starting a different anti-inflammatory drug to avoid gastrointestinal problems including stomach ulceration. Medications for many medical conditions influence the choice of perioperative drugs. Dietary supplements, such as glucosamine chondroitin, calcium, and vitamins, affect patients' health and food needs.

Patient's Lifestyle

Clients have different expectations for patients leading a sedentary life versus working or service animals. If a dog's main job is to sit on the couch most of the day, recovery from a ruptured cranial cruciate ligament and its attending arthritis is much different from a search and rescue animal. If a patient lives in a city-dwelling apartment, it will have different experiences during recovery than a dog living in the country, with acres of freedom. If the patient is a working animal, an extensive rehabilitation regimen may be recommended to regain/maintain strength, flexibility, and endurance [2]. The same holds true for an indoor cat versus an outdoor cat. Will the client be able to medicate a mostly outdoor cat postoperatively? Do they have the ability to keep them inside for a short time?

Medical History

A complete medical history begins with confirming the signalment with the owner: age, breed, sex (intact or neutered), and presenting complaint. A preconceived diagnosis may affect physical exam findings; therefore, it is important to ask open-ended questions. (For example, a patient presented with hip dysplasia may actually have a cranial cruciate rupture causing more lameness than poor

O = Onset
L = Location
D = Duration
Ch = Character (better/worse/static)
A = Alleviating/Aggravating factors
R = Rx (medications, other therapies)
T = Temporal pattern
S = Symptoms associated

Figure 1.2 Old charts: a mnemonic device to remember important aspects of a patient's history.

hip conformation.) Carefully interviewing the client provides the much-needed information to aid in the diagnosis. In addition to the presenting complaint, e.g. lameness, the entire patient is taken into consideration with inquiries into coughing (C), sneezing (S), vomiting (V), diarrhea (D), increase in thirst or urination, polyuria/polydipsia (PU/PD), and appetite (A). These parameters are easily recorded in the medical record as C, S, V, D, PU/PD, and A with notations made accordingly. Note all current and previous medical problems as they may influence the surgical experience. Form questions to prevent leading a client into a specific "yes or no" answer. For instance, asking a client "Is Lily more lame today?" provides a yes or no answer as opposed to asking, "When do you see Lily's lameness increase?" Another example, asking a client "Is Sam vomiting more today?" versus "Did you see Sam eat anything unusual prior to the vomiting?" With the second questions, the client needs to give a more detailed answer providing the clinician with better historical information. Record all prior surgical procedures and outcomes. A patient may present for a second opinion of a recurrent problem. Historical knowledge influences the treatment plan.

The current exercise regimen may determine the client and patient's ability or lack of ability to provide appropriate postoperative rehabilitation. This may influence the surgical plan. A mnemonic for obtaining a history is using the old charts method (Figure 1.2).

Client Expectation

Although delicate to obtain, a client's personal situation and expectations (time, financial commitment, lifestyle, recovery, and other obligations) also influence the surgical plan. A client with many commitments may not have the time required for extensive post-op rehabilitation. For this person, a more conservative plan or an inpatient program may better fit the client's lifestyle. In addition, if the patient requires multiple procedures and/or treatments based on the current plan, alternative treatment plans may be more desirable. An example may be an open, traumatic, fracture with bone destruction that the client would like to repair. However, repairing the fracture requires a lengthy recovery with multiple surgeries and the likelihood of many different types of complications. Their financial and time commitment would be substantial so amputation may be elected.

Another example would be a mass removal, and for the best outcome, chemotherapy is recommended postoperatively. However, the client is not interested in pursuing additional treatments. These realities may need to be considered prior to moving forward with any surgery.

Physical Exam

A complete physical exam covers the patient from the tip of the nose to the tip of the tail. Failure to recognize patients' underlying medical problems can lead to devastating consequences. (The extent of the exam performed by a veterinary technician varies with individual veterinary practices.) A complete physical exam includes all parameters:

- Temperature, pulse, respiration, and weight
- Body condition score
- General appearance
- Attitude
- Locomotion
- Head and face
- Oral pharynx
- Lymph nodes
- Integument
- Musculoskeletal
- Perineum
- Abdominal cavity
- Respiratory
- Cardiovascular
- Nervous system

Use of a paper or electronic physical exam form serves as a reminder to examine all body systems. Many products exist for record keeping and they continue to evolve. Clinics generally search for a system that works best for them.

Temperature, Pulse, Respiration, and Weight

Obtain a temperature, pulse, and respiration (TPR) and weight at every visit. Clients appreciate knowing if their pet's TPR is in the normal range (Table 1.1). Knowledge of a patient's presurgical TPR influences the anesthetic protocol. Changes in TPR affect intra-operative and postoperative care. Accurate weight provides proper medication dosing including preanesthetic medication. If the patient is obese, calculating medications from an ideal weight should be considered. Monitoring obese patients, at each visit, aids in weight management.

Body Condition Score

Many charts help determine a patient's body condition score (BCS). Determining a patient's level of obesity or thinness influences treatment plans. Body condition scores (BCS) vary with the source, one style of chart uses a scale of 1 to 9, with 1 being emaciated and 9 being extremely obese.

Table 1.1 Normal feline and canine TPR.

Parameter	Feline	Canine
Temperature	101–102.5 °F	101–102.5 °F
Pulse	160–240 beats/min	70–160 beats/min
Respiration	20–30 breaths/min	10–39 breaths/min

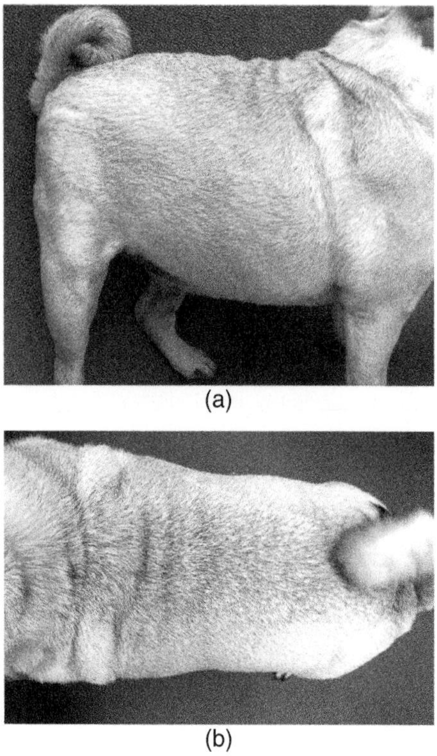

Figure 1.3 (a) An obese pug (BCS 7) shown in lateral view, (b) an obese pug (BCS 7) shown in dorsal view.

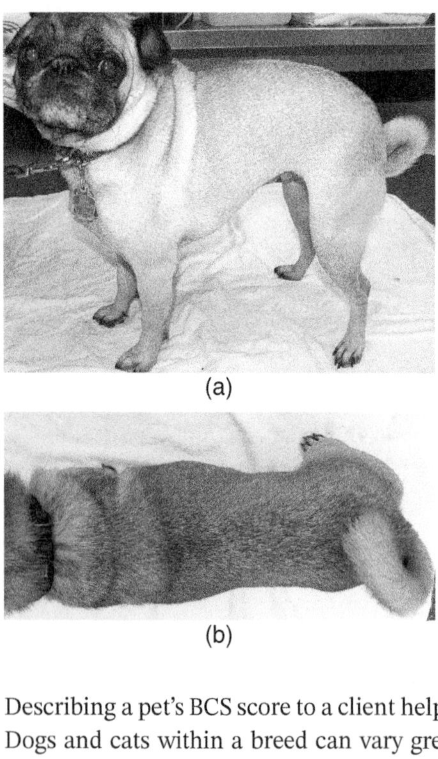

Figure 1.4 (a) A thin pug (BCS 4) shown in lateral view, (b) a thin pug (BCS 4) shown in dorsal view.

Describing a pet's BCS score to a client helps in understanding the nutritional needs of the animal. Dogs and cats within a breed can vary greatly (Figures 1.3a,b and 1.4a,b). Printing copies of the BCS images and providing them to clients allow for a visual reminder of a healthy state. See Chapter 8, *Aftercare and Home Care,* for examples of BCS charts.

General Appearance

A patient's general appearance may be a sign of their overall health. Unwell patients often have an unkempt appearance, poor hair coat, etc. They generally do not groom themselves as normal or maybe overgroom a painful or irritating area. Obese or hypothyroid patients may be sluggish. Emergent patients may be obtunded, comatose, painful, etc. Alternatively, a patient may be in perfect condition except for its presenting complaint.

Attitude

Patients come with all personalities. They may be bright, alert, and responsive (BAR) or quiet, alert, and responsive (QAR). Unusual environments and pain can produce fear and concern or may cause aggression. Careful reading of a patient's attitude prevents misunderstandings and provides a safe working environment. Dogs, by nature, hide their pain. Cats are often over-aroused in an unfamiliar environment.

Maintaining a calm, quiet environment alleviates patients' fears and client concerns. Keeping cats in crates helps them to feel safe. Often time, much of the initial exam can be carried out with a cat within the crate. Providing a mat or blanket on the floor for a dog may help it to relax. Dogs, unlike cats, prefer to be at ground level. Performing a physical exam on the floor alleviates dogs' fears of being off the ground. Patients can also "get away" if too stressed instead of leaping from an exam table and possibly sustaining an injury. Performing physical exams on the floor also helps to maintain a healthy working environment by avoiding back injuries from lifting heavy dogs, and providing an easy way to back away from aggressive patients. Small dogs, however, are more used to lifting and carrying by their owners. Physical exams on tables are useful for these patients provided they are safe and the client or an assistant can aid in restraint. Providing a mat on the floor or table provides sturdy footing for the patient. A mat or blanket also adds comfort and cushioning for the patient and staff (Figure 1.5).

Medications prior to arrival at the clinic can help with fear, aggression, and anxiety. Feline patients can benefit from gabapentin prior to appointments if they are prone to anxiety on

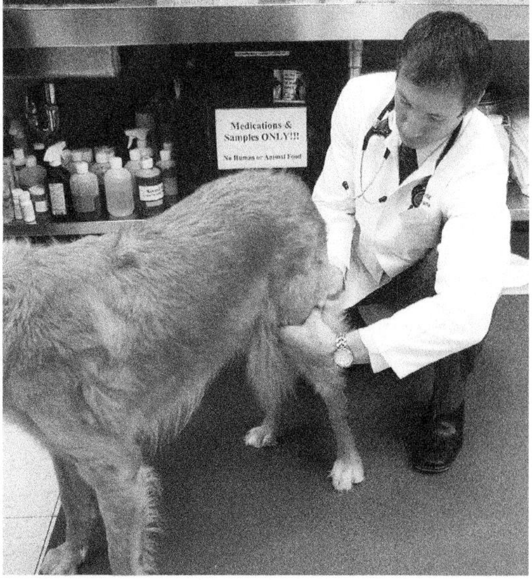

Figure 1.5 A physical exam on a comfortable floor mat provides patient and staff stability and comfort.

Table 1.2 Dosing and timeline of administration of sedative agents [4].

Drug	Dose	When to administer	Contraindications
Acepromazine	Tablets: 1–2 mg/kg Recommended: Injectable (administered via oral transmucosal [OTM]): 0.01–0.05 mg/kg Note: Small volumes can be diluted with 0.9% saline for easier administration	Time of onset is about 20–30 min, so it is best given orally 30–60 min prior to the hospital visit.	Patients with significant cardiovascular or kidney disease, liver failure, trauma, critically ill, pediatrics, and geriatrics
Gabapentin	10–20 mg/kg Use the upper end of the dose in very hard-to-handle dogs and the lower end of the dose in geriatric patients	Give orally the night prior to the hospital visit and repeat the same dose in the morning of hospital visit, at least two hours prior to arrival.	Patients with liver failure, critically ill, and pediatric.
Melatonin	By patient's body weight, total dose (not per kg): • <5 kg, give 1 mg • 5–15 kg, give 1.5 mg • 15–50 kg, give 3 mg • >50 kg, give 5 mg	Give orally on the morning of the hospital visit, two hours prior to arrival.	None
Trazodone	5 mg/kg	Give orally the night prior to hospital visit, then repeat same dose the morning of hospital visit at least two hours prior to arrival.	Patients with pre-existing arrhythmias, taking monoamine oxidase inhibitors (MOAIs), and patients with seizure history/epilepsy.

Timing recommendations are based on morning appointments. If appointment falls in the afternoon or evening, morning-administered medications are likely to have little effect. Timing regimen must be adjusted based on patient's appointment time.

transport and in the clinic setting at 100 mg/cat 2 hours prior to transport [3]. Table 1.2 provides guidelines for canine dosage and timing [5]. These can aid in providing a more comfortable patient experience (Table 1.2).

Locomotion

Allowing a patient to roam the exam room during history taking provides an assessment of a patient's uncontrolled movement. (Assure that all doors are closed.) Note any lameness or gait abnormalities. If a hallway or outside area is available, ask the client to walk the dog on a leash. Try to minimize distractions by eliminating unnecessary personnel and closing hallway doors. Request a variety of speeds, as lameness may be more prevalent at faster or slower speeds. For example, a patient with hip dysplasia may walk relatively normally but "bunny hops," with both rear feet moving as one, when at a rapid gait. Some lameness may only be observed after working the patient. If this is the case, having them worked prior to the appointment will aid in diagnosis. Observe the patient sitting in the exam room. Patients with cranial cruciate rupture may sit with one leg slightly extended due to pain induced when flexing the stifle (Figure 1.6) [6].

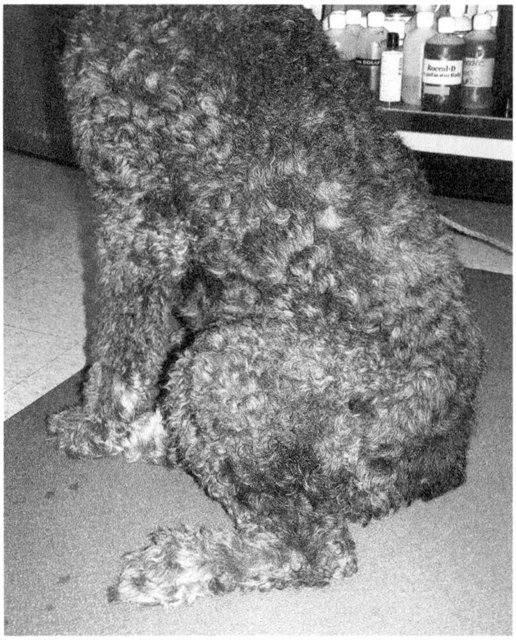

Figure 1.6 The "sit test" often indicates a ruptured cranial cruciate ligament as the patient does not want to flex the stifle fully.

Most cats do not walk on a leash which provide a challenge in locomotion assessment. Placing a crate or box at one end of a closed exam room and the cat at the other end provides the cat with a destination. It may run or slink to the crate or box allowing for gait evaluation. Keep all people away from the crate to aid in letting the cat think it is "getting away." Having the client provide a video of the abnormality at home can also be a helpful tool with cats or intermittent lameness in any species.

Always ask the client if, and when, they note any lameness at home. Patients in an unfamiliar setting or on slippery hospital tiled floors may walk differently than at home. Doing a gait analysis on different surfaces may be helpful such as concrete or a rug runner. Ask clients which leg they believe is causing the problem but do not assume they are correct, confirm the leg of concern by pointing it out in the exam room. Patients with front leg lameness drop their head when putting weight on the unaffected limb [7]. The degree of lameness is graded on a scale of 0–5 as follows [8]

- *Grade 0/5*: No lameness, stands normally
- *Grade 1/5*: Stands with abnormal posture, no lameness
- *Grade 2/5*: Mild lameness
- *Grade 3/5*: Moderate lameness
- *Grade 4/5*: Severe lameness
- *Grade 5/5*: Consistent non-weight-bearing lame

Head and Face

Assess all parts of the head and neck. Palpate the bone and musculature of the head for asymmetry and/or muscle wasting. Neuromuscular diseases may cause muscle atrophy on one or both sides of the face. Trauma of the head may cause fractures. Young patients may have an open fontanel at the top of the skull. Monitor the patient for any pain or discomfort when moving the head and neck from side to side and up and down.

Observe the eyes for nystagmus, symmetry, pupil dilation and constriction, light response, eyelid masses, tear production, scleral color, ectropion, and entropion. Examine the ears for debris, odor, masses, aural hematoma, intact tympanic membrane, discharge, and color change. Palpate and observe the nose for changes including masses, deviated septum, stenotic nares, and discharge. Check for a cough while palpating the trachea. Palpate the thyroid gland for size abnormalities.

Oral Pharynx

Begin the oral exam by lifting the lip, if the patient does not protest, continue the exam with caution to avoid personal injury. Assess the teeth for correct number (42 teeth in the adult dog and 30 in the adult cat), retained deciduous teeth, calculus and plaque, mobility, and color. Observe the gingiva and oral mucosa for color (red, pink, or various shades of black), moisture, gingivitis, periodontal disease, alignment, masses, and bleeding. The gingivae should be pink and moist. (Pigment may be dark in some breeds making assessment difficult.) If the gingiva is tacky, it may indicate dehydration, and if dark red/blueish, it can indicate cyanosis. Check capillary refill time by pushing on the mucosa to blanch the color. Normal color should return in one to two seconds. Assure the tongue is normal color and does not contain any masses. The tongue may be dark pigmented in addition to the normal pink color. If possible, look at the tongue for abnormalities and check the gag reflex. Check the tonsils for inflammation and location within their crypts. Check the palate for elongation, redness, and ulceration.

Lymph Nodes

Palpate lymph nodes for enlargement. Feel all lymph nodes to assess size differences. The most accessible nodes are submandibular (not to be confused with the submandibular salivary glands), prescapular, axillary, inguinal, and popliteal. Lymph node enlargement may be an indication of inflammation or neoplasia.

Integument

The skin can indicate underlying conditions. Allergic patients may bite or lick any part of the body; however, feet and legs are especially vulnerable. Check for alopecia, redness, or irritation from self-trauma. Check the skin for erythema, rashes, excess moisture, dryness, or flakiness. These may indicate conditions ranging from allergies to fleas to Lyme disease. Observe any parasites such as fleas and ticks. If present, treat and provide the client with prevention and control information.

Discern any indication of pyoderma. It may be indicated by the presence of pustules, rash, or skin odor. Skin infections present at the time of surgery can lead to surgical site infections. Pyoderma must be treated appropriately. If possible, delaying the procedure until after the skin has healed may be indicated, especially on elective procedures. Alternatively providing antibiotic therapy at the time of surgery may prevent bacterial infection of the surgery site.

Musculoskeletal

Patients presenting for lameness receive a complete orthopedic exam. This includes all legs not just the injured area. If an exam begins with a painful leg, the patient anticipates discomfort and may react to minimal stimulus of other legs creating false exam findings. Beginning the exam with the unaffected side provides for a more comfortable patient. Ideally, a musculoskeletal exam is

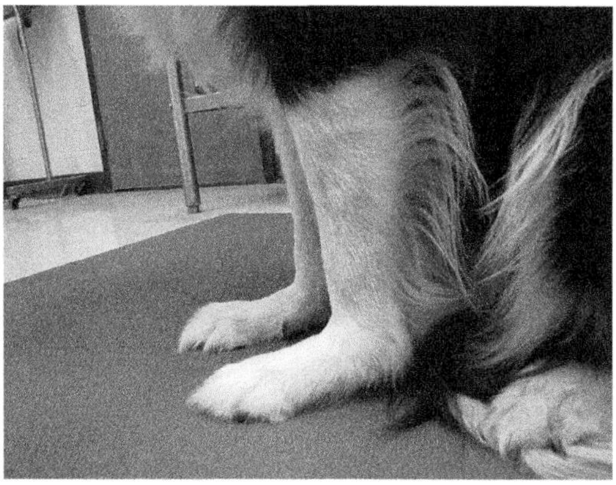

Figure 1.7 A Border Collie with carpal hyperextension.

performed with the patient in lateral recumbency to provide a non-weight-bearing exam. However, uncooperative patients may be examined while standing or may need sedation to complete manipulation of all limbs.

The orthopedic exam begins with the toes, feeling for any swelling, tenderness, or pain. Look between the toes for foreign materials, redness, or injuries. Each toe is moved, checking for normal range of motion (ROM). Examine the toenails for abnormal or asymmetric wear indicating an unusual gait or dragging the foot. Observe the bottom and between the pads for injuries or foreign objects such as glass shards, sticks, grass awns, or thorns.

Examine the carpus for swelling and pain. Discern the range of motion. (See *Table 8.1 Normal Rang of Motion*, in Chapter 8, *Aftercare and Home Care.*) Normally a dog or cat can flex its carpus until the toes touch the caudal side of the ulna. The normal degree of extension is 10–12° [7]. Extending beyond this range indicates damage to the palmar fibrocartilage (Figure 1.7).

Deviation from standard is a cause for concern and may indicate an acute or chronic condition. Carpal valgus is present when the carpus deviates laterally. Carpal varus indicates medial deviation of the carpus. Both conditions may result from trauma or genetics. They often occur with bowing of the radius due to premature closure of the distal ulna growth plate [7]. Some breeds of dogs have naturally occurring carpal valgus such as the Shih Tzu, Lhasa Apso, and English Bulldog. Other conditions to monitor in the carpus are fractures and luxations. (Note: if the forelimb is the area of concern, begin the exam on the rear limb.)

Inspect the elbow for pain and swelling. Edema of the elbows is more easily palpated while the patient is standing to allow for comparison of left and right sides. Observe the elbow range of motion. Normal elbow flexion permits the carpus to almost touch the cranial area of the shoulder. Decreased flexion is indicative of osteoarthritis [9]. Pain on hyperextension of the elbow may indicate an ununited anconeal process while pain on rotation can be indicative of osteochondritis dissecans.

Evaluation of the shoulder is more difficult due to its extensive muscle mass. Begin by checking the range of motion and observing for any pain response. Examine for pain in the biceps tendon by fully flexing the shoulder and extending the elbow (Figure 1.8). Lameness caused by biceps injury exacerbates with this maneuver.

Moving to the rear legs, examine the toes and foot as with the front legs. The tarsus is palpated for pain and swelling. Observe range of motion. Hyperflexion of the tarsus can accompany an avulsion or laceration of the common calcaneal tendon (Achilles mechanism) (Figure 1.9). Palpate the full length of the tendon for swelling, pain, and laxity.

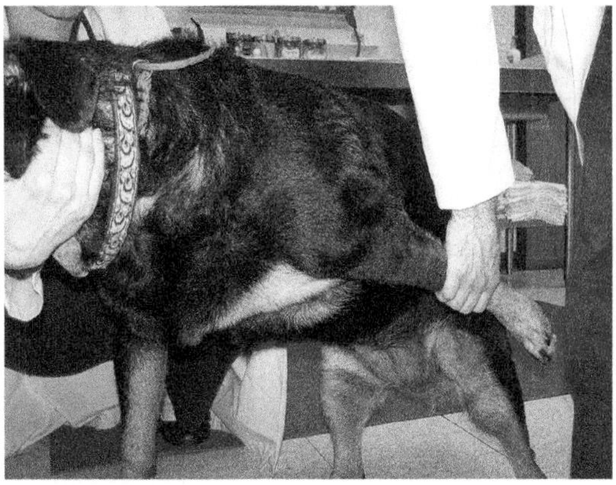

Figure 1.8 Patients with biceps tendon conditions become more lame after performing the biceps flexion test as shown. The shoulder is flexed for two minutes, leg is released, and patient is allowed to walk.

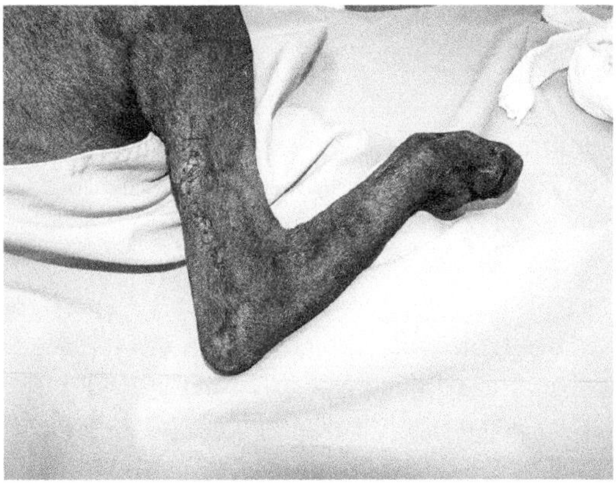

Figure 1.9 Labrador Retriever showing breakdown of surgical repair of lacerated Achilles tendon; note hyperflexion of the tarsus.

Palpate the stifle for pain and effusion. Swelling of the medial side of the stifle is often indicative of cranial cruciate ligament (CCL) rupture. Move the stifle through a full range of motion observing for discomfort. To assess joint stability, perform a cranial drawer test. Grasp the distal femur with one hand and the proximal tibia with the other, and attempt to move the tibia cranially. If movement is present, the cranial cruciate may be torn (Video 1.1). Another test for CCL problems is the tibial thrust. Place a hand over the stifle with the forefinger resting on the tibial crest, with the other hand flex the tarsus. If the CCL is torn, the tibia moves cranially (Video 1.2) (Figure 1.10a,b).

Assess the location of the patella. Determine if it lays within the patellar groove or if it lays medially or laterally to normal. If outside the normal location, ascertain the patella's ability or inability to return to a normal position and stay there. Patella luxation has four levels:

- *Grade 1*: Patella intermittently luxates but spends most of its time in the normal position
- *Grade 2*: Patella easily luxates but is readily put back into place, spends most of its time in normal position
- *Grade 3*: Patella often luxates but can be put back into place with effort, spends most of its time out of place
- *Grade 4*: Patella is always luxated and is unable to be moved back into a normal position (Figure 1.11a,b)

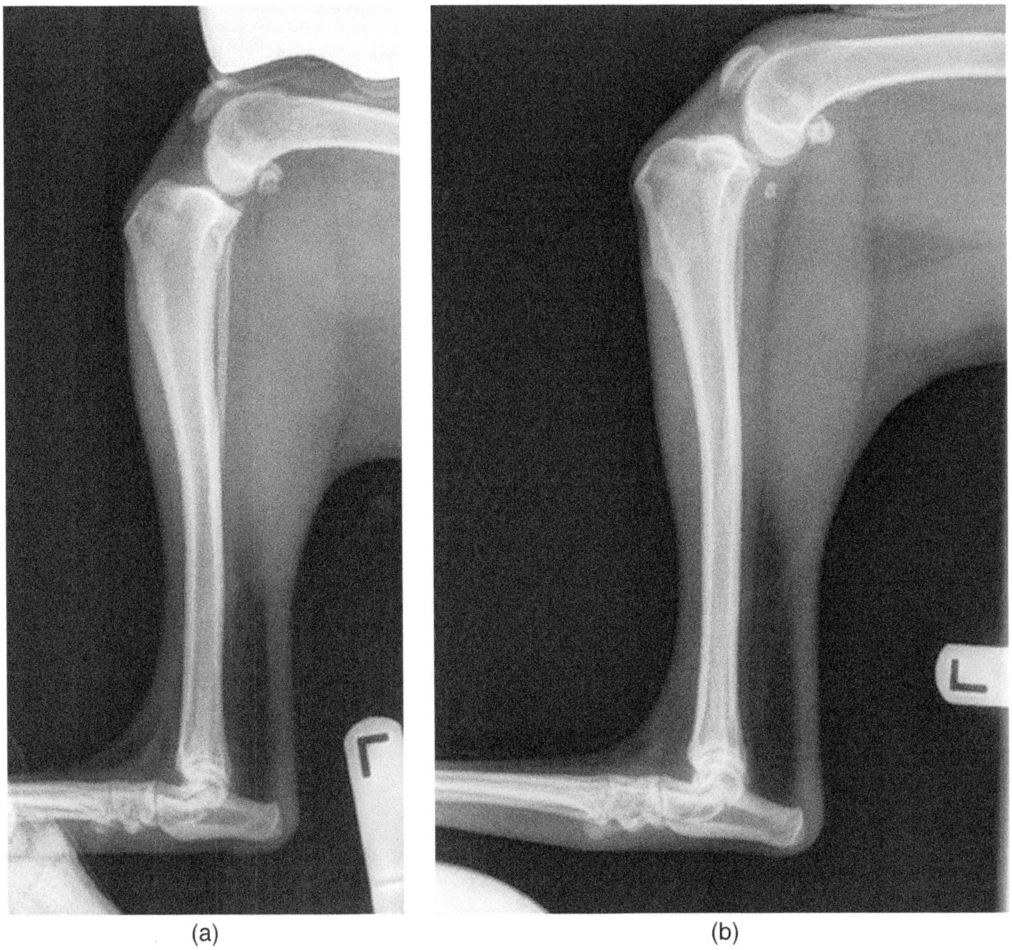

Figure 1.10 (a) Lateral radiograph of a normal left stifle, (b) lateral radiograph of a left stifle demonstrating cranial tibial thrust.

As with the shoulder, the deep musculature of the hips prevents palpation of swelling. Evaluate the range of motion of the hips and determine if pain is present on flexion or extension. Place a hand over the hip while taking it through a ROM to help evaluate if a hip luxation is present. A sedated exam is indicated to evaluate a patient completely for hip dysplasia by performing the Ortolani maneuver to check for hip laxity, the angle of subluxation, and the angle of reduction [9].

Perineum

Evaluate the external urogenital system. Examine the prepuce for swelling and discharge. The scrotum in neutered animals should be flat. Intact dogs and cats' testes are symmetrical. Note any abnormalities. Altered animals normally display minimal to no drainage, however, record any vaginal swelling or secretions. Examine the rectum for irritation, masses, ulcerations, and swelling. Palpate the anal glands to determine fullness. Perform a digital rectal exam to check for masses or hernias.

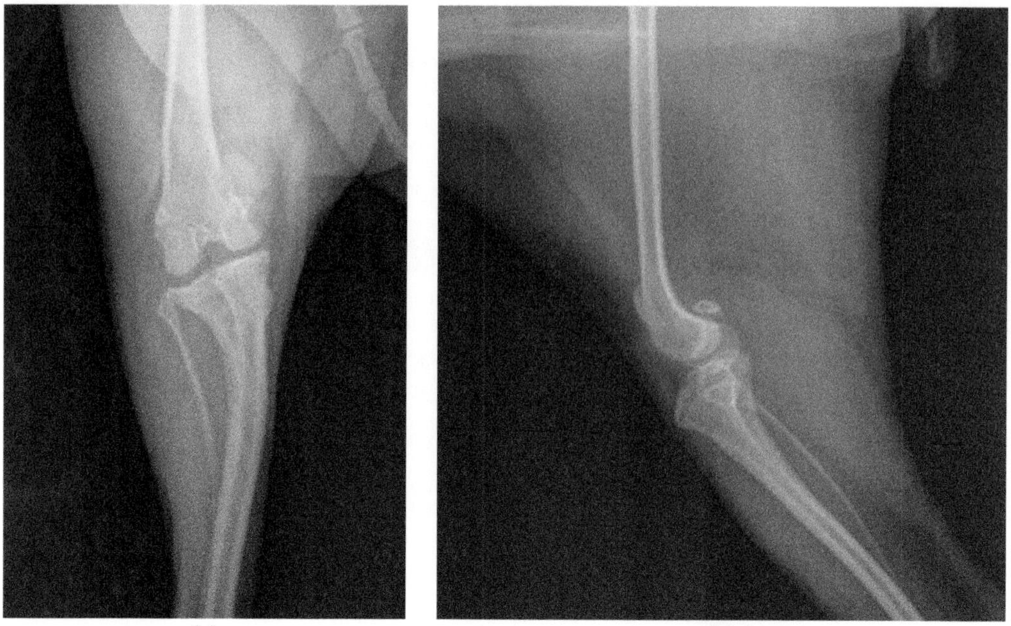

Figure 1.11 (a) Cranial radiograph of a right stifle showing Grade 4 medial patella luxation, (b) lateral radiograph of a right stifle showing Grade 4 medial patella luxation and cranial displacement.

Abdominal Cavity

Systematically palpate the abdominal cavity using the flats of both hands to examine each organ. (It may be better to palpate small dogs and cats with one hand, cupping the abdomen between the thumb and fingers.) Begin just behind the ribs feeling for masses, distension, and abnormal positioning of the liver, stomach, spleen, kidneys, bladder, small intestine, and bowel. An irritated and enlarged gall bladder or pancreas may also be palpable. Observe the patient for a pain response. They may display tension, flinching, restlessness, biting, and/or vocalizing. Pain may also be associated with pupil dilation. Palpate the mammary chain for any masses. Pregnant and nursing animals may discharge milk upon examination. Normal milk is white or cream colored. Examine the abdomen for inguinal or umbilical hernias.

Respiratory System

Listen to all lung quadrants and the trachea for breath sounds. Cats normally have quieter lung sounds than dogs. Cat lung sounds are only heard during inspiration [10]. Abnormal breathing may express as wheezing, gasping, crackling, coughing, or lack of breath sounds. Note if breathing difficulty is on inspiration or expiration. If panting, close the animal's mouth to assess true lung noises.

Cardiovascular System

Auscultate the heart for murmurs, arrhythmias, and muffled heart sounds. All four quadrants should be assessed. Sinus arrhythmia is a common finding, where the heart rate changes during breathing. While this is noted in the medical record, it is not a sign of cardiac pathology. Palpate the femoral pulse while listening to the heart. A pulse should be present for every heartbeat, if not, it indicates a pulse deficit. Areas of the heart to listen for murmurs are the aorta, mitral, and pulmonic valves on the left side and the tricuspid valve on the right side. Record murmurs in quality (Grade I–VI), location of intensity, timing, and radiation. Turbulent blood flow not only produces a heart murmur but also a thrill that is palpable on the chest wall with higher-intensity murmurs (V–VI) [11].

Nervous System

Along with examining locomotion for lameness, neurologic disorders are also noted. Observe the patient for scuffing or dragging the feet, inability to bear full weight (knuckling), and the inability to lift itself fully when rising. It is often difficult to determine if weakness or lameness is the result of an orthopedic or neurologic condition. Evaluate the patient's brain and mental status by observing its reaction to:

- Strong smells (e.g. alcohol)
- Menace, nystagmus, pupillary light response, and ability to follow the movement of a finger
- Corneal and palpebral reflexes
- Noise reaction
- Moving head normally by self and ability to "right" itself
- Gag and laryngeal reflexes
- Tongue retraction

Assessment of the spinal cord involves testing the spinal reflexes, postural reactions, and pain response. Use a reflex hammer to tap the appropriate tendon to check for a response. The triceps tendon behind the elbow, the patellar tendon of the stifle, and the gastrocnemius tendon of the hock are the most often tested reflexes. Note if the reflex is normal, hyper-reflexive, or not present. Check for conscious proprioception of the limbs by turning each of the feet under, thus forcing the patient to stand on the dorsal area of the foot. A patient with a normal postural reaction will immediately move the foot into a typical plantar/palmar position. This test is often repeated to confirm the response. Delayed response indicates a neurologic condition (Figure 1.12).

Other postural reactions include hopping – holding three legs in the air and walking the animal sideways toward one leg on the ground to allow the animal to move the leg laterally. Wheel barrowing is holding the rear legs in the air and allowing the patient to walk forward and maintain weight,

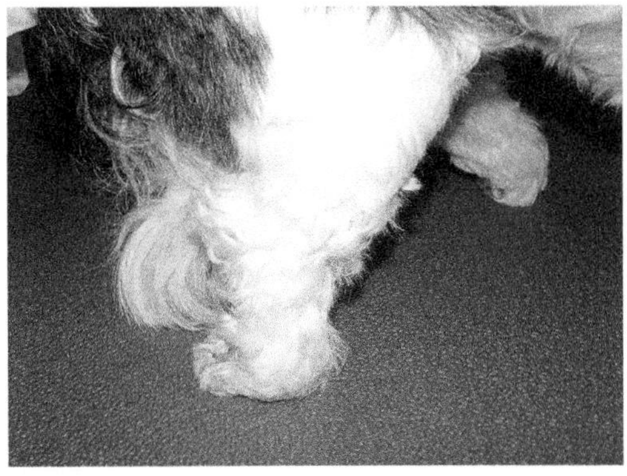

Figure 1.12 Patient with intervertebral disc disease demonstrating absent conscious proprioception or CP deficits.

and hemi-standing or hemi-walking is holding both legs of one side in the air while allowing the patient to walk with the other two legs. Any abnormality of the above may indicate a neurologic condition.

Evaluate pain response by pinching the toes. Gauge the response as a reflex (pulling the leg away) or a true pain response noted when the patient turns to look at the source of pain, vocalizes, and/or the pupils dilate. The panniculus aids in localizing the area of a spinal lesion. Pinch the skin of the back just off midline beginning at the tail and slowly moving forward to the head. Watch for contractions of the skin (Video 1.3). The spinal lesion is located in one vertebra caudal to the location of the first skin contraction [10].

Complete the neurologic exam by observing the anus for tone, it is normally closed and gap free. Evaluate the perineal reflex by stimulating the skin around the anus and watching for a contraction of the sphincter. The complete history and physical exam provide the veterinarian and client with much-needed information for creating a surgical plan.

References

1 Kaplan, J.L., Stern, J.A., Fascetti, A.J. *et al.* (2018) Taurine deficiency and dilated cardiomyopathy in golden retrievers fed commercial diets. *PLoS One*, 13(12), e0209112.

2 Goldberg, M.E. & Tominson, J.E. (2018) *Physical Rehabilitation for Veterinary Technicians and Nurses*. Wiley Blackwell, Hoboken, NJ.

3 Haaften, K.A., Eichstadt Forsythe, L.R., Stelow, E.A. *et al.* (2017) Effects of a single preappointment dose of gabapentin on signs of stress in cats during transportation and veterinary examination. *Journal of the American Veterinary Medical Association*, 251(10), 1175–1181.

4 James, S.P. & Mendelson, W.B. (2004) The use of trazodone as a hypnotic: a critical review. *The Journal of Clinical Psychiatry*, 65(6), 752–755.

5 Cummings, K. (2022) Pre-hospital sedation options for aggressive and anxious dogs. http://MSPCA.orgl/angell [accessed on 28 July 2023].

6 Zeltzman, P. How to confirm partial ACL tear veterinary practice news, September 2009 https://www.veterinarypracticenews.com/how-to-confirm-partial-acl-tear/ [accessed on 28 July 2023].

7 Piermattei, D., Flo, G. & DeCamp, C. (2006) *Handbook of Small Animal Orthopedics and Fracture Repair*, 5th edn. Saunders-Elsevier, St. Louis, MO.

8 Kerwin, S.C. Tips and tricks for the orthopedic exam at http://www.dcavm.org/12febnotes.pdf [accessed on 24 February 2023].

9 Fossum, T.W. (2019) *Small Animal Surgery*, 4th edn. Mosby, Inc, St. Louis, MO.

10 McCurnin, D. & Bassert, J. (2002) *Clinical Textbook for Veterinary Technicians*, 5th edn. WB Saunders, St. Louis, MO.

11 Kittleson, M.D. & Kienle, R.D. (1998) *Small Animal Cardiovascular Medicine*. Mosby Inc., St. Louis, MO.

2

Preoperative Planning

Gerianne Holzman[1] *and Lana Bishop*[2]

[1] *University of Wisconsin, School of Veterinary Medicine, Emerita, Madison, WI, USA*
[2] *Blue Pearl Pet Hospital, Des Moines, IA, USA*

Preparation for surgery includes evaluation of the entire patient, not just the specific area of concern. Assuring the patient is otherwise healthy for anesthesia and surgery, performing laboratory and imaging tests all provide a comprehensive assessment of the patient's health status. Assessing the need for perioperative antibiotic therapy depends on the type of procedure, its duration, and the patient's general condition. Planning for the patient's pre-, intra-, and postoperative pain control is an essential aspect of patient care. Veterinary technicians play an important role in preoperative planning by performing tests and providing the veterinary surgeon and anesthesia staff with the results. They also follow the veterinarian's orders by calculating the medication dosage, filling prescriptions, and administering medications.

Laboratory Tests

A preoperative assessment is performed on each individual patient to determine its anesthetic risks and general physiologic status. Knowledge of a patient's condition aids in creating an anesthetic protocol. Common preoperative tests include complete blood count (CBC), serum chemistry panel, and urinalysis. A database of a packed cell volume (PCV), total protein, and blood urea nitrogen (BUN) performed with a chemistry strip and blood glucose via a glucometer provides the minimal information required prior to surgery. A patient's age, physical condition, and surgical procedure determine the need for more extensive testing. Patients suffering a traumatic event, undergoing a complicated operation, or in a debilitated condition also lend themselves to additional laboratory tests. Certain breeds may signify a need for other tests. For example, Doberman Pinschers may carry the trait for von Willebrand disease, indicating the need for a buccal mucosal bleeding time or other clotting tests.

Surgical Patient Care for Veterinary Technicians and Nurses, Second Edition.
Edited by Gerianne Holzman and Teri Raffel Kleist.

Companion website: www.wiley.com/go/holzman/patient

Table 2.1 Complete blood count reference values.

Test	Units	Canine	Feline
RBC	$\times 10^6/\mu l$	4.95–7.87	5.0–10.0
Hemoglobin	g/dl	11.9–18.9	9.8–15.4
Hematocrit	%	35–57	30–45
MCV	fl	66–77	39–55
MCH	Pg	21.0–26.2	13–17
MCHC	g/dl	32.0–36.3	30–36
Reticulocyte	%	0.0–1.0	0.0–0.6
Platelets	$\times 10^3/\mu l$	211–621	300–800
MPV	fl	6.1–10.1	12–18
WBC	$\times 10^3/\mu l$	5.0–14.1	5.5–19.5
Segs	$\times 10^3/\mu l$	2.9–12.0	2.5–12.5
Bands	$\times 10^3/\mu l$	0.0–0.45	0.0–0.3
Lymphocytes	$\times 10^3/\mu l$	0.4–2.9	1.5–7.0
Monocytes	$\times 10^3/\mu l$	0.1–1.4	0.0–0.9
Eosinophils	$\times 10^3/\mu l$	0.0–1.3	0.0–0.8
Basophils	$\times 10^3/\mu l$	0.0–0.14	0.0–0.2

Reference values derived from University of Georgia College of Veterinary Medicine as examples only; reference values are not appropriate for interpretation for other laboratories.
Source: Adapted from Latimer [1].

Complete Blood Count

A complete blood count (CBC) measures the actual number and percent of specific blood cellular components: red blood cells (including cell morphology), white blood cells (including all cell types), hemoglobin, hematocrit, packed cell volume, and platelet count/estimate. This test is performed on whole blood collected with an anticoagulant. Normal values are determined for each individual analyzer machine (Table 2.1).

Serum Chemistry Panel

A serum chemistry panel or metabolic panel determines the current level of chemicals within the body [2]. These establish the health of the liver, kidneys, and pancreas as well as the body's electrolyte status. The test is preferably run on serum but may be performed on plasma. Normal values are determined for each individual analyzer machine (Table 2.2).

- *Alkaline phosphatase (ALP)*: An enzyme that may be elevated in certain cancers and muscle and liver diseases.
- *Alanine aminotransferase (ALT)*: An enzyme involved in liver function, elevations of which indicate liver damage or disease.
- *Aspartate aminotransferase (AST) or serum glutamic oxaloacetic transaminase (SGOT)*: An enzyme associated with liver parenchymal cells as well as red blood cells and cardiac and

Table 2.2 Serum chemistry reference values.

Test	Units	Canine	Feline
Albumin	g/dl	2.3–3.1	2.8–3.9
ALKP	U/l	1–114	0–45
ALT	U/l	10–109	25–97
Ammonia	µg/dl	19–120	0–90
Amylase	U/l	226–1063	550–1458
AST	U/l	13–15	7–38
Bile acids (fasting)	µmol/l	0–8	0–5
Bilirubin, total	mg/dl	0.0–0.3	0.0–0.1
Calcium	mg/dl	9.1–11.7	8.7–11.7
Chloride	mEq/l	110–124	115–130
Cholesterol	mg/dl	135–278	71–156
CK	U/l	52–368	69–214
Creatinine	mg/dl	0.5–1.7	0.9–2.2
Globulin, total	g/dl	2.7 4.4	2.6–5.1
Glucose	mg/dl	76–119	60–120
Iron	mg/dl	94–122	68–215
Lipase	U/l	60–330	0–76
Magnesium	mg/dl	1.6–2.4	1.7–2.6
Phosphorus	mg/dl	2.9–5.3	3.0–6.1
Potassium	mEq/l	3.9–5.1	3.7–6.1
Sodium	mEq/l	142–152	146–156
Total CO_2	mEq/l	14–26	13–21
Total protein (serum)	g/dl	5.4–7.5	6.0–7.9
Triglycerides	mg/dl	40–169	27–94
Urea nitrogen (BUN)	mg/dl	8–28	19–34

Reference values derived from University of Georgia College of Veterinary Medicine as examples only; reference values are not appropriate for interpretation for other laboratories.
Source: Adapted from Latimer [3].

skeletal muscle. The ratio of AST to ALT may differentiate causes of liver damage but is also a cardiac marker.

- *Blood urea nitrogen (BUN)*: A by-product of protein breaking down in the body is urea compounds containing nitrogen. The kidneys excrete these by-products. Kidney malfunction due to disease or urine blockage causes the compounds to remain in the blood resulting in an elevated BUN. Dehydration can reduce kidney function and cause a rise in this test. Liver disease may demonstrate below-normal blood urea nitrogen.
- *Calcium*: An abundant mineral that aids in bone growth, muscle contraction, blood vessel expansion and contraction, and secretion of hormones and enzymes.

- *Cholesterol*: A lipid or fat produced by the liver; cholesterol is vital for normal body function. Although elevated cholesterol contributes to arteriosclerosis in people, this is not a concern in the small animal patient. Poorly functioning thyroid glands may show an elevated cholesterol level.
- *Creatinine kinase (CK)*: An enzyme expressed in many tissues and cells which helps to evaluate tissue damage, particularly in muscles.
- *Creatinine (CREAT)*: A by-product of muscle metabolism, which is excreted by the kidneys; elevations of this chemical indicate kidney malfunction.
- *Glucose*: A monosaccharide or sugar; carbohydrates convert to glycogen in the body when an animal's energy level dictates, and glycogen converts to glucose. Glucose monitors metabolism and physiology. Low blood sugar (glucose) or hypoglycemia may manifest as weakness, incoordination, or even seizures. High blood sugar or hyperglycemia can come about from stress, but in certain disease conditions, particularly diabetes mellitus, excess glucose is excreted in the urine. Blood glucose levels above 180 mg/dl must be investigated further.
- *Magnesium*: An electrolyte involved in muscle, nerve, and enzyme function; it helps to move other electrolytes into and out of cells.
- *Phosphorus*: A non-metallic chemical element; phosphorous helps to build and repair bones and aids in nerve function and muscle contraction. Phosphorous works in combination with calcium: if calcium levels rise, phosphorous levels decline. Phosphorous levels increase in patients with renal dysfunction.
- *Total bilirubin*: A by-product of the breakdown of hemoglobin; elevations occur when excess red blood cells break down, when the liver is diseased and unable to clear the bilirubin, or if the bile duct is occluded keeping it from sending bilirubin into the intestine.
- *Total protein*: A combined measurement of albumin (produced in the liver) and globulin (produced in the immune system); these proteins can be elevated or decreased in infectious diseases. They may elevate when a patient is dehydrated.
- *Triglycerides*: A type of fat that stores energy and provides energy to the muscles.
- *Electrolytes*
  - *Sodium (Na)*: A chemical element; it controls the amount of water in the body. The transmission of sodium into and out of cells generates electrical signals. These signals control body processes within the brain, nervous system, and muscles. Increased sodium levels can indicate dehydration and kidney disease. Decreased sodium can be found in patients with liver, kidney, and heart disease.
  - *Potassium (K)*: A chemical element inside of cells; it regulates heartbeat and muscle functions. Increased potassium (hyperkalemia) and decreased calcium (hypokalemia) can be found in patients with kidney disease. Either condition may manifest in patients taking certain medications. Angiotensin-converting enzyme (ACE) inhibitors, digoxin, and cyclosporine are examples of drugs that may cause hyperkalemia. Diuretics, aminoglycosides, insulin, and other drugs may lead to hypokalemia
  - *Chloride (Cl)*: An ion formed from the element chlorine; it is found in fluid outside of cells and helps to maintain normal fluid balance in the body. Increased chloride levels can be found with diarrhea, kidney disease, and hyperparathyroidism. Decreases in chloride can occur with vomiting, adrenal, and kidney disease.
  - *Carbon dioxide (CO_2)*: A chemical compound; it is a by-product of cellular metabolism which travels through the body with the hemoglobin and leaves the body through the lungs. Poor respiratory function, kidney disease, and metabolic conditions affect its level.

Coagulation Tests

Coagulation tests are recommended for liver-associated procedures and thrombocytopenia. The majority of hepatic procedures have a risk of hemorrhage that can be life-threatening. The liver is essential for production of procoagulant and anticoagulant substances. Hepatic disease can increase the risk of hemorrhage and thrombosis [4]. Prothrombin time (PT) and activated partial thromboplastin time (aPTT) assess secondary hemostasis via reagents that activate coagulation through the extrinsic or intrinsic pathway, respectively. Prolongation of the PT indicates defective extrinsic and/or common pathways, whereas aPTT prolongation indicates defective intrinsic and/or common pathways [5].

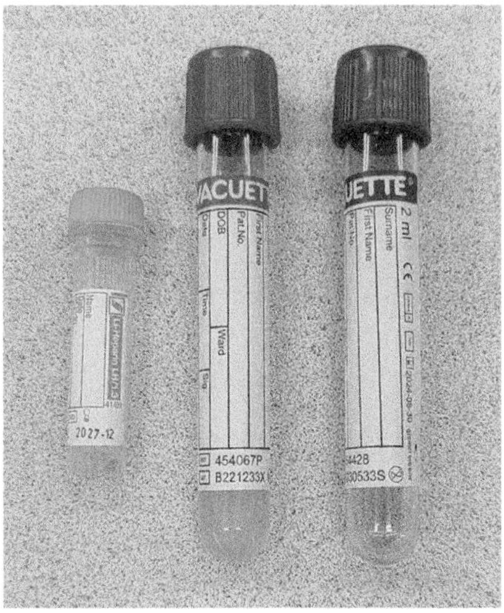

Figure 2.1 Left to Right: green (heparin), red (plain, no additive), and purple (EDTA) blood collection tubes.

Blood Collection Tubes

To obtain the most accurate results from blood tests, the proper blood collection tube is required. The colors of the tops of the tube indicate the type of additive, if any, contained in the tube. It is imperative to gently rotate the tubes after collection to properly mix the blood with the additive, if present (Figures 2.1 and 2.2; Table 2.3).

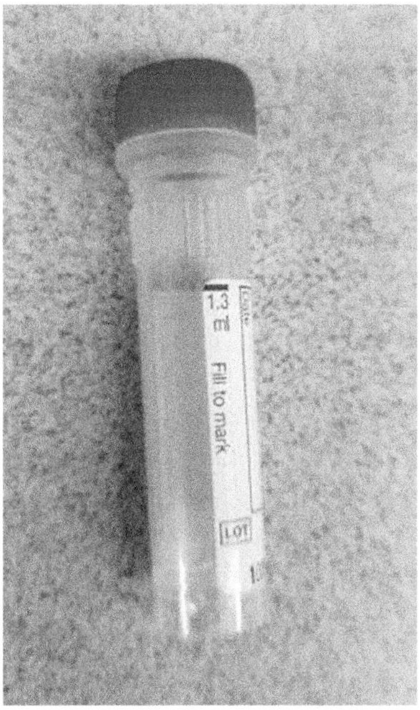

Figure 2.2 Blue (sodium citrate) blood collection tube.

Urinalysis

Urine for testing is obtained by free catch, manual expression, catheterization, or via cystocentesis. For samples requiring a culture and sensitivity test to check for urinary tract infection, cystocentesis is preferred to avoid urethral or catheter contamination. To perform a cystocentesis, the patient may lay in lateral or dorsal recumbency. The sample may also be obtained with the patient standing, but this position is difficult for the technician working underneath the dog, whereas cats are not likely to stand still. Samples are easily obtained from female dogs laying in dorsal recumbency. The patient needs to be held comfortably on its back by one or two assistants. Alcohol is poured onto the caudal abdomen to form a "pool" along the midline (Figure 2.3).

Using a 22 ga × 1–1½″ needle on a 10 ml syringe, the needle is inserted straight perpendicular (90° angle) to the body, directly through the pool of alcohol. Often, one can feel the needle puncturing the bladder. The syringe is aspirated slightly to check for successfully obtaining urine. If present, the syringe is filled, suction released, and the syringe is removed. If blood is noted in the

Table 2.3 Common blood collection tubes.

Color	Additive	Product/tests
Green	Heparin	Plasma – ammonia, electrolytes, etc.
Red	No additive or clot activator (separator tubes)	Serum – chemistry panels
Purple	EDTA	Whole blood – complete blood count
Blue	Sodium citrate	Whole blood/plasma – coagulation panel

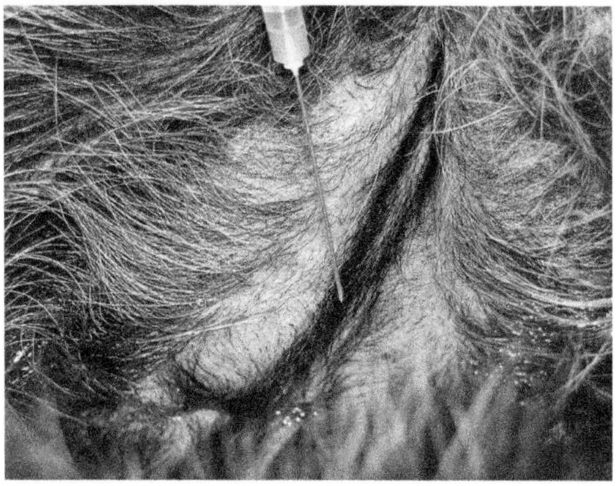

Figure 2.3 "Puddle" of alcohol on a female dog prior to performing a cystocentesis. The needle is directed perpendicular to the body through the puddle and into the bladder.

syringe, aspiration ceases and the needle is withdrawn. (Blood contaminates the sample and may cause a false-positive blood reading on a urinalysis.) Moving cranially or caudally to the original site depending on the expected size of the bladder may yield success. Full bladders tend to be more cranially located while smaller-diameter bladders tend to reside nearer to the pelvis. Palpating the bladder may help in locating it but sometimes this is difficult in patients with distended abdomens. Ultrasound is a useful tool for imaging the bladder and obtaining urine samples for all patients (Figures 2.4 and 2.5).

A similar technique is useful in male dogs; however, the prepuce keeps the alcohol from pooling. The needle is inserted at more of an angle to the body aiming for the midline below the prepuce. Another technique is to move the prepuce to the side and insert the needle directly perpendicular to midline.

Small dogs and cats have more easily palpable bladders. The patient is laid in lateral recumbency with an assistant holding the front and back legs while the patient is stretched in a comfortable position. Using one hand to palpate the bladder, the hair is smoothed down with alcohol. Keeping the bladder isolated in one hand, the needle is inserted directly perpendicular to the body and into the bladder. Urine is aspirated into the syringe. If blood is seen, the procedure is stopped and tried in another location.

Free catch and expressed samples are acceptable for routine urinalysis without a bacterial culture. Non-absorbent litter in a plastic litter pan aids in collecting free-catch urine from cats. For dogs, walk them outside and use a ladle or cup to collect urine. After obtaining the sample, transfer the urine to a sterile container for testing.

Urine catheterization is obtained through a variety of catheters. Red rubber and Foley catheters create less urethral trauma and have a decreased risk of bladder perforation than polypropylene catheters. Catheters are inserted using aseptic technique. The penis or vulva is cleaned with a

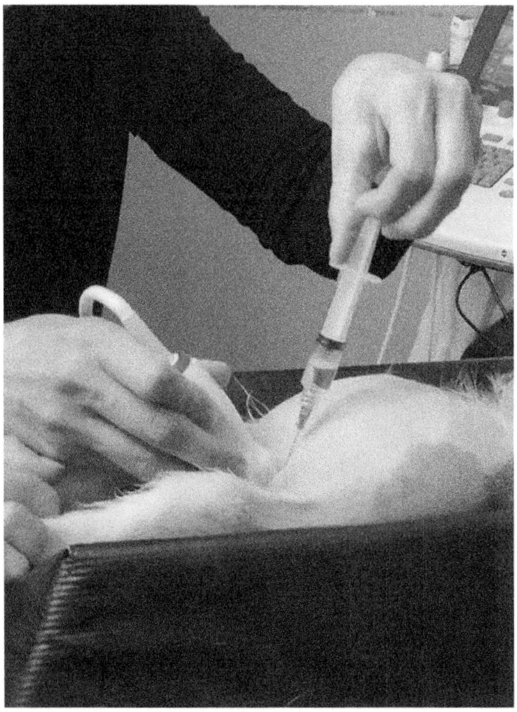

Figure 2.4 Ultrasound-guided cystocentesis. *Source:* Courtesy of Heather Vaske.

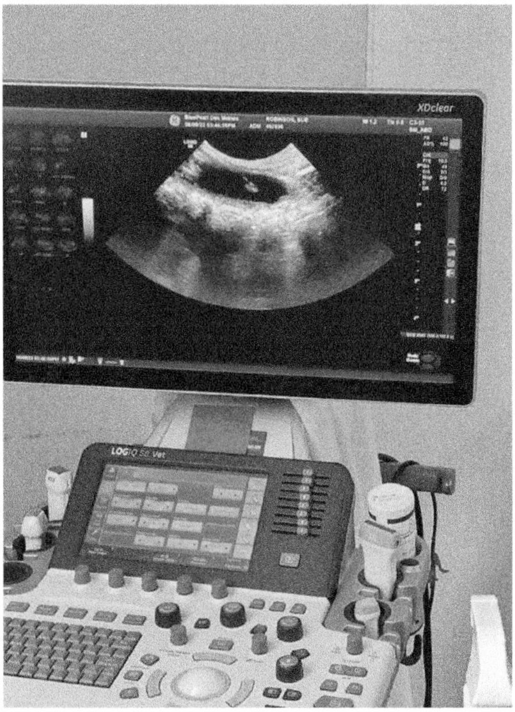

Figure 2.5 Ultrasound image showing the urinary bladder (dark gray or hypoechoic) with a needle (bright or hyperechoic) inserted to collect urine. *Source:* Courtesy of Heather Vaske.

dilute antiseptic of choice. After applying sterile lubricant to the tip of the urinary catheter, the technician (wearing sterile gloves) inserts the catheter. Success is evident when urine flows out of the catheter. If planning for an indwelling (Foley) catheter, the catheter's balloon is filled with the appropriate volume of media (saline or air) depending on the manufacturer's recommendation. For short-term catheterizations, either to obtain a urine sample or to empty the bladder one time, the catheter is removed immediately following the procedure. Urine from a catheter may be used for bacterial testing but may contain urethral contaminants.

Urinalysis tests include the following [6]:

- *Specific gravity (SG)*: Using a refractometer determines the urine's concentration. Dilute urine may indicate renal disease, adrenal problems, high calcium, diabetes, or hyperthyroidism. High specific gravity may be a sign of dehydration. Normal feline SG range: 1.020–1.040; canine SG range: 1.016–1.060.

The following tests are all performed using a urine dipstick:

- *pH*: Measures the acidity level of the urine; bacterial infections create alkaluria, struvite crystals form in alkaline urine, and cystine crystals in acidic urine. Normal pH values: feline (6.0–7.0) and canine (6.0–7.0)
- *Protein*: May indicate inflammation, hematuria, or glomerular disease. Normal protein values in dogs and cats are "negative to trace."
- *Glucose*: Indicates the presence of sugar in the urine; it may be indicative of diabetes. (If positive, perform a blood glucose test to confirm.) Normal urine glucose test for felines and canines is "negative."
- *Ketones (acetone)*: Checks for the presence of acetate and acetoacetate; it may be present in diabetes or starvation. Normal value for cats and dogs is "negative."
- *Bilirubin*: A positive test may indicate liver dysfunction; bilirubin (old blood cells) normally metabolizes through the liver into the colon – when the liver does not function properly, the bilirubin is discharged through the kidneys. Normal urine bilirubin value for canines and felines is "trace – 1+." (Higher readings are more often seen in concentrated urine.)
- *Blood*: Indicates hematuria; it may be an artifact of cystocentesis or catheterization. Urine sediment examination confirms or disputes this finding. The normal value for dogs and cats is "negative – trace."

Urine sediment examination looks for microscopic components in the urine, which may be crystals, casts, red blood cells, white blood cells, epithelial cells, or bacteria. If present, these entities may be indicative of a medical condition and are investigated along with clinical signs and other tests such as bloodwork and urine cultures.

Other Diagnostic Tests

In addition to the common blood and urine tests, a variety of conditions benefit from preoperative sampling. These include fine needle aspirates (FNAs) of joints, abdomen, pulmonary spaces, masses, cysts, and abscesses for cytologic exam. Prior knowledge of the condition of a surgical site (joint, mass, etc.) aids the surgeon's preoperative planning and prognosis. Blood clotting (coagulation) tests may be indicated if excessive bleeding is expected during surgery such as liver-associated procedures.

Abdominocentesis

This test may be performed with the patient standing or in lateral recumbency. Sampling from a standing position allows gravity to move any fluid to the most ventral aspect of the abdomen for ease of sampling. After clipping and prepping the area to tap, a needle (attached to a syringe) is inserted through the abdominal wall to obtain the sample. Some patients may need evacuation of large quantities of fluid. For these animals, insertion of an intravenous catheter with the stylet removed, attached to extension tubing, and a three-way stopcock decreases potential for organ trauma. One person holds the catheter in place while an assistant uses the stopcock and a syringe to remove the abdominal fluid. Fluid is analyzed for blood or urine as well as a microscopic examination.

Arthrocentesis

Arthrocentesis provides the surgeon with valuable information for diagnosis, presurgical planning, and postoperative complications. Combined with radiographs, the joint fluid may indicate the need, or lack of need, for surgery. Bacterial presence indicates a septic joint while a high cell count may indicate immune-mediated polyarthritis (IMPA). These two conditions are treated very differently – one with antibiotics and the other with steroids. Joint taps are readily performed on the carpi, elbows, tarsi, and stifles. It is more difficult to accomplish an arthrocentesis of the shoulder or hip due to the depth of the joint and the overlying musculature.

Arthrocentesis is most often carried out on a sedated or anesthetized patient with added pain control medications. Usually, the patient is in lateral recumbency to facilitate access to the joints. The affected side is up except when tapping the elbow which is accessed from the medial side. The joint(s) of choice is clipped and surgically scrubbed (Figures 2.6 and 2.7). A towel or drape beneath the leg provides a clean surface to avoid contamination from the patient's hair and surroundings. An assistant holds the leg in the desired position (Figure 2.8). The technician or doctor dons sterile gloves to avoid contaminating the arthrocentesis site. A needle is inserted into the joint and may or may not be attached to a syringe (Figure 2.9). It is personal preference on which technique to employ. The gauge and length of the needle are determined by the joint being sampled and by the size of the patient. After inserting the needle into the joint and fluid is seen in the needle hub, the fluid is slowly aspirated (Figure 2.10). If blood is noted, the procedure is immediately stopped to avoid sample contamination and thus false-positive readings of blood in the synovial fluid. (However, depending on the patient's condition, blood may be present in the course of the disease.)

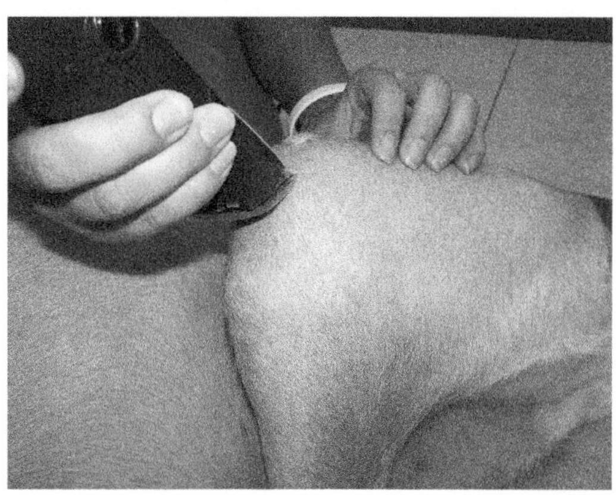

Figure 2.6 Arthrocentesis of a stifle step 1: clipping the hair.

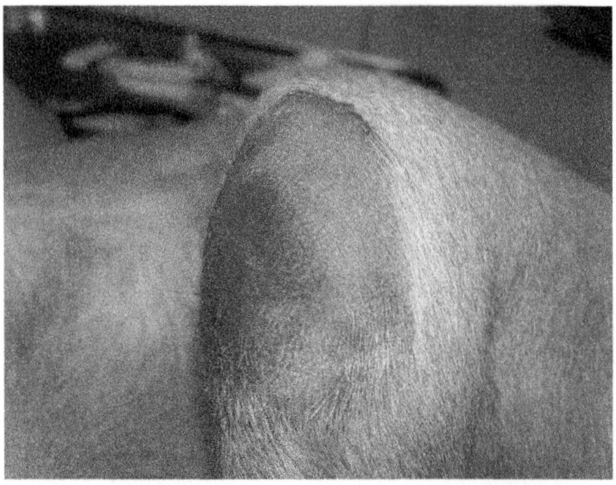

Figure 2.7 Arthrocentesis of a stifle step 2: prepping the skin.

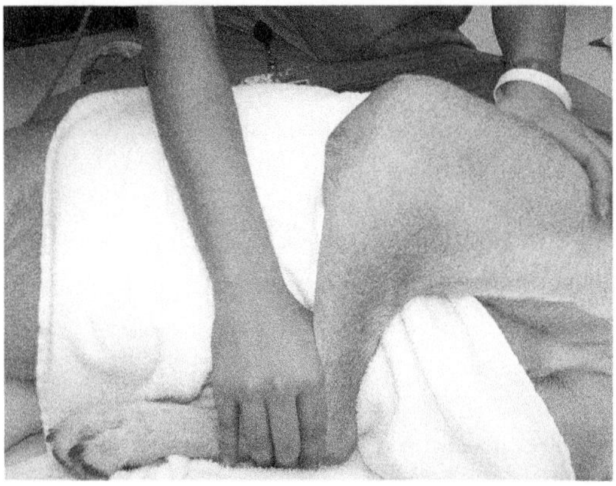

Figure 2.8 Arthrocentesis of a stifle step 3: positioning the leg.

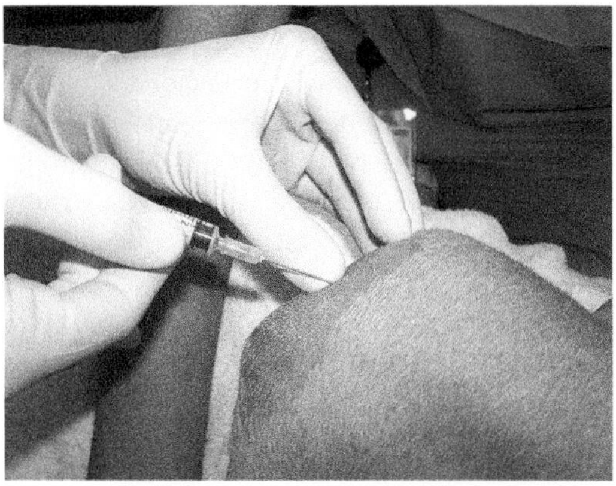

Figure 2.9 Arthrocentesis of a stifle step 4: inserting the needle two-third distally between the patella and the tibial crest.

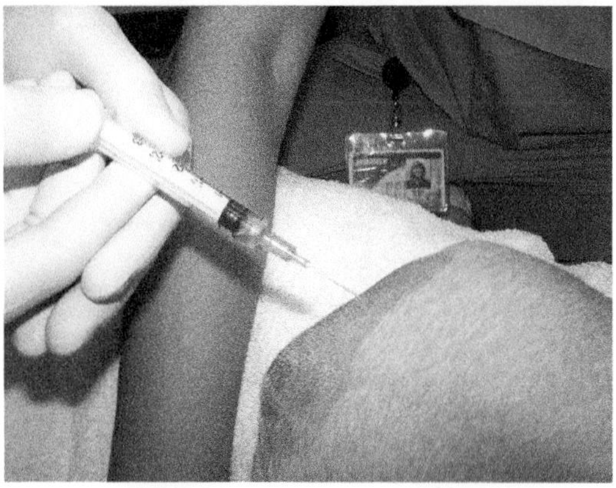

Figure 2.10 Arthrocentesis of a stifle step 5: aspirating synovial fluid.

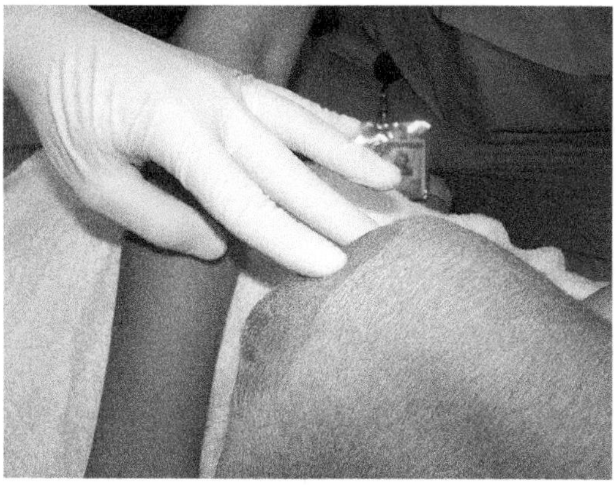

Figure 2.11 Arthrocentesis of a stifle step 6: applying pressure to the tap site.

After obtaining the desired sample, aspiration is stopped prior to removing the needle and digital pressure is applied to the arthrocentesis site if drainage is present (Figure 2.11). The syringe and needle are disconnected and air is drawn into the syringe. After reconnecting the needle and syringe, the sample is squirted onto a microscope slide. Small amounts of fluid are smeared on a slide and examined for its cytologic properties. Larger quantities of fluid are put into an EDTA (purple top) Microtainer for cytology and fluid analysis. EDTA prevents clotting of the synovial fluid. If a culture is desired, a quantity of fluid is kept separate from the EDTA preservative by placing it in a non-additive tube (red top).

Arthrocentesis of the most common joints are performed through the following techniques [7]. Effusive joints provide easier access.

1) *Carpus*: Palpate the joint at the base of the accessory carpal bone; flexion and extension of the joint aid in localizing this access space and the needle is inserted from the dorsal cranial aspect – occluding the cephalic vein avoids inadvertent venipuncture
2) *Elbow*: A variety of techniques are described for accessing the elbow – medially, laterally, caudally, and with the elbow flexed and extended – personal preference comes with experience; however, the goal is to gain access to the joint between the humeral condyles
3) *Tarsus*: The joint is hyperextended and the needle is inserted lateral or medial to the fibular tarsal bone aiming for the middle of the joint
4) *Stifle*: The stifle is flexed to open up the joint space and the needle is inserted medially or laterally into the patella ligament about two-thirds of the way distally between the patella and the tibial crest – the needle is at a slight angle to the stifle with the goal to insert it caudal to the patella

Whenever performing an arthrocentesis, if bone is encountered, the needle is "walked" off the bone to enter the joint space. Repeated attempts increase the likelihood of blood contamination of the sample.

Fine Needle Aspirate

Fine needle aspirates obtain samples for cytologic examination to aid in diagnosis and treatment plans. Sites to be tested include masses, cysts, surgery sites, abscesses, etc. If infection or fluid is expected, the FNA site is clipped and cleaned with an antiseptic solution. When aspirating a solid mass, minimal prep, by wetting the hair with alcohol, better visualizes the mass. While steadying the mass with one hand, a needle alone or attached to a syringe is inserted into the desired site.

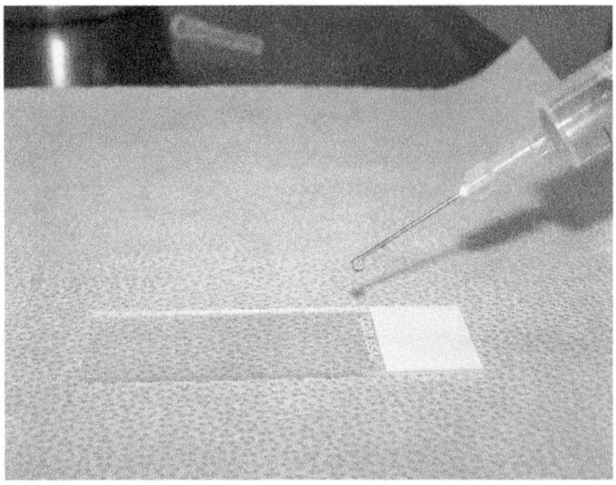

Figure 2.12 Applying needle aspirate to a slide for cytology.

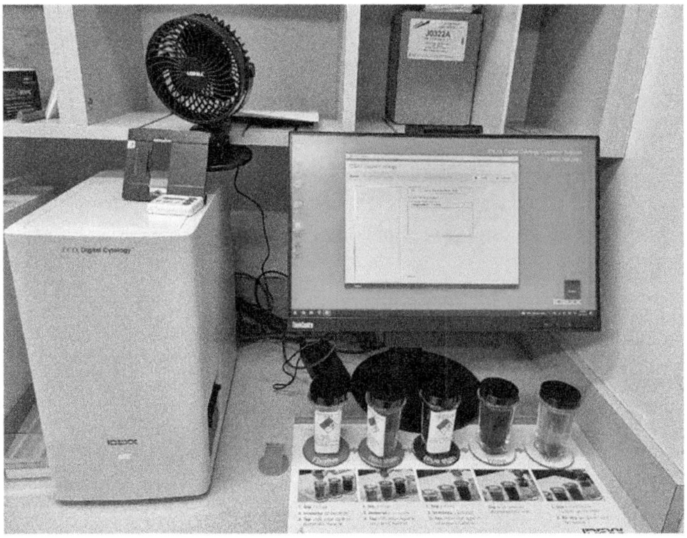

Figure 2.13 Idexx™ digital cytology instrument.

If fluid is seen, it is immediately aspirated and treated in the same manner as synovial fluid described under arthrocentesis. When performing an FNA on a solid mass, after inserting the needle into the mass, the needle is moved in several directions to increase the likelihood of obtaining a diagnostic sample. There may be enough cells within the bore and hub of the needle without aspiration. The rest of the technique for cytologic examination is as previously described (Figure 2.12).

An IDEXX Digital Cytology instrument takes high-resolution images of a slide to allow for in-hospital fine needle aspirates to be read by a veterinary clinical pathologist. This provides a comprehensive report, with images, in two hours or less (Figure 2.13).

Imaging

Preoperative, intra-operative, and postoperative imaging – radiographs, computed tomography (CT), magnetic resonance imaging (MRI), contrast studies, and ultrasound – aid in diagnosis, surgical planning, and evaluation. Individual and combined modalities provide the surgeon and veterinary technician with specific information. For metastatic staging, multiple modalities may be used, i.e. three-view chest radiographs and an abdominal ultrasound or a full-body CT scan.

Personal Protection

X-rays produce radicals in exposed cells that may break or change chemical bonds within molecules. Cells may be damaged, die, or mutate. Parameters that contribute to biological effects include radiation dose rate, total dose received, energy of the radiation, part of body exposed, individual sensitivity, and cell sensitivity. The blood-forming, reproductive, and digestive organs are most sensitive to radiation effects. The nervous system, muscles, and connective tissue are less sensitive.[1]

Veterinary technicians performing radiographs must take precautions to assure their own safety. The level of exposure is minimized with proper safety measures. The X-ray tube is the primary source of radiation exposure. Elimination of direct contact with the primary beam is essential. The most common source of X-ray exposure is scattering radiation bouncing off the patient. The amount of scatter increases when a patient receives a high dose of radiation. Therefore, keep patient dosing to the minimum needed to achieve desired results. Collimating the beam to the focus area reduces scatter and improves image quality. Maintaining a distance from the patient while taking a radiograph is ideal but this usually requires sedation or full anesthesia to retain proper positioning. Even standing straight with your gloved hands restraining the patient instead of bending over the patient reduces exposure. Many positioning aids are commercially available such as weighted sandbags, radiolucent V-troughs, and foam wedges at multiple angles. Other items commonly used for non-manual positioning include towels, Velcro straps, leashes, and white porous tape. Standing behind shielding provided by a specially reinforced wall or window and lead curtains and screens provides the best protection. If patient contact is required, personal safety is essential. Lead aprons come in a variety of shapes and thicknesses. Depending on its lead equivalence, an apron can block 90% or more of scattered radiation [8]. Thyroid shields must always be in place. The lens of the eye is also sensitive to radiation. Protective eyewear with side protection can reduce scatter to the eyes by 90%. Gloves provide excellent protection but care must be still taken to keep hands out of the primary beam as they are designed to protect from scatter radiation only. Proper positioning of the patient and the use of the aforementioned devices help to keep hands away from the primary beam.

Gloves, aprons, and lead shields must be periodically examined for cracks, bite marks, and tears that limit their effectiveness. Replace any damaged protection device as it is ineffective.

All personnel responsible for taking radiographs or monitoring patients during an imaging procedure must wear a dosimeter to track occupational exposure. Individual dose limits must not be exceeded. Calibrated dosimeters, provided by a monitoring service, record exposure. An evaluation is provided on a routine basis (Figure 2.14).

Individuals routinely exposed to scatter radiation wear one dosimeter under the apron to assess the effectiveness of the protective clothing. Another dosimeter worn at shoulder or collar level provides information on exposure of unprotected body parts. A combination of the two readings provides an accurate measurement of the effective dose. When hands are routinely near the primary beam such as fluoroscopy, ring or bracelet dosimeters may also be employed. The current occupational dose limits according to the United State Nuclear Regulatory Commission (USNRC) are provided in Table 2.4[2].

1 2011. http://xrayweb.chem.ou.edu/notes/safety.html.
2 https://www.nrc.gov/about-nrc/radiation/health-effects/info.html#dose.

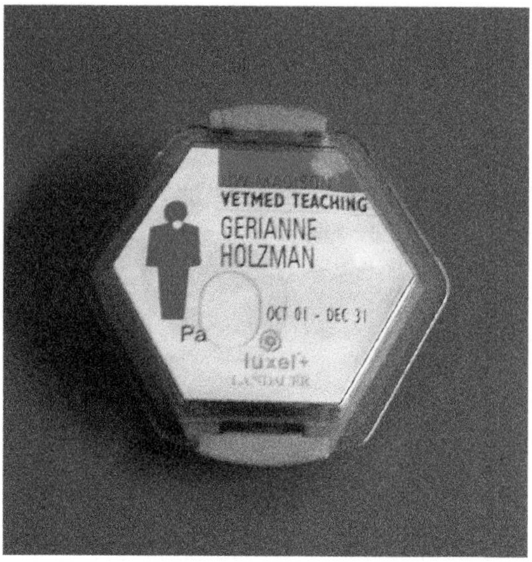

Figure 2.14 Dosimeter for measuring radiation exposure.

Table 2.4 United States Nuclear Regulatory Commission occupational dose limits.

Body part	Dose limit
Whole body	5000 mrem/yr*
Any organ	50,000 mrem/yr
Skin	50,000 mrem/yr
Extremity	50,000 mrem/yr
Lens of eye	15,000 mrem/yr
Embryo/fetus of worker	100 mrem/yr

* 1000 mrem = 1 rem.

Radiographs

Radiographs are created when either a cassette or digital plate is struck by X-ray photons. X-rays are, according to Roentgen, highly penetrating invisible rays that are a form of electromagnetic radiation. These rays are produced in a circuit containing a cathode and anode contained within the X-ray tube. When the circuit is closed, it supplies power to the cathode side of the X-ray tube. This causes the filament in the cathode to heat up, producing electrons and converting the electrons into X-ray photons. The anode directs the X-rays toward the patient while dissipating heat from their production [9].

Digital radiography revolutionized the process by drastically decreasing processing time and dose. It still requires proper technique and positioning but the image quality is better and more adjustable in postprocessing. Digital radiographs are still prone to distortion and movement artifacts [9].

Exceptional detail is required for orthopedic imaging to allow for evaluation of osteoarthritis, degenerative changes, implant measuring, multiple fracture lines, osteochondritis dissecans (OCD) lesions, etc. The films need to be of high contrast – bones white, background black, and soft tissue gray. Peak kilowatt voltage (KVP) is set lower than for a thorax or abdomen. Enough mA is used to provide a diagnostic amount of blackness on the image. A technique chart is created for

Table 2.5 Sample radiograph technique chart.

All American Animal Hospital

With grid — Regular screens

Thorax

cm	10	11	12	13	14	15	16	17	18	19	20	21	22	23	24	25	26	27	28	29	30
kVp	68	70	72	74	76	78	80	82	85	88	91	94	97	100	103	106	109	112	115	118	121
mAs	2.5 mAs*																				
mA × time	300 mA × 8.33 ms*																				

*For obesity or fluid increase to 5 mAs. For very thin pts decrease to 240 mA and 2.0 mAs

Abdomen

cm	10	11	12	13	14	15	16	17	18	19	20	21	22	23	24	25	26	27	28	29	30
kVp	66	68	70	72	74	76	78	81	83	86	89	83	85	87	89	81	83	85	87	89	91
mAs	7.5 mAs											15 mAs				30 mAs					
mA × time	300 mA × 25 ms											300 mA × 50 ms				300 mA × 100 ms					

For VD abds on deep-chested or thin pts, you may need a decrease in kVp by 10% or decrease time by half

Spine/skull, pelvis, large extremities

cm	10	11	12	13	14	15	16	17	18	19	20	21	22	23	24	25	26	27	28	29	30
kVp	61	63	65	67	69	71	73	75	77	79	81	77	79	81	83	85	87	90	92	94	96
mAs	25 mAs											45 mAs									
mA × time	300 mA × 83.3 ms											300 mA × 150 ms									

For VD pelvis decrease lateral pelvis technique by 4 kVp

Non-grid — Fine screens

Thorax

cm	4	5	6	7	8	9	10	11	12	13
kVp	47	49	51	53	55	57	59	61	63	65
mAs	8 mAs									
mA × time	240 mA × 33.3 ms									

Abdomen

cm	4	5	6	7	8	9	10	11	12	13
kVp	50	52	54	56	58	54	56	58	60	62
mAs	8 mAs					16 mAs				
mA × time	240 mA × 33.3 ms					240 mA × 66.7 ms				

Spine/skull pelvis

cm	4	5	6	7	8	9	10	11	12	13
kVp	50	52	54	56	58	54	56	58	60	62
mAs	15 mAs					30 mAs				
mA × time	300 mA × 50 ms					300 mA × 100 ms				

Extremities* (and turtle bodies)

cm	0.5	1	2	3	4	5	6	7	8	9	10	11	12
kVp	42	44	46	48	50	52	54	56	58	54	56	58	60
mAs	15 mAs									30 mAs			
mA × time	300 mA × 50 ms									300 mA × 100 ms			

*For avian and reptile extremities, subtract 3 kVp

Avian and reptile whole bodies

cm	2	3	4	5	6	7	8	9	10	11	12
kVp	46	48	50	52	54	56	58	54	56	58	60
mAs	15 mAs							30 mAs			
mA × time	300 mA × 50 ms							300 mA × 100 ms			

Use the extremity chart above –3 kVp for extremities

This chart was designed for Kodak lanex regular and fine screens with green film.

Source: Courtesy of Amy Lang, RTR.

each individual radiography unit (Table 2.5). Radiography texts are best referenced for specific patient positioning information and will not be covered here.

Computed Tomography Scan and Magnetic Resonance Imaging

All radiographic imaging aids in the determination of a structure's normalcy or pathology [10]. The advantage of computed tomography (CT) and magnetic resonance imaging (MRI) is the

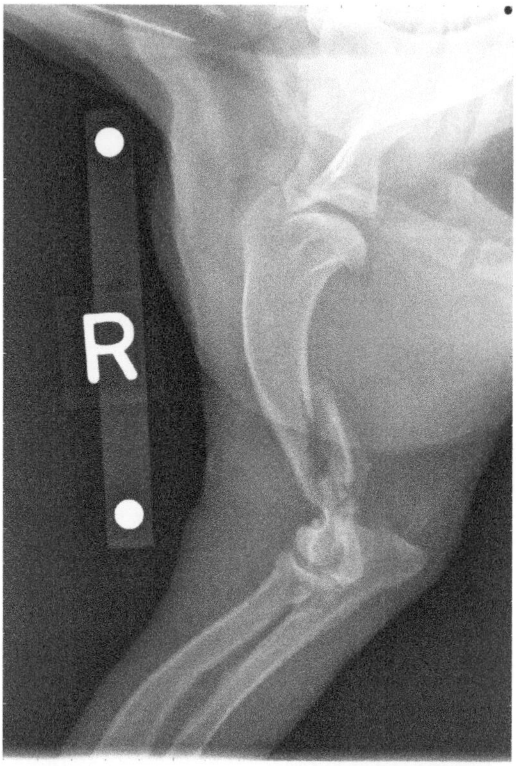

Figure 2.15 Radiograph showing the lateral view of a severely comminuted distal humeral fracture.

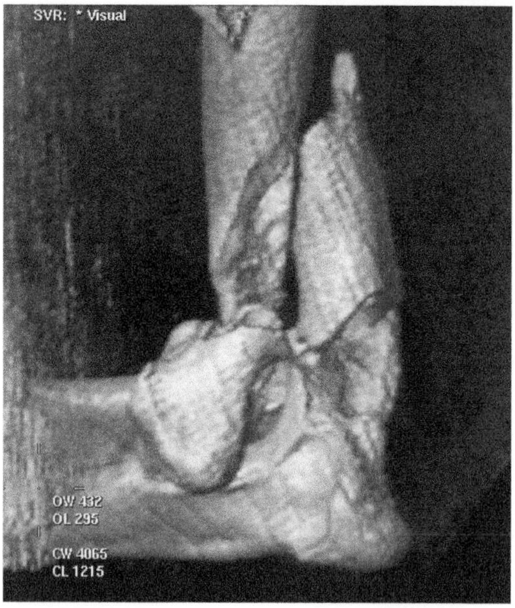

Figure 2.16 Computerized Tomography (CT) 3-D reconstruction of the same fracture seen in Figure 2.15. When viewed in motion, the reconstruction aids in planning the surgical repair.

tomographic nature of the images. This allows for cross-sectional, three-dimensional, and anatomic localizations of lesions. Comparisons can be made between radiographs and CT scans for preoperative planning (Figures 2.15 and 2.16).

Cross sections eliminate the superimposition of structures inherent in a two-dimensional "flat" film/routine radiograph. CT and MRI provide images of greater contrast than traditional films due to the computer technology providing deeper blacks, brighter whites, and more intense grays. The biochemical environment creating the MR image also provides greater contrast and better diagnostics.

Computed tomography and magnetic resonance images are created with electronic technology. Flowing electrons carry information about the subject to a screen creating an image. During an MRI, the patient's hydrogen protons – which possess magnetic fields – directly induce voltage in a conductor by electromagnetic induction. In CT, X-ray photons pass through the patient and convert to electric signals. A computer then processes these signals to create a digital image. MRI has better subject contrast than CT and is superior in demonstrating the brain, spinal cord, and soft tissue structures such as ligaments and cartilage in joints [9].

Ultrasound

Ultrasound imaging supports many diagnostic needs. Most common areas of ultrasound are abdomen (including all organs), heart, tendons, and joints. Ultrasounds guide the diagnostician in obtaining biopsies and fine needle aspirates of organs and masses. Prior to undergoing an ultrasound procedure, the patient's hair is shaved. Insufficient shaving allows hair to interfere with the contact between the ultrasound transducer and the skin. For abdominal ultrasounds, shave the patient cranially to the sternum and caudally to the pubis. The lateral sides are shaved dorsally to midway between the ventral midline and the spine (Figure 2.17). This provides full imaging of the entire abdominal contents.

Ultrasound is defined as sound waves greater than 20,000 Hz/s. Human hearing range is 20–20,000 Hz. Diagnostic ultrasound employs frequencies of 2–15 MHz (1 MHz = 1,000,000 Hz). To create the ultrasound wave, electricity is sent to piezoelectric crystals within an ultrasound transducer where it is converted into sound creating a pulse [11]. The pulse travels to the body part

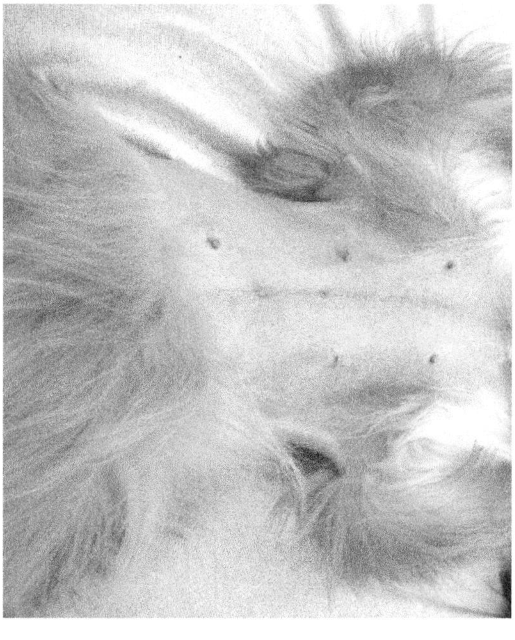

Figure 2.17 Shaving a patient for an abdominal ultrasound covers the distance from the sternum to the pubis and halfway up the sides.

being viewed creating an echo. The echo returns to the transducer where it is converted back to electricity creating an image on the ultrasound machine. Ultrasound works best in soft tissue, as they do not penetrate air (lungs) or bones well. Unlike other diagnostic imaging, no radiation is used in ultrasounds, only sound waves. Thus, no personal or patient protection is required (Figure 2.18).

Transducers come in a variety of frequencies – higher frequencies create better image resolution. However, the higher frequency allows less penetration of deep tissues. Transducers are mechanical or electronic. Mechanical transducers contain single or multiple crystals within an acoustic coupling medium. The crystals oscillate or rotate within the transducer heading creating the ultrasound wave and receiving the echo. Mechanical transducers are subject to wear. Electronic transducers contain piezoelectric material arranged in arrays: linear or sector (curved or phased).

a) Sector array
   i) Parallel or concentric rings of crystals
   ii) Curved transducer face (Figure 2.19)
   iii) Sector or pie-shaped image (Figure 2.20)
   iv) Used for deep application or narrow areas, e.g. intercostal spaces for thoracic images

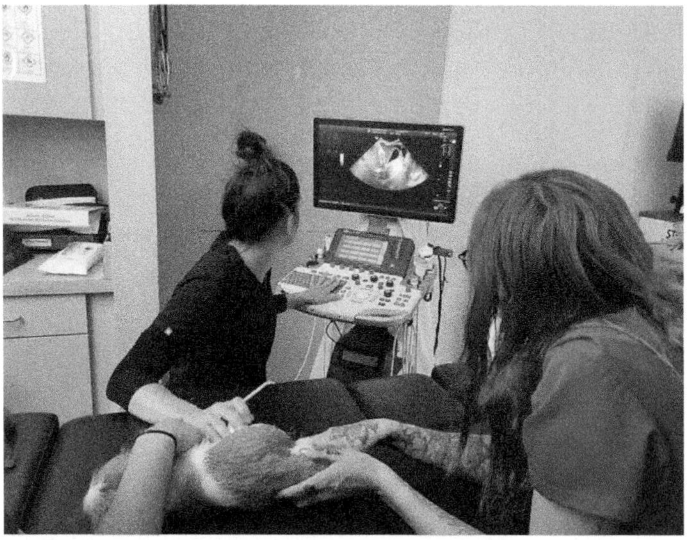

Figure 2.18 Performing an abdominal ultrasound with the patient in lateral recumbency.

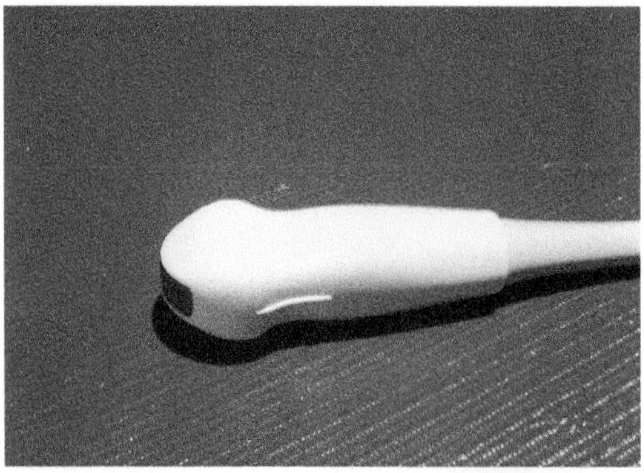

Figure 2.19 Sector ultrasound transducer.

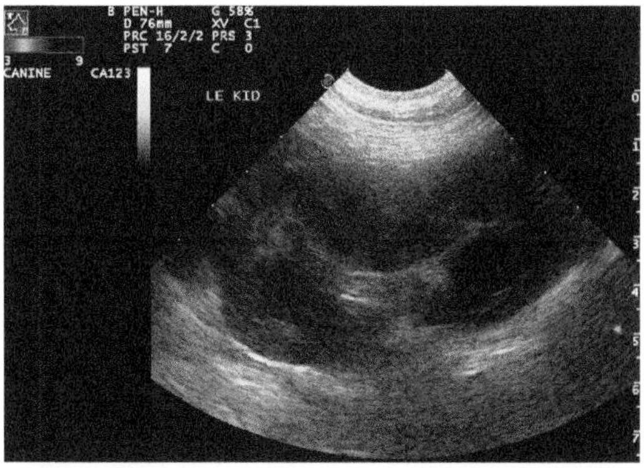

Figure 2.20 Left kidney ultrasound image using a sector transducer. *Source:* Courtesy of Fern Delaney.

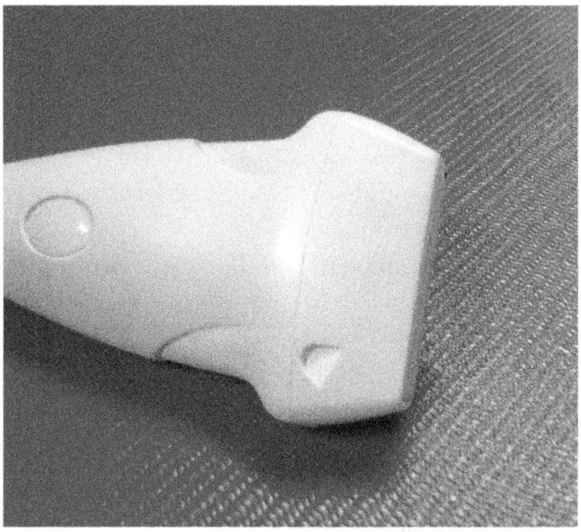

Figure 2.21 Linear ultrasound transducer.

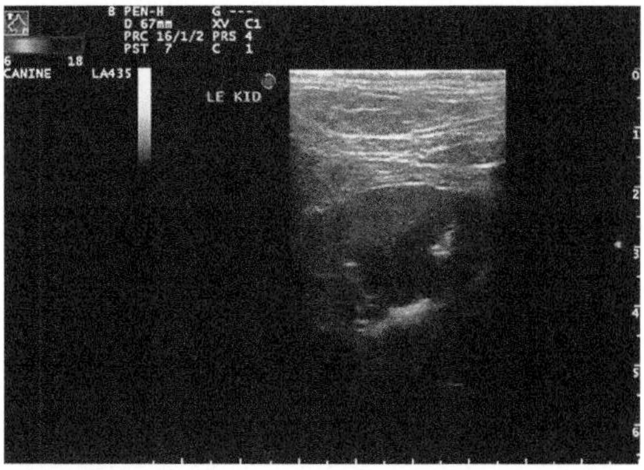

Figure 2.22 Left kidney (same as in Figure 2.20) ultrasound image using a linear transducer. *Source:* Courtesy of Fern Delaney.

b) Linear array
   i) Parallel crystals
   ii) Flat transducer face (Figure 2.21)
   iii) Rectangular image (Figure 2.22)
   iv) Used for superficial application or to cover larger areas

Ultrasound is performed in two modes: brightness mode (B-mode) or motion mode (M-mode). B-mode is a single point in time. M-mode is monitoring an ultrasound over time such as an echocardiogram.

In traditional radiographs, artifacts are undesired. However, in ultrasound, artifacts can be used to enhance imaging of certain tissues. For example, ultrasounds travel well through fluid-filled structures, e.g. bladder, and can create better visualization of structures located distally, e.g. uterus.

Contrast Studies

Varieties of radiographic contrast studies are performed to diagnose potential surgical conditions. The insertion of contrast media or air into organs can aid in diagnostics. Prior to performing any contrast radiographs, survey images are taken to view any gross abnormalities.

Cystogram

1) Indicated for dysuria, polyuria, and hematuria.
2) May diagnose cystic calculi, neoplasia, rupture, ectopic ureters, and urethral or ureteral damage.
3) Procedure: Fast the patient, perform an enema to empty the colon, use sterile catheterization technique, empty the bladder, inject the contrast material to moderate bladder distension, and radiograph the patient.
4) Contrast media: Carbon dioxide or nitrous oxide (negative contrast) or water-soluble organic iodide in 20% iodine solution (positive contrast – preferred); the volume is based on patient's weight (Figure 2.23).

Esophagram

1) Indicated for dysphagia.
2) May diagnose neoplasia, functional swallowing abnormalities (with fluoroscopy), foreign body, strictures, or megaesophagus.
3) Procedure: Avoid sedation to maintain swallowing, administer the contrast media to patient orally by eating/licking or via oral syringe, and perform a series of radiographs to assess transport of the media through esophagus.
4) Contrast media: Barium paste, barium liquid, oral aqueous iodine, or non-ionic organic iodine agents. Depending upon the study, contrast may be given in food boluses.

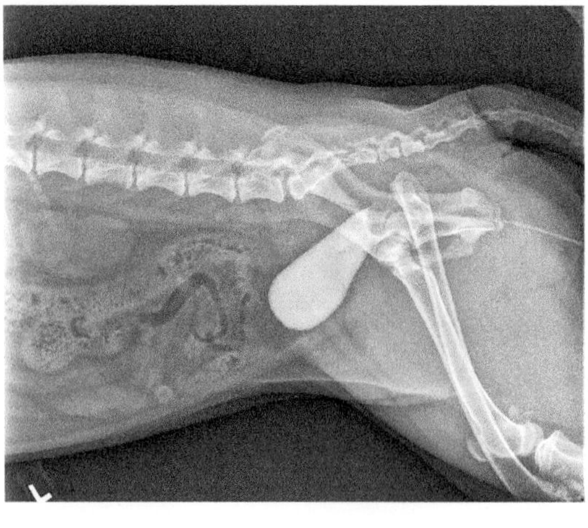

Figure 2.23 Contrast cystogram of patient hit by a car resulting in pelvic and femur fractures. Radiograph is to determine if bladder trauma is present.

Arthrogram

1) Indicated for enhanced visualization of articular cartilage and synovium.
2) May diagnose osteochondritis dissecans, lesions associated with trauma, joint mice, biceps tenosynovitis, or fragmented medial coronoid process.
3) Procedure: Sterilely prep joint, perform arthrocentesis using sterile technique to assure positioning within joint, inject contrast, and perform imaging.
4) Contrast media: Dilute isotonic iodine (positive contrast), sterile air, or carbon dioxide through a filter (negative contrast).

Enterogram

1) Indicated for vomiting, palpable mass, pain, weight loss, or melena; **do not** perform if bowel obstruction or leakage is suspected.
2) May diagnose foreign bodies, decreased or increased intestinal lumen size, intestinal content, mucosal abnormalities, or peristaltic speed.
3) Procedure: Fast patient for 24 hours, administer enema 2–4 hours prior to imaging if patient's condition is stable, acute crisis may not permit intestinal emptying, and feed or stomach tube appropriate dose of contrast media to patient assuring esophageal not tracheal placement of media.
4) *Sedation*: Avoid medications that affect gastrointestinal motility such as fentanyl, dexmedetomidine, and xylazine. If sedation is required, ketamine (2.7 mg/kg) mixed with diazepam (0.09 mg/kg) given intramuscularly 20 minutes prior to the procedure for cats and acepromazine (0.05 mg/kg) intravenously for dogs are appropriate tranquilizers [10].
5) *Contrast media*: Barium sulfate (preferred for routine studies), ionic organic iodine, and nonionic organic iodine (use if perforation is suspected).

With the increased use of endoscopy, clinicians perform less gastrointestinal contrast studies. Endoscopic and colonoscopy exams assess all structures of the stomach and small and large intestine while potentially removing foreign material causing a blockage. Serial contrast radiographs, however, still aid in evaluating stomach and intestinal motility. The contrast media are monitored and timed as it passes through the gastrointestinal system.

Medications

Antibiotics

The use of perioperative antibiotics is a controversial subject. Overuse or misuse of antibiotics can lead to resistant bacterial infections. Patients on continuous courses of antibiotics may cause a mutation of the specific organism leading to its resistance to that particular antibiotic.

The currently accepted guidelines for perioperative antibiotics are to provide injectable broad-spectrum antibiotics (e.g. Cefazolin 22 mg/kg) at the beginning of a procedure and every two hours until the surgery is completed. The use of antibiotics is not usually required in surgeries expected to last less than two hours [12].

Common examples of short procedures are routine ovariohysterectomy or castration. In the face of obvious infection – contaminated wounds, abscesses, and septic joints – the wound should be sterilely swabbed for bacterial culture and sensitivity prior to administering antibiotics. This procedure allows for maximum culture results, thus providing specific information on drug susceptibility. Highly infected patients may be maintained on a very short course of a broad-spectrum antibiotic while awaiting culture findings.

Analgesics

Pain control is an important aspect of every surgical patient's care. All patients undergoing any procedure will have some discomfort ranging from mild and tolerable to unbearable pain. Veterinary patients cannot describe their pain level but subtle signs can determine a patient's pain score (Figure 2.24).

Nociception or pain is defined as "an unpleasant sensation which may be associated with actual or potential tissue damage and which may have physical and emotional components." In nature, as a survival technique, animals do not readily display pain. However, they will learn to avoid a stimulus that causes a painful response [13].

Pathophysiology of Pain

In order to manage pain, it is important to have a basic understanding of the complex interactions coming together to create the pain response. This allows for formation of a plan to control pain prior to a procedure, during surgery, and postoperatively. Nociception is the processing of a noxious stimulus resulting in the perception of pain by the brain. Nociception divides into three parts: transduction, transmission, and modulation (Figure 2.25). *Transduction* is the conversion of the unpleasant sensation into electrical impulses by a free afferent nerve ending. *Transmission* transports these impulses along nerve fibers to the nucleus caudalis of the brain. These trigeminal afferent nerves subdivide into two categories:

- A-delta or fast fibers, responsible for sharp stabbing pain as in a fracture
- C or slow fibers, responsible for dull throbbing pain as in a chronic condition

Modulation is the synapse of the neurons in the nucleus caudalis in the medulla of the brain. This leads to the perception of pain. The goal of patient analgesia is to block this perception.

Where to Control Pain

Different modalities of treatment can be combined, or used alone, to produce the desired analgesic effect in a specific area. Local and regional anesthetics and alpha-2 agonists block the transmission of pain. Anti-inflammatory drugs work at the site of transduction and also modulate the pain response. Opioids modulate pain perception centrally and locally.

When to Control Pain

It is documented that preventing pain will decrease the total volume of required analgesics [14]. If pain control is not started until after a patient is showing discomfort, a higher level of drugs is needed to stop this increased sensitivity to noxious stimuli in the central nervous system. This is also known as "wind-up." A multi-modal approach to pain management before, during, and after a procedure will reduce "wind-up" and provide a more comfortable patient. Combining pain medications and sedatives in the pre-anesthetic protocol will decrease the need for a high concentration of inhalation anesthetics. Providing anti-inflammatory drugs at the beginning or end of a procedure will reduce the local pain response due to tissue manipulation. Providing patients with postoperative pain relief aids in healing. Instructing clients to follow the suggested dosing schedule of postoperative oral medication will help to eliminate the chance of overdosing a patient.

University of Wisconsin pain scale

0–1 No pain to probably no pain Dog or, cat demonstrates normal behavior for a score of 0
A score of 1 demonstrates normal behaviors but with anxiety being more of an issue

- Sitting and walking normally, sleeping comfortably, normal affectionate responses, normal gromming, and normal posture

2- Mild discomfort

- Patient will eat
- Dogs will sleep but may not dream
- Cats may sleep for short periods of time
- Patient may resist palpation of suspected area of discomfort (surgical wound, abdomen, ect.)
- Animal is not depressed

3- Mild pain or discomfort

- Patient gaurds suspected area of discomfort
- Dogs look slightly depressed and are unable to get comfortable
- Dogs may tremble or shake
- Cats may sit in a sphinx-like position for extended periods
- Characteristic of respiration may change for both species
- Dogs may be interested in food but only eat small amounts (may be picky)

4- Mild-to-moderate pain

- Patient resist palpation of suspected painful area
- Patient may lick or chew at wound
- Patient my site or lie in an abnormal position (not curled up or relaxed)
- Patient may be slow to rise and appear somewhat depressed
- Dogs may not appear interested in food they may take a few bites and then stop
- Cats are not usually interested in food
- Dogs may whimper or cry occasionally (animal may respond to quite voice and petting)

5- Moderate pain

- Patient may be reluctant to move and may be recumbent for hours without moving
- Patient may be depressed
- Patient may be inappetant
- Patient may bite or attempt to bite when painful area is approached
- Dog may vocalize when attempts are made to move it or when it is approached
- Cats may growl, hiss, and attempt to hide or escape
- Abdominal splinting is present (in abdominal cases)
- No interest in food, minimal sleep, and decreased activity
- Dogs may tremble or shake with head held low

6- Moderate pain+

- Same criteria as above but dog vocalizes more frequently and without provocation
- Cats may not move from one position for extended periods of time
- Cats may face the back of cage
- Patient may have glazed eyes
- Cats may squint their eyes
- Respiratory character may be increased with an abdominal lift
- Pupils may be dilated

7- Moderate to severe pain

- Same criteria as 5 or 6 but patient is also depressed and uninterested in its surroundings.
- Dogs will cry out when moved and will spontaneously or continuously whimper (although some dogs may not vocalize)
- Cats appear frozen, frightened, and attempt to hide, growl, hiss, or bite when approached
- Dogs may urinate/defecate without attempting to move

8- Severe pain

- Same criteria as for a score of 7 but vocalizing may be more of a feature
- Grunting on expiration may be appreciated
- Patient may thrash around the cage intermittently
- Patient may be so consumed With pain that they do not notice caretaker's presence

9- Severe-to-excruciating pain

- Same criteria as for a score of 8~ but dog is also hyperesthetic, hyperalgesic, or allodynic
- Cats may growl, freeze, bite, or attempt to escape
- Patient may attempt to escape or bite if picked up
- Patient may tremble involuntarily when any part of the body near the painful area is touched

10- Excruciating pain

- Same criteria as a score of 9 but dog or cat is emitting semi-conscious or continuous sounds unless the dog is almost comatose
- The patient is hyperesthetic or hyperalgesic or allodynic
- The patient's entire body is trembling and sign of pain are elicited whenever the dog is touched or approached

Observe patient, interact with them, palpate the suspected painful area, and communicate with others who have been working with the patient (technicians, students, interns ...). Take into account the patients physiologic parameters like heart rate, respiratory rate and blood pressure but do not base the presence or absence of pain on those factors alone (opioids and vagal tone can decrease heart rate while hypovolemia and anxiety can increase it). Consider the species and breed; cats and certain dog breeds are more stoic (Newfoundlands, Pitbulls) than others (Northern breeds). Dogs will often wag their tails in response to commands or touch and many cats will continue to purr even when they are experiencing moderate to severe pain. Tail wagging and purring should not be used as an indication that an animal is not in pain. Scores of 0–3 may not require additional analgesics but may benefit from low–dose anxiolytics. Scores of 4–7 will likely benefit from a multi-modal approach to analgesia. Scores of 8–10 should consider additional analgesics and an alteration in the pain management plan. If the patient exhibits most of the behaviors in a certain category but also exhibits a behavior in a higher category, the patient gets bumped up to the higher score (dog is moderately painful and scores a 5 but is also hyperesthetic, that dog gets a pain score of 9). Use multi-modal or balanced analgesia for the best results. Please consult with the Anesthesia and Pain Management Department if you have questions or concerns.

Figure 2.24 University of Wisconsin (UW) – Veterinary School Pain Scale. *Source:* courtesy of Lesley Smith, DVM, DACVA, and the staff of the UW Veterinary Care Anesthesia and Analgesia Section.

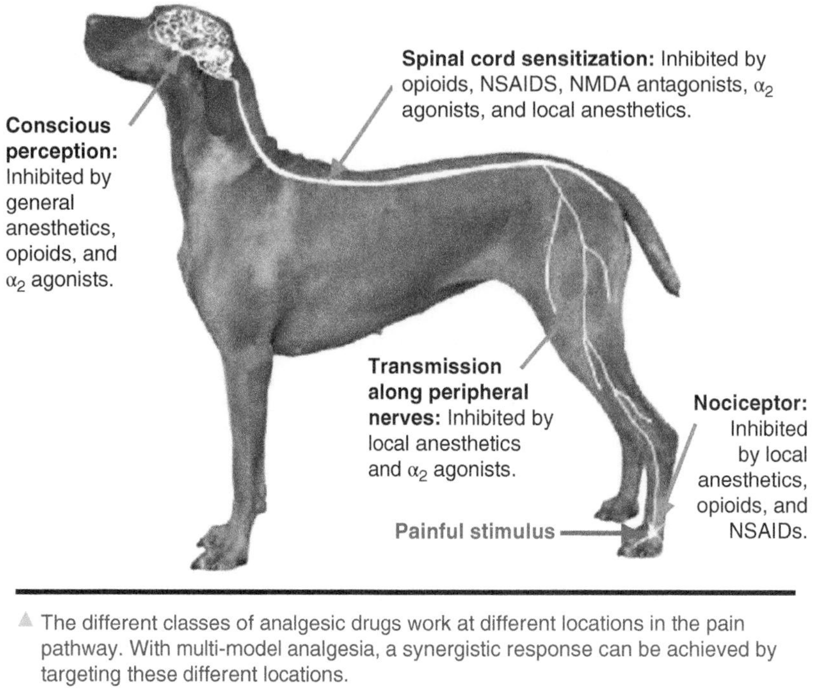

Figure 2.25 Pain pathway. *Source:* Courtesy of http://peakvas.com/peak-pain-management.

1) Preoperative

   A wide variety of drugs exists for aiding in systemic pain control prior to anesthetizing a patient. These include hydromorphone, butorphanol, morphine, dexmedetomidine, etc. All of these drugs work differently in the brain. The drug of choice is determined by many factors, including:

   - *Patient's condition*: assess age, body score, underlying medical conditions, etc.
   - *Cost*: some drugs are prohibitively expensive to use in large patients
   - *Procedure*: length and invasiveness, e.g. renal transplant versus bladder stone removal
   - *Hospital policy*: clinics "get in the habit" of using certain drug protocols

   Assess each patient, in consultation with the surgeon, to determine the best choice of medication for its individual situation.

2) Perioperative

   Regional and local anesthetic blocks are often used in veterinary dentistry to control pain at the site of the procedure. Local blocks, in combination with sedation, may be used for a minor laceration repair in general surgery. More commonly, using an epidural spinal block preoperatively maintains a patient's comfort at a lower anesthetic plane. Epidurals provide complete anesthesia to the caudal half of the body. They are contraindicated in patients with elevated intracranial pressure and clotting disorders (due to the chance of causing an epidural hematoma), decreased blood volume, as well as animals with pyoderma at the injection site and with abnormal anatomy creating difficulty locating the epidural landmarks [15].

3) Postoperative
   Upon recovery from anesthesia, it is important to keep patients comfortable and slowly encourage return to normal habits as soon as they are awake and walking. The most commonly used medications are non-steroidal anti-inflammatory drugs (NSAIDs) and opioids.

Non-steroidal Anti-inflammatory Drugs (NSAIDs)

NSAIDs treat pain and extreme sensitivity associated with inflammation. Most NSAIDS used in veterinary medicine are COX-2 selective. The breakdown of arachidonic acid by cyclooxygenase (COX) enzymes released at the site of surgery produces prostaglandins. Further production is created by the development of cytokines and growth factors at the site. Prostaglandins are a component of the inflammatory cascade and contribute to sensitizing neurons to noxious stimuli. Inhibition of COX enzymes limits prostaglandin production and thus reduces painful inflammation (Figure 2.26).

The choice of anti-inflammatory medication is dependent upon the patient's current medication, general health, and condition to be treated as well as clinician and client preference (Table 2.6).

Opioids

Opioids provide consistent, effective pain management. Opioid receptors are found throughout the body, particularly in the central and peripheral nervous system. Desired effects and undesired side effects vary depending upon the drug type and the particular receptor stimulated. Desired results are pain suppression through peripheral, spinal, and supraspinal analgesia with minimal sedation. Potential side effects include respiratory depression, bradycardia, ileus, urine retention, excitement, delirium, tachycardia, hypertension, and temperature reduction.

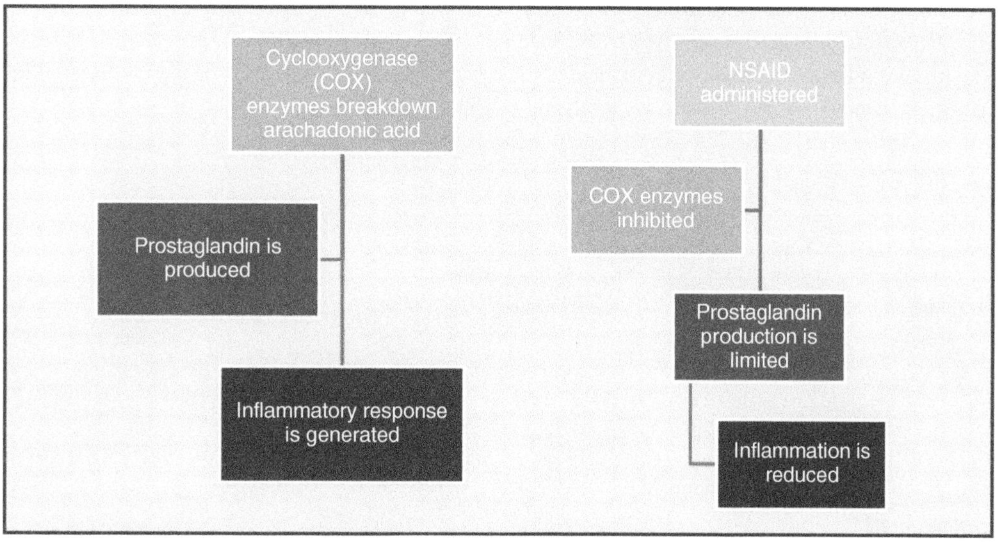

Figure 2.26 Simplified inflammatory cascade diagram.

Table 2.6 Non-steroidal anti-inflammatory drugs (NSAID) doses.

Drug	Route	Canine dose	Feline dose
Carprofen	Injectable/oral	4.4 mg/kg q 24 h or 2.2 mg/kg q 12 h	Not applicable
Deracoxib	Oral	1–4 mg/kg q 24 h, max 7 d	Not applicable
Etodolac	Oral	10–15 mg/kg q 24 h	Not applicable
Firocoxib	Oral	5 mg/kg q 24 h prn for 3 d for post-op pain or prn for osteoarthritis	Not applicable
Grapiprant	Oral	2 mg/kg q 24 h (not for use under 3.6 kg, 9 mo, or pregnant/nursing)	Not applicable
Ketoprofen	Injectable/oral	1 mg/kg q 24 h IV or PO up to 5 d	1 mg/kg q 24 h IV or PO up to 5 d
Meloxicam	Injectable/oral	0.2 mg/kg once PO then 0.1 mg/kg q 24 h PO	0.05 mg/kg single, one-time SQ dose
Robenacoxib	Oral	Not applicable	2 mg/kg q 24 h, once then 1–2 mg/kg for up to 6 d

Abbreviations: h = hours, d = days, IV = intravenous, SQ = subcutaneous, PO = per os (oral).
Dosing schedule is taken from medication inserts provided by their manufacturers.

The major classes of opioids are agonists, partial agonist/antagonists, partial agonists, and antagonists. Agonists produce the best effect by binding to a given receptor. Partial agonists bind to a receptor but give less effect than agonists give. Partial agonists/antagonists bind to more than one receptor but do not affect both receptors. Antagonists have no effect on opiate receptors and are often used to reverse the effects of agonist drugs (Table 2.7).

Patients must be monitored closely when using any controlled substance. All agonists are reversible if the patient displays undesirable side effects. A fentanyl constant rate infusion (CRI) can be stopped but its effects will continue for about 30 minutes. Fentanyl patches take effect within 12–24 hours of application. Fentanyl will remain in the body for 12–24 hours after patch removal.

Controlled substances are required to be stored in a secure location. Meticulous records must be kept following Drug Enforcement Agency (DEA) guidelines. Clients should be counseled regarding proper disposal of any unused medication.

Table 2.7 Opioid drug doses.

Drug	Type	Route	Canine Dose	Feline Dose
Morphine	Agonist – Class II narcotic	IV,IM or SQ	0.1–2.0mg/kg q 4-6h	0.1–0.5mg/kg q 4–6h (Note: only 50% of cats create the metabolite that provides analgesia)
Hydromorphone	Agonist – Class II narcotic	IV, IM, SQ	0.05–0.2mg/kg q 2–4h	0.025–0.2mg/kg q 2–4h
Oxymorphone	Agonist – Class II narcotic	IV,IM, SQ	0.05–0.2mg/kg q 2–4h	0.025–0.1mg/kg q 2–4h
Fentanyl	Agonist – Class II narcotic	IV (CRI) of Transdermal Patch	CRI: 2–40µg/kg/hr Patch: 3–5µg/kg/hr for 3–5 days	CRI: 2–40µg/kg/hr Patch: 3–5µg/kg/hr for 3–5 days

Table 2.7 (Continued)

Drug	Type	Route	Canine Dose	Feline Dose
Methadone	Agonist/NMDA receptor Antagonist Class II narcotic	IV, IM	0.3–1.0mg/kg q 4–5 hours	0.3–0.5mg/kg q 4–5 hours
Butorphanol	Partial Agonist/ Antagonist Class IV narcotic	IV, IM, SQ	0.1–0.5mg/kg q 1–2h	0.1–0.5mg/kg q 1–2h
Buprenorphine	Partial Agonist Class IV narcotic	IV, IM, SQ	Inj:0.005–0.02mg/kg q 4-8h	Inj: Inj:0.005–0.02mg/kg q 4–8h SL: 5–30μg/kg q 12h
Naloxone	Antagonist	IV, IM, SQ	0.002–0.04mg/kg given to effect for reversal of agonist (Note: duration of action is 30–60 minutes)	0.002–0.04mg/kg given to effect for reversal of agonist (Note: duration of action is 30–60 minutes)

Source: Dosing schedule derived from Merck Manual, Veterinary Manual, online, updated November, 2022. https://www.merckvetmanual.com/veterinary/management-and-nutrition/pain-assessment-and-management/analgesic-pharmacology, from Kristen Cooley, BA, CVT VTS (Anesthesia and Analgesia) and https://www.aaha.org/globalassets/02-guidelines/2020-anesthesia/aahaanesthesiaguidelines_opioids.pdf.

A multi-modal approach to analgesia is desired. The duration and extent of a procedure will help to determine the desired drug protocol. The goal is to have a patient that is comfortable, eats well, returns to normal activity, and heals quickly.

References

1 Latimer, K.S. (2011) *Duncan and Prasse's Veterinary Laboratory Medicine: Clinical Pathology*, 5th edn. Wiley-Blackwell, p. 372.

2 Foster, R. (Doctors Foster and Smith). peteducation.com [accessed on 24 February 2023].

3 Latimer, K.S. (2011) *Duncan and Prasse's Veterinary Laboratory Medicine: Clinical Pathology*, 5th edn. Wiley-Blackwell, pp. 374–375.

4 Prins, M., Schellens, C.J.M.M., van Leeuwen, M.W. *et al.* Coagulation disorders in dogs with hepatic disease. *The Veterinary Journal*, 185(2), 163–168, 210.

5 Tobias, K.M. & Johnston, S.A. (2012) *Veterinary Surgery Small Animal*. Elsevier.

6 Kahn, C.M. (2011) *The Merck Veterinary Manual*, 9th edn. Merck Sharp & Dohme Corporation, Whitehouse Station, NJ.

7 Piermattei, D.L., Flo, G.L. & DeCamp, C.E. (2006) *Handbook of Small Animal Orthopedics and Fracture Repair*, 4th edn. Saunders-Elsevier, St. Louis, MO.

8 Le Heron, J., Padovani, R., Smith, I. *et al.* (2010) Radiation protection of medical staff. *European Journal of Radiology*, 76, 20–23.

9 Brown, M. & Brown, L. (2014) *Radiography for Veterinary Technicians*, 5th edn. Elsevier.

10 Thrall, D.E. (2007) *Textbook of Veterinary Diagnostic Radiology*, 5th edn. Saunders-Elsevier. Chapter 4 Amy S. Tidwell.

11 Lopchinsky, R.A., VanName, N.H. & Kattaron, M. (2000) *Physical Principles of Ultrasound*. UIC. webinar.

12 Johnson, A.L. (2007) Fundamentals of orthopedic surgery and fracture management. In: Fossum, T.W. (ed), *Small Animal Surgery*, 3rd edn. Mosby, St. Louis, MO.

13 Holzman, G. (2009) *Pain Control in Dentistry and Oral Surgery*. Annual Veterinary Dental Forum, Phoenix, AZ.

14 Shaffran, N. Managing difficult pain cases: neuropathic pain and wind-up phenomenon on https://www.vin.com/apputil/content/defaultadv1.aspx?pId=11372&meta=generic&catId=35310&id=5709881&ind=207&objTypeID=17 [accessed on 28 July 2023].

15 Egger, C. and Love, L. (2009). Local and regional anesthesia techniques, part 4: epidural anesthesia and analgesia https://www.dvm360.com/view/local-and-regional-anesthesia-techniques-part-4-epidural-anesthesia-and-analgesia [accessed on 28 July 2023].

3

Asepsis and Infection Control

Teri Raffel Kleist[1] *and Cassandra Simmons*[2]

[1] *Madison College, retired, Madison, WI, USA*
[2] *College of Veterinary Medicine, Purdue University, West Lafayette, IN, USA*

Surgical Suite Preparation

There are many factors that influence the outcome of any surgical procedure. The patient is an obvious contributor to the outcome. The patient's health status at the time of surgery, the ability of the patient to heal, and the invasiveness of the procedure will affect success. The personnel involved in the surgical procedure will also influence the outcome. Anesthesia personnel have the responsibility of keeping the animal alive while under anesthesia and guiding the patient through recovery with as little incident as possible. The surgeon and any member of the sterile surgical team have the potential for introducing pathogens that may compromise the success of the case. Finally, the environment of the operating room can contribute to potential contamination if not properly cared for.

Maintaining and controlling the operating room environment is a critical step in protecting the patient and personnel from contamination. Areas to be considered include air handling, attire, traffic, air particles, cleaning products' contaminants, and standardization of operation room cleaning procedures.

Theater Design

Air Exchanges

Currently, the Center for Disease Control (CDC) recommends 15 air exchanges per hour for operating rooms. In addition, operating rooms should have a laminar airflow system. Studies have shown that laminar airflow significantly reduces the number of particles in the air. If a laminar air system is not possible, a positive airflow (air flows out when the door is opened) will aid in keeping irritants out of the operating suite. Incoming air should be at ceiling level while outgoing air should be at floor level. Whatever type of system is used, proper care and maintenance are critical in achieving optimal efficiency. Cleaning of the system (ducts, grates, filters, and drain pans) will increase the efficiency of the system. Annual assessment of air quality in the operating room should also occur.

Surgical Patient Care for Veterinary Technicians and Nurses, Second Edition.
Edited by Gerianne Holzman and Teri Raffel Kleist.

Companion website: www.wiley.com/go/holzman/patient

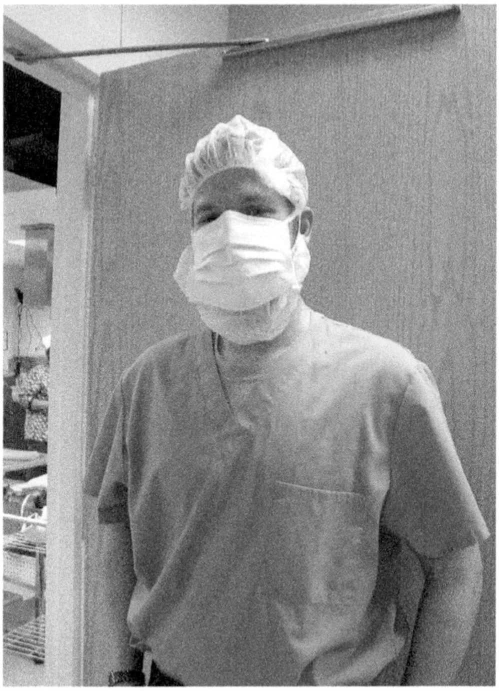

Figure 3.1 Bouffant hat.

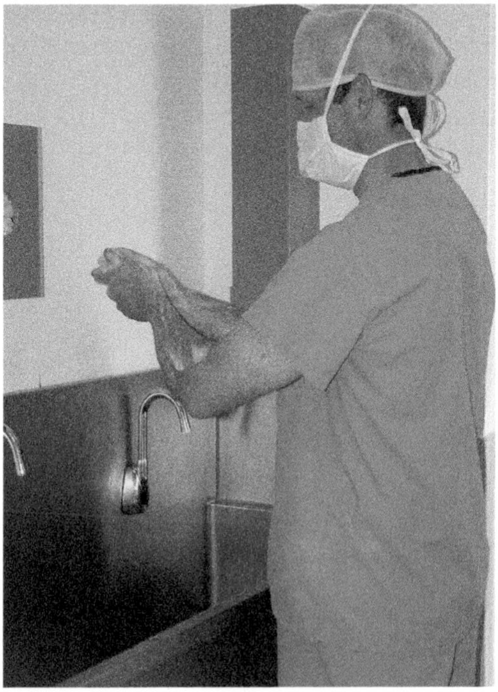

Figure 3.2 Surgeon's cap.

Surgical Attire

Proper surgical attire is critical in reducing the potential for the introduction of contaminants to the surgical suite. Facility-approved, freshly laundered scrub suits are most commonly used. According to Association of Operating Room Nurses (AORN), clothing to be worn in restricted areas of the hospital (operating rooms) should not be worn to the facility from outside areas (i.e. home). Tops must be tucked into pants to avoid skin cell shedding at surgical table height. Scrubs should not be laundered at home due to increased risk of cross-contamination. Once soiled or at the end of the day, the scrubs should be put in a designated hamper for laundering by the facility. Street clothes must never be worn underneath scrubs. Undershirts or tank tops can be worn for added warmth, but no article of clothing should extend beyond the sleeves or pant legs of the scrubs. Another "attire" to be worn is some type of hair coverage device (Figure 3.1). Most commonly used is a bouffant hat. It must be large enough to cover all hair for both men and women. There are surgeon's caps available for those individuals who have very short hair that will be covered by this smaller type of cap (Figure 3.2). Beard covers are also available for those with facial hair that needs to be covered. Beard covers have elastic loops on either end and those loops fit over the ears. A head covering must be worn in addition to the beard cover. There is the option of wearing a surgical hood if facial hair is present and a beard cover is not available. The surgical hood is designed to cover head hair as well as facial hair (Figure 3.3). Most often head covers are of a disposable, single-use nature. Some facilities will allow cloth head covers as an option. Cloth head covers need to be laundered at the end of each day.

The use of shoe covers is still debated among facilities. Some require dedicated shoes for the operating rooms and that shoe covers be worn when *leaving* the restricted area of the operating rooms. Other facilities require shoe covers

Figure 3.3 Surgical hood.

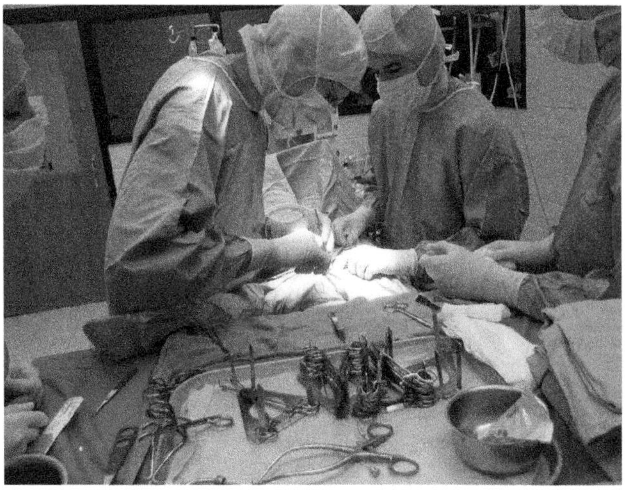

to be worn in order to enter the restricted area of the operating rooms. At any rate, the policy that is established by the facility must be adhered to and enforced by the veterinary technician in the operating room area. Surgical masks are the final piece of attire to be addressed. Masks should be worn whenever sterile packs are open or when there is a surgery in progress. Masks are designed to filter exhaled air, so it is imperative that they be worn correctly. Some manufacturers even print the work "inside" on the side that should be toward the face. There are two styles of surgical face masks available. First, the most common style is the double-tie face mask. The ties are secured at the crown of the head and the back of the neck. Ties should not be crossed behind the head (lower ties tied at the crown of the head and upper ties secured behind the neck) and then secured as this leaves too large a gap on the side of the face for particles to escape. This style of mask is also offered with ear loops instead of ties. Either is acceptable, however ties are preferred. Masks frequently have a malleable metal band that runs across the bridge of the nose if the mask is put on correctly. This band is intended to be molded to the bridge of the nose for a conforming fit – again in an effort to reduce the number of expired particles from escaping. Another style of face mask is a preformed cup style that does not cover as much of the face as the tie style. With the elastic strap instead of ties, it offers a speedier application and removal but does not cover as much surface area of the face, thus increasing the risk of aerosolized particles.

Traffic

Traffic in the operating room is an often-overlooked situation. People just "sticking their head in" to ask a quick question, anesthesia personnel entering and exiting the room frequently, and circulating technicians being unprepared for a case and having to leave and re-enter the room numerous times with equipment are all examples of traffic that can be avoided. Minimal movement in and out of the operating room is obviously the ideal. Once the patient has been moved into the room, positioned on the table, and has received the final sterile prep, people moving around should be minimized. Especially true with joint arthroplasty, no opening of the operating room door should occur unless there is an emergency. Since joint replacement cases are extra sensitive to surgical site infections, every effort to reduce the introduction of potential pathogens needs to be observed.

Cleaning

Before the First Case of the Day

Before the first case of the day, the furniture in the operating room needs to be arranged so a good traffic flow is possible. Back tables should be pushed up against the walls, and electrosurgery units and suction units should be plugged in and ready for use but pushed back away from the surgery table. The anesthesia machine should be placed where it will be used; in most cases, that will be at the head of the table. For some cases (i.e. ophthalmic procedures or other head/facial procedures), however, that may mean placing the anesthesia machine at the back of the table. The surgery table should be at the height of the transport table for ease of transferring the patient. The height of the surgery table for the surgeon can be adjusted after the patient is positioned. All flat surfaces including overhead lights should be damp dusted with a lint-free rag and 70% isopropyl alcohol or commercially available disinfectant wipes.

In Between Cases

Gross debris (blood and fluids) should be cleaned up with paper towels or mopped up as soon as the case is finished. All flat surfaces should be disinfected. It is best to avoid applying disinfectants with a spray bottle as they aerosolize particles in the operating room. Either spray the cleaning rag outside of the operating room or use commercially available disinfectant wipes. The broadest-spectrum disinfectant available would be a wise choice to reduce exposure of potentially harmful bacteria to already compromised patients. If the surgery table has a split top, cleaning the drain tray under the split must be done. Elevate one side of the table to allow access to the drainage tray to remove any contaminants that may have fallen into the tray (i.e. blood, urine, hair, sutures, etc.). Some surgery tables will have trays that can be pulled from one end or another to allow cleaning (Figure 3.4). If necessary, mopping the floor with a clean mop head may be done between cases, otherwise spot cleaning would be sufficient.

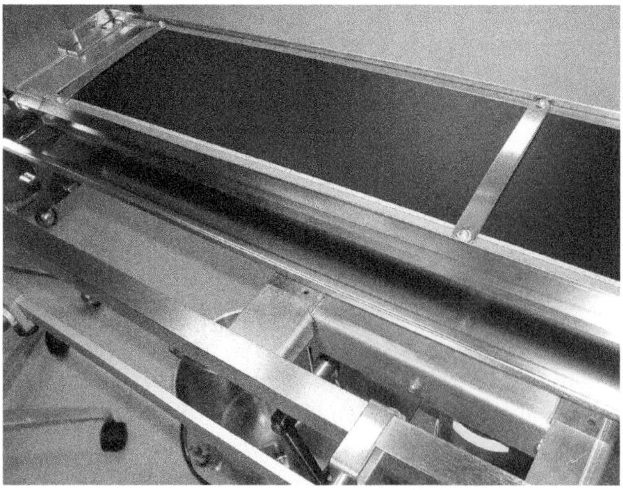

Figure 3.4 Surgical table with split top open for cleaning.

Terminal Cleaning – End of Day

After the last case of the day, the surgical suite should undergo a more vigorous cleaning. All furniture should have a physical scrubbing done. All surfaces, including wheels or casters, should be freed of any debris (hair, suture ends, etc.). All shelves of equipment should be scrubbed as well. All equipment such as electrosurgery, laser, and suction machines should be wiped down with a disinfectant. Linen hampers, kick buckets, sponge basin stands, etc. should be wiped down and disinfected as well. Floors should be wet vacuumed. Mopping should be avoided unless clean mop heads and fresh solution are used in each room to prevent the spread of bacteria. Air intake grills, door handles, and windowsills should be wiped down. Walls and ceilings should be checked and spot cleaned as needed.

Solutions to Use for Cleaning

There is no perfect disinfectant available for use in the veterinary hospital, so facilities need to decide, based on their needs, what will work the best.

Sodium Hypochlorite

A dilute bleach solution of 1:32 (1 oz. in 32 oz. of tap water) is an effective disinfectant. While inexpensive, the disadvantages may outweigh the cost-effectiveness. Once mixed it is highly unstable and light sensitive so it needs to be made fresh every day and stored in an opaque spray bottle. It is not a good cleaner, so areas need to be cleaned before being disinfected. Bleach does not perform well in the presence of detergent or organic material, so surfaces must be free of those products. Finally, as is true with many products, it requires a 10-minute contact time to reach full effectiveness (Figure 3.5).

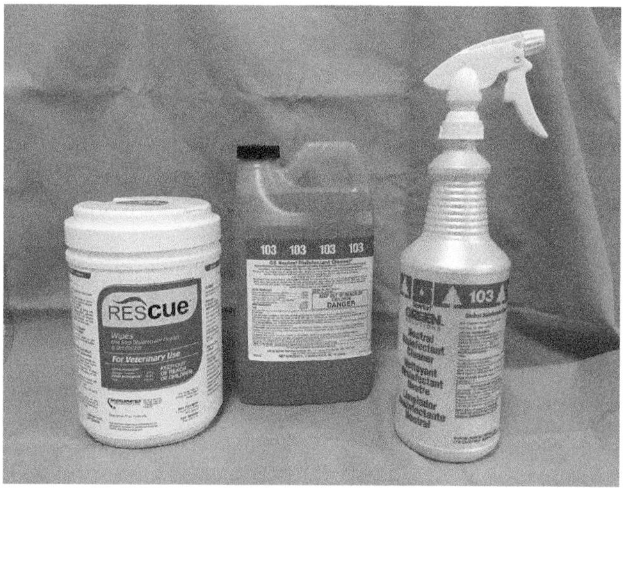

Figure 3.5 Disinfectants for cleaning the surgical suite.

Potassium Peroxymonosulfate

Potassium peroxymonosulfate (Trifectant®) is used as a 1% solution. It claims bactericidal, virucidal, and fungicidal capabilities. Once mixed with the 1% solution, it is stable for 10 days. It also requires a 10-minute contact time but is an effective cleaner as well as disinfectant. Some references claim unreliable performance against dermatophytes.

Quaternary Ammoniums

Quaternary ammoniums are commonly used due to their cleaning and disinfection properties. They also require a 10-minute contact time and strict attention to dilution/mixing directions from the manufacturer. One common mistake is diluting the product with tap water when the manufacturer specifically indicates distilled water. Tap water generally contains too many minerals and contaminants that interfere with the product's performance. Some discussion has been had regarding the ineffectiveness of these types of chemicals against non-enveloped viruses (canine parvovirus, feline panleukopenia, and feline calicivirus). The addition of diluted bleach to these cleaning products produces an effective cleaning/disinfecting combination, but the instability of bleach may prove to be an inefficient and costly alternative.

Accelerated Hydrogen Peroxide

The use of accelerated hydrogen peroxide products (Rescue™) has become increasingly popular in veterinary facilities. These products are effective against many pathogens including *Canine parvovirus, Canine influenza,* and *Microsporum canis.* Formulations available include concentrate, ready-to-use spray bottles, and saturated wipes making use very convenient.

Regardless of the type of disinfectant chosen, there are some very important things to remember. First and foremost is to read and follow the directions on the label! All too often in veterinary medicine, we inaccurately dilute chemicals due to shortage of time, no measuring device readily available, or historical visual assessment ("make it a light blue color"). Improper dilution can affect the health and safety of both workers and patients, as well as the overall efficacy of the products. Disinfectants will not act the way they are expected to act when improperly diluted. This inaccuracy can lead to the unintentional spread of potentially lethal organisms.

Application of the disinfectant must be done as directed by the manufacturer in order to achieve the expected outcome. Whether sprayed on, wiped on, mopped on, or foamed on, inappropriately applied products are ineffective.

To achieve microorganism kill/control, the chemical must also be left on the surface for the directed time. Spraying a tabletop and wiping it right away does practically nothing. Following the manufacturer's instructions is imperative. Many chemicals are required to be in contact with the surface for 5–10 minutes in order to function as they are tested and intended. Reading the instructions for use (IFU) will identify required duration of contact. Upon completion of contact time, completely drying the surface is important. If left damp, the moisture can counteract the efficacy of the products since it may promote bacterial growth.

Patient Preparation

Proper preparation of the surgical patient is a critical step in the surgical case and is related to the outcome and subsequent potential infection of the surgical site. Improper patient preparation can have catastrophic consequences for the surgical procedure and incision integrity [1].

Clipping

Surgical prep of veterinary patients consists of two steps: clipping (removal) of the hair/fur and skin cleansing with an antiseptic. Clipping and prepping of the patient must be done outside of the surgery room. Loose hair, dermal flora, and splashing solutions greatly increase the risk of contamination of the area. A smock must be worn over scrubs to protect the clothing underneath whenever clipping a patient. When clipping surgical patients, the use of a size 40 clipper blade with an electric clipper is a standard approach. Various other sizes of clipper blades are available but do not provide the close removal of hair that is achieved with the 40 blade. It is also imperative that the hair be shaven *against* the grain of the hair to ensure the closest cut of the hair that is possible. Even with longhaired patients, it is ill-advised to clip with the grain (growth) of the hair. Helpful hints that ensure a symmetric, neat, nontraumatic shave include: pulling the skin tight and moving the clipper blade away from the opposite hand (Figure 3.6); using the toothed edge of the clipper blade – at a 90° angle to the hair – to create a straight edge for the margins of the clipped area (Figure 3.7); and always using a clean, sharp clipper blade to provide the cleanest, shortest cut of the hair shaft. Clipper blades with missing teeth or that feel dull should not be used and should be replaced or repaired.

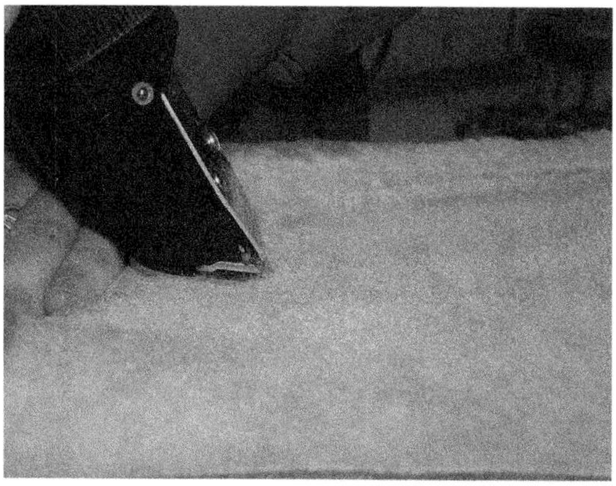

Figure 3.6 Proper angle of clipper blade to skin.

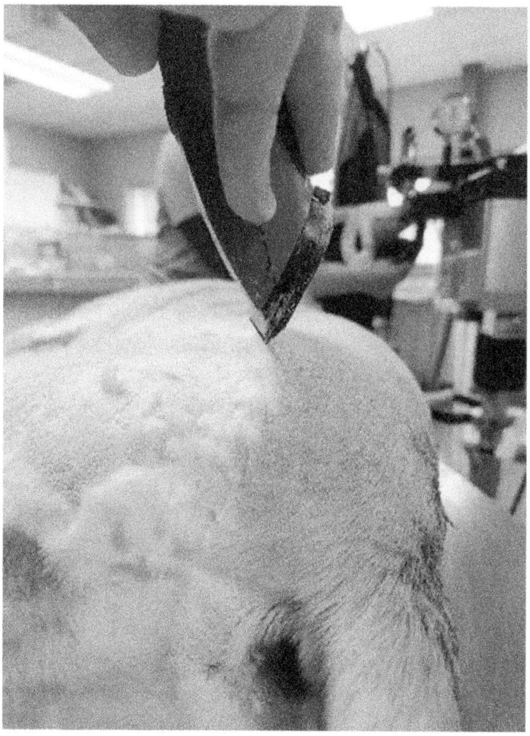

Figure 3.7 Angle of clipper blade to achieve a straight clipped edge.

Knowing the anatomic landmarks and margins for clipping a patient for a surgical procedure is the responsibility of the technician. Having a skilled, knowledgeable person handling this task is an invaluable peace of mind for the surgeon. Good communication between the technician and the surgeon is critical for this step of the process. The technician should check with the surgeon to be sure the site of the incision is understood. In addition, the technician should check with the surgeon to see if any additional areas need to be clipped for the procedure (i.e. graft site for a fracture repair or a chest tube exit site for a thoracic procedure). Technicians must have a thorough knowledge of the procedure being performed and possible intra-operative complications in order to adequately prepare the patient. The following guidelines for clipping of the surgical patient are merely guidelines. Each case must be treated individually in the event unusual circumstances are present.

Abdominal

In general, abdominal procedures for both male and female patients will be fairly standard. An abdominal clip will extend from either mid-sternum or the xiphoid to the pubis and laterally to the ventral edges of the ribs. Surgical procedures that are more focused on the cranial abdomen may necessitate a more cranial clipped margin to mid-sternum. More caudal abdominal procedures may require the extension of the caudal margin back to the scrotum/vulva of the patient. It is recommended that when clipping an abdomen, the clipper blade always moves away from the umbilicus, as this will create a cut against the grain of the hair and will provide as close a clip as possible. Short hair left on the skin, from an inadequate clip, could potentially be incised by the blade and end up as foreign body in the abdomen. Infection could result from the presence of a foreign body. Table 3.1 shows recommended guidelines for clipping margins for abdominal procedures. Whether or not the prepuce of a male is to be included in the surgical field, the hair on the prepuce should be completely removed and the prepuce flushed with a weak povidone-iodine or chlorhexidine solution mixture. Adding 1 ml of full-strength povidone-iodine solution to 20 ml of tap water will be adequate. If using chlorhexidine, add 6.3 ml of 2% chlorhexidine solution to 250 ml of 0.9% sodium chloride. After clipping is completed and vacuuming of the hair has occurred, the prepuce can be flushed with the chosen solution. Then, insert the tip of the 35 ml syringe into the prepucial opening (Figures 3.8–3.11) and pinch the tissue around the tip of the syringe (to trap fluid within the prepuce) and dispense ~10 ml of the solution. Gently massage the prepuce. Place a towel on the abdomen and pull the prepuce to either lateral side, release the pinch grip on the prepuce, and allow the fluid to escape from the prepuce onto the towel. The entire procedure should be repeated until all the dilute solution has been used. Modifications in volume of dilute solution made and administered must be considered if the patient is either a very small or a very large dog.

Thoracic

Thoracic procedures require either the lateral side or the ventral side of the chest to be clipped (Figure 3.11). Depending on the surgical procedure and the approach the surgeon will use, clipping margins can vary greatly. Communication with the surgeon is imperative in order to certain the correct area of the patient is clipped. An additional special circumstance is true with thoracic cases, which does not occur with any other type of surgical procedure; more often than not, a chest tube will be placed in patients that have undergone thoracic surgery. The exit site of the tube must be known

Table 3.1 Abdominal procedures' clipping guidelines.

Procedure	Cranial edge	Caudal edge	Lateral edge
Gastrotomy, gastropexy, splenectomy, liver biopsy/lobectomy, gall bladder, and kidney	Mid-sternum	Cranial edge of pubic bone	Ventral edge of ribs
Urinary bladder, duodenum, jejunum, and pancreas	Xiphoid	Cranial edge of pubic bone	Ventral edge of ribs
Prostate, ileum, and colon	Xiphoid	Scrotum/vulva	Ventral edge of ribs

Figure 3.8 Infusing prepuce with dilute povidone-iodine solution.

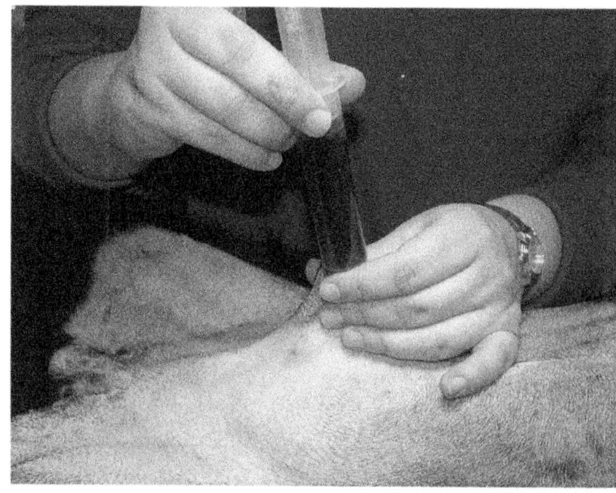

Figure 3.9 Gently massaging prepuce.

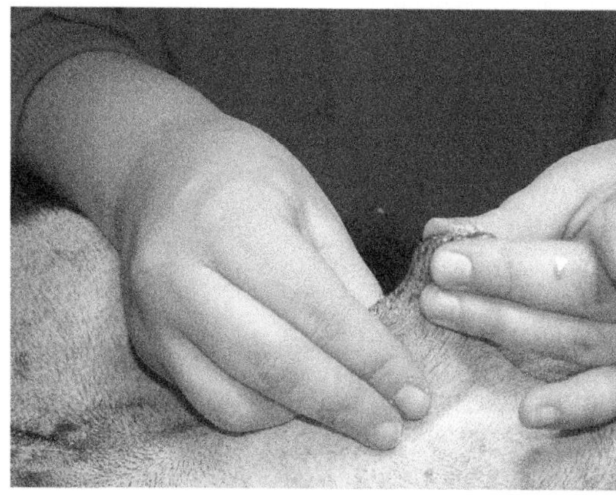

Figure 3.10 Releasing solution from prepuce.

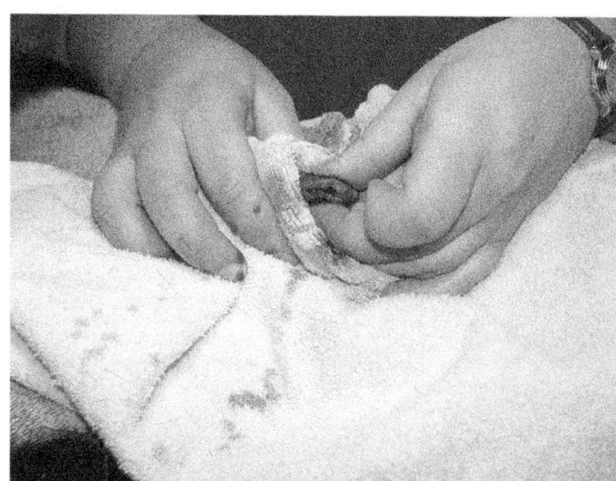

Figure 3.11 Patient clip for lateral thoracotomy. *Source:* Courtesy of Cassandra Simmons.

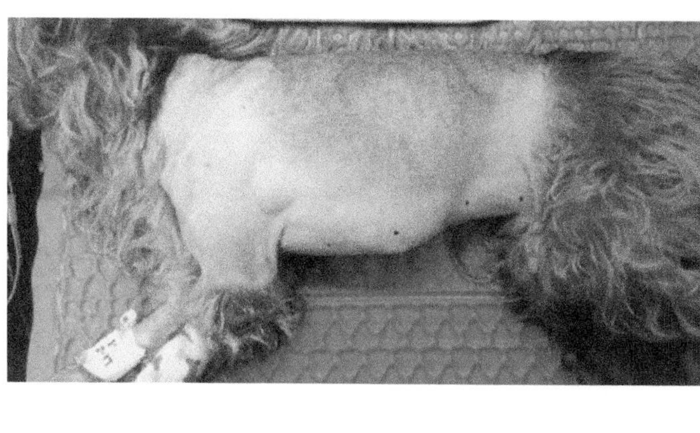

Table 3.2 Thoracic procedures' clipping guidelines.

Procedure	Clipping guidelines
Ventral approach via sternotomy – (lung lobectomy and heart base tumor)	Cranially to the base of the ventral neck, caudally 2–3 clipper widths caudal to the xiphoid process, and laterally to halfway between the dorsal and ventral midlines
Lateral approach (4–5 intercostal space usually) – (PDA ligation, lung mass, and chylothorax)	Cranially to the base of the neck, caudally 2–3 clipper blade widths caudal to the last rib, dorsal, and ventral midline

by the technician clipping the patient in order to guarantee enough hair has been clipped to accommodate the surgeon's intentions for the chest tube. Again, communication with the surgeon prior to clipping is critically important. Table 3.2 identifies guidelines for clipping for thoracic procedures.

Orthopedic

Prepping a patient for an orthopedic procedure is generally quite extensive (Figure 3.12). Even if the procedure is a single joint arthroscopy, the potential of an arthrotomy being performed necessitates a wide clip. The standard rule of thumb when clipping for an orthopedic procedure is to clip from the joint proximal to the incision to the joint distal to the proposed incision site. In the event of a proximal joint surgery (hip or shoulder), the clip extends a minimum of two clipper blades beyond the dorsal midline. Especially with orthopedic procedures, like an arthrodesis or fracture repair, the technician must be certain to communicate with the surgeon regarding the need for clipping for an autogenous cancellous bone graft harvest. Procedures on the forelimb generally use the head of the humerus or

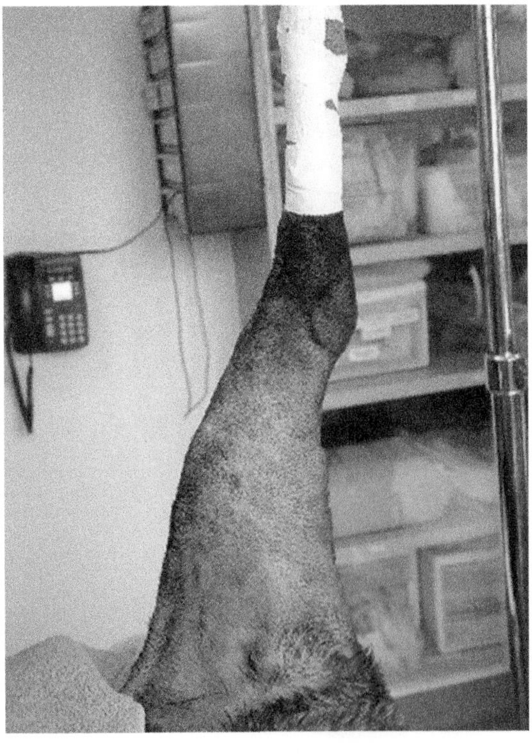

Figure 3.12 Orthopedic clip for stifle surgery.

Table 3.3 Forelimb orthopedic procedures' clipping guidelines.

Procedure/location of surgery	Proximal margin	Distal margin
Phalange and metacarpal procedures	Shoulder	Toenails – including hair in interdigital space
Carpal arthrodesis, distal radius/ulna fractures, angular limb deformity, and mid-shaft radius/ulnar fracture	Shoulder	First phalanx
Elbow surgery, distal humeral fracture, ununited anconeal process repair, and fractured coronoid process repair	Dorsal midline and ventral midline	Carpus
Proximal humeral fracture repair and Scapular fracture repair	Two clipper widths beyond dorsal midline and ventral midline	Mid-radius
Forelimb amputation	Two clipper widths beyond dorsal midline; ventral midline; caudal to last rib; and cranial to base of neck	Mid-radius

In addition to proximal and distal margins, all hair should be removed circumferentially on the limb.

Table 3.4 Hindlimb orthopedic procedures' clipping guidelines.

Procedure/location of surgery	Proximal margin	Distal margin
Phalange, digits, and metatarsal	Mid-femur	Toenails – including hair found in interdigit space
Tibia/fibula fracture repair	Hip	First phalanx
Stifle surgery (cruciate ligament repair, arthroscopy, and medial patellar luxation repair)	Hip	Tarsus
Femur (distal fracture repair)	Hip	Tarsus
Femoral head osteotomy and proximal femoral fracture repair	Two clipper widths beyond dorsal midline	Tarsus
Total hip arthroplasty	Ventral midline; two clipper widths beyond dorsal midline; caudally to tuber ischii; and cranial to last rib	Tarsus

In addition to proximal and distal margins, all hair should be removed circumferentially on the limb.

the proximal tibia as a graft site unless that bone is involved in the surgery. For hind limbs, the wing of the ilium is the most common bone graft-harvesting site. Large margins should be clipped for the graft, and due to wide variations in animal size, exact measurements cannot be provided. A good rule of thumb is to clip two to three clipper blade widths in all directions from the graft site incision. Tables 3.3 and 3.4 show recommended guidelines for clipping margins for orthopedic procedures.

Neurologic

Patients having a neurologic procedure performed have one of the easiest clipping situations. The recommended margins are to clip three to four vertebral spaces cranial and caudal to the suspected space. This allows ample room for the surgeon to extend the incision should other vertebral spaces need to be explored. As with other clipping guidelines, the technician must communicate with the

Table 3.5 Neurologic procedures' clipping guidelines.

Procedure	Cranial/caudal margins
Cervical ventral slot[a]	Clip 3–4 vertebra cranial and caudal to suspected vertebral space.
Cervical dorsal laminectomy	On the dorsal midline – clip 3–4 vertebra cranial and caudal to suspected vertebral space.
Cervical dorsal laminectomy – suspect site C_1–C_2	Clip mid-cranium to C_5
Thoracic laminectomy/hemi-laminectomy and lumbar laminectomy/hemi-laminectomy	On the dorsal midline; clip 3–4 vertebra cranial and caudal to suspected space (i.e. if suspect space is T_{13}–L_1, clip from T_{10} to L_4)

[a] This clip occurs on the ventral neck.

surgeon to be sure the appropriate area is clipped. Additionally, if a cervical procedure is being performed, be sure to ask the surgeon if a dorsal or ventral approach will be utilized. Much time can be wasted if the dorsal cervical area is clipped and prepped only to find out the surgeon planned on a ventral approach. Table 3.5 displays suggested clipping guidelines for neurologic cases.

Miscellaneous Sites

Patients having a surgical procedure that involves the sensory organs – eyes, ears, tongue, or facial bones – are more challenging to prep. Special anatomic configurations as well as extra sensitive tissue require a special approach.

Ophthalmic

Ophthalmic procedures should never have a clipper involved in the surgical site prep unless the procedure to be performed is an enucleation. This type of extra-ocular procedure requires the removal of the entire eye and therefore any accidental trauma to the eye from the clipper is a non-issue because the eye is being removed anyway. Any intra-ocular procedure should have fine-bladed scissors (i.e. baby Metzenbaum) used to remove eyelashes and/or any fine hair on the eyelid margins that need to be removed. Applying a water-soluble lubricant to the blades of the scissors prior to trimming the hair will have the hair adhere to the blades rather than falling into the eye. The blades of the scissors should be wiped with clean gauze frequently, and lubricant reapplied each time the blades are cleaned. Table 3.6 shows recommended guidelines for ophthalmic procedure clipping.

Table 3.6 Ophthalmic procedures' clipping guidelines.

Procedure	Margins
Ophthalmic cases – intra-ocular – corneal laceration repair and foreign body removal	Using a fine-bladed scissors with water-soluble lubricant on blades, trim eyelashes and hair on eyelids near conjunctival margin
Ophthalmic cases – extra-ocular – enucleation	A clipper blade width from eyelid margins (dorsal and ventral direction) and a clipper blade width from medial and lateral canthus.

Note: Eyelids should be sutured closed prior to beginning clipping for an enucleation.

Aural

Aural surgeries vary greatly in nature and as such, so does the clipping. Procedures of the ear canal and inner ear require a much different clip than those just involving the pinna. As a word of caution, bulla osteotomy procedures also require clipping of the ventral neck to facilitate the approach the surgeon will make to the surgical site. Table 3.7 describes recommended clipping margins for various aural procedures.

Head and Mouth

Procedures of the mouth and head can be intra-oral or extra-oral. Intra-oral dental surgery is generally performed by veterinary dentists and will not be addressed in this text. Intra-oral procedures involving the removal of a mass may be performed by a soft tissue surgeon. Suffice to say, however, that intra-oral procedures generally require little to no clipping. If the mass is entirely within the mouth, there is no need to clip any hair. Procedures that are extra-oral in nature do require some caution when clipping so as not to injure or traumatize either of the eyes, depending on where the incision is to be made. Table 3.7 describes recommended clipping margins for cranio/facial procedures.

Perineal

Perineal procedures are also a unique clipping situation. Whether a perineal hernia repair, an anal sacculectomy, or a perianal tumor removal, the margins for clipping are fairly standard. One additional step in the patient prep that is unique to any perineal procedure is the placement of a purse string suture in the anus. The method of a purse string suture placement will be described in the patient prep section of this chapter. In most states, this should be considered a task that can be delegated to technicians as it is not a primary closure of a wound but rather a step in a nursing procedure. It is advisable to check with the Practice Act in the state to determine eligibility to perform this task. Table 3.8 outlines the recommended hair removal margins for various perineal procedures.

Table 3.7 Facial/aural procedures' clipping guidelines.

Procedure/location of surgery	Margins
Mandibular mass removal, mandibulectomy, and fracture repair	Rostral edge of mandible caudally to ramus of mandible; dorsally to commissure of lip; and ventrally to ventral midline
Maxillectomy and maxillary fracture repair	Rostral edge of maxilla caudally to ear and dorsally to lateral canthus of eye.
Aural procedures[a] – pinna hematoma lancing, mass removal, and laceration repair	Clip entire pinna from tip to dorsal attachment to head.
Aural procedures – lateral ear canal resection and total ear canal ablation	Remove hair from medial and lateral sides of pinna; dorsally to dorsal midline; ventrally to ventral midline; rostrally to lateral canthus of the eye; and caudally to base of neck
Aural procedure – ventral bulla osteotomy	Laterally to the base of the affected ear and entire ventral mandible from mandibular symphosis to the mid-cervical neck.

[a] Check with surgeon to find out if both medial and lateral sides of pinna need to be clipped.

Table 3.8 Perineal procedures' clipping guidelines.

Procedure	Cranial edge	Caudal edge	Lateral edge
Anal sacculectomy	Base of tail	Ventral side of tail	To the level of tuber ischii on both sides
Perineal urethrostomy	Base of tail	Ventral side of tail and ventrally on limbs to stifle. Only medial aspect of limbs needs be clipped	To the level of the tuber ischii
Perineal hernia	Base of tail or cranially to lower sacral vertebrae	Ventral side of tail and ventrally to the level of abdomen	To the level of tuber ischii

Amount of hair to be clipped is dependent on size of hernia.

Open Wound Clipping

Open wounds are considered contaminated but still require special attention when clipping. The main focus when prepping an open wound is to prevent any more contamination (hair) from entering the wound. A couple of options are available to achieve this goal. First of all, a saline-soaked sponge can be placed over the wound. Be sure to leave all wound edges visible so removal of hair can be accomplished on the edges. Any hair that may fly or fall into the wound will land on the sponge and will be much easier to remove than if it had landed on the tissue. Once clipping has been completed, simply fold the corners of the sponge(s) to the middle and lift it out of the wound.

Another option is to cover the open wound with a thick layer of water-soluble lubricant. Once the wound is covered with lubricant, clipping may begin. It is always best to clip away from the wound, but clipping against the grain of the hair must also be observed. Care should be taken to avoid, as much as possible, depositing any clipped hair in the wound. Once clipping is completed, the wound must be flushed well with sterile saline before the prepping begins, to remove the lubricant and any hair that may have fallen into the wound.

With regard to clipping for any surgical procedure, a complete vacuuming of all the removed hair must occur. Ensure stray clumps of hair under the patient or on the towel the patient is lying on are removed. If the technician's smock has large amounts of hair on it, do not forget to vacuum the smock as well. Holding the vacuum hose with one hand permits the other hand to be free to manipulate the animal's skin or the towel to avoid having those items sucked into the hose. Placing one finger (of the hand holding the vacuum hose) over the end of the hose will cut the suction to aid in avoiding traumatizing tissue with excessive suction power (Figure 3.13).

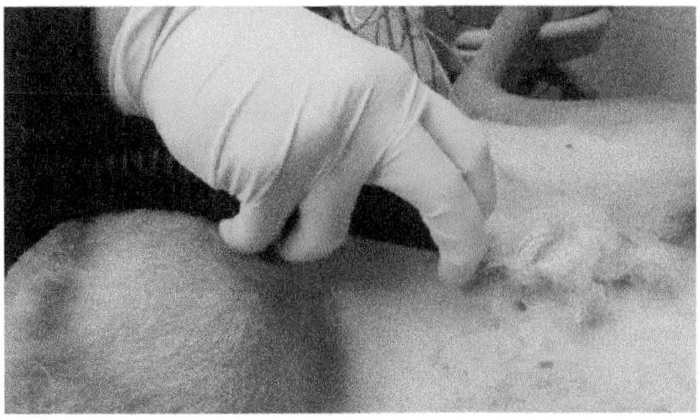

Figure 3.13 Vacuuming with hand over end to control suction. *Source:* Courtesy of Michelle Jaeger.

Clipper Care

After each patient has been clipped, the blade should be evaluated. If any teeth are missing from the blade, the blade should be removed and thrown away. If the blade appears to be intact, it needs to be cleaned and lubricated. After each use, clipper blades must be disengaged from the clipper head, removed, and cleaned. Using a stiff plastic (not metal) bristle brush, remove the hair from the blade, the teeth, and the clipper head. Reattach the blade, but do not snap the blade into place when the clipper is not running. Once the clipper has been turned on, snap the blade into position being certain to properly engage the blade. If the teeth are not moving or there is a knocking or rattling sound, the blade is not properly positioned. Once the blade is running smoothly, spray a commercially available clipper blade lubricant on the teeth and allow it to run for at least one minute. After a minute of running, take a paper towel or gauze and blot away any excess lubricant. If a new clipper blade is placed on the clipper head, before it is used on a patient, it must be cleaned with a commercial blade wash. With the clipper running, submerge just the teeth in the blade wash for a minute or so. Remove the blade from the solution, turn off the clipper, and blot away any excess solution on the blade. This step will remove oils from the factory and will improve the longevity of the blade.

Patient Skin Preparation

Preparation of the skin of the surgical patient has been a long-debated issue. Information used as a guideline for human surgical patients does not translate exactly for veterinary patients. Efficacy of products on animal skin differs from human skin due to the different thickness (i.e. bovine skin vs. human skin), fat content (i.e. porcine skin vs. human skin), and that fact that animal skin, for the most part, is covered by fur. Nonetheless, often references with a human surgical patient base are utilized as standards of care with veterinary patients. Smocks worn while clipping should be removed for the prep. A surgical head covering, mask, and exam gloves should be worn to decrease the risk of cross-contamination of the surgical site.

Surgical Scrub Products

There are two basic options of surgical scrub products available for use for surgical patient preparation. Each has redeeming qualities of its own, but overall, one is superior when all categories are considered.

Chlorhexidine

Chlorhexidine scrub is a 2 or 4% detergent-based product that can be used to cleanse the surgical site of veterinary surgical patients. It has a rapid onset of action, persistent effectiveness in the presence of bodily fluids, and excellent residual effect. Chlorhexidine requires a three-minute contact time to maximize the benefits of the product. It can be rinsed with sterile water or 70% isopropyl alcohol. Generally, the 2% product is rinsed with 70% isopropyl alcohol and the 4% product is rinsed with sterile water. Care should be taken to supplement body heat with an external device as much as possible as rinsing agents can cause hypothermia.

Povidone-Iodine

The other option for patient prep is povidone-iodine (Figure 3.14). Although less expensive than chlorhexidine, it is inactivated in the presence of organic material, has significantly lower residual activity, and when rinsed with isopropyl alcohol, has lower effectiveness.

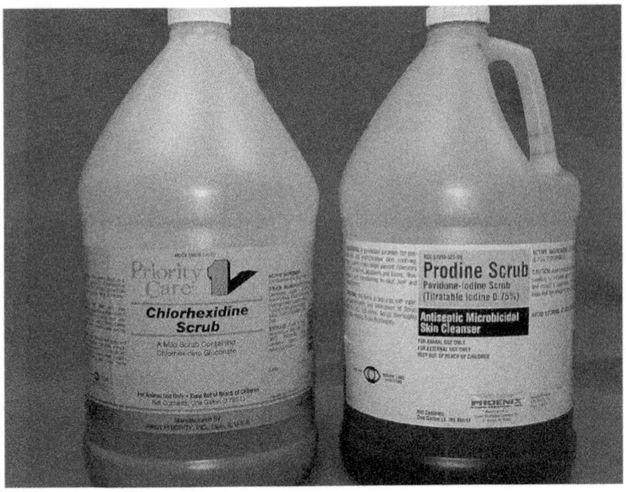

Figure 3.14 Scrub products available for patient prep.

Because it is an iodine-based product, the orangish/brown color is appreciated by some as an indicator of what area has been covered.

There is a recent study with human surgical patients, comparing the rate of surgical site infections and the skin preparation product used, that proves helpful when choosing between options. The patients were either prepped with 2% chlorhexidine gluconate and rinsed with 70% isopropyl alcohol or 10% povidone-iodine scrub and painted with 10% aqueous povidone-iodine solution. The study showed that those patients prepped with 2% chlorhexidine had a significantly lower rate of surgical site infections (SSI) 30 days postoperatively. The findings concluded that due to chlorhexidine's many redeeming qualities, the skin flora of the patient was reduced, thus lowering SSI. It would seem reasonable to translate this same application to veterinary medicine and veterinary surgical patients.

Rinsing Agents

Rinsing agents have traditionally been either 70% isopropyl alcohol or sterile water/saline (Figure 3.15). While alcohol does add some antiseptic qualities, some feel that the hypothermia caused by evaporating alcohol outweighs any antiseptic benefits. Using sterile water/saline to rinse the detergent product from the animal's skin has less of a hypothermic effect but offers no additional antiseptic value. Additionally, sterile water/saline may increase the sudsing action of the scrub product which means special attention must be paid to ensuring complete removal of the scrub agent is attained. Determining which product to use may be based on the size of the patient having surgery, the product used to cleanse the skin, the type of surgery being performed, and the estimated length of the anesthetic episode. All these factors can contribute to hypothermia and the benefits must be compared to the consequences.

Final Paint Solutions

Final painting of the clipped and scrubbed area needs to happen as a final step in the skin preparation process. Whichever chemical base (chlorhexidine or povidone-iodine) is used for the scrub should also be used for the final paint (Figure 3.16). Because chlorhexidine and povidone-iodine

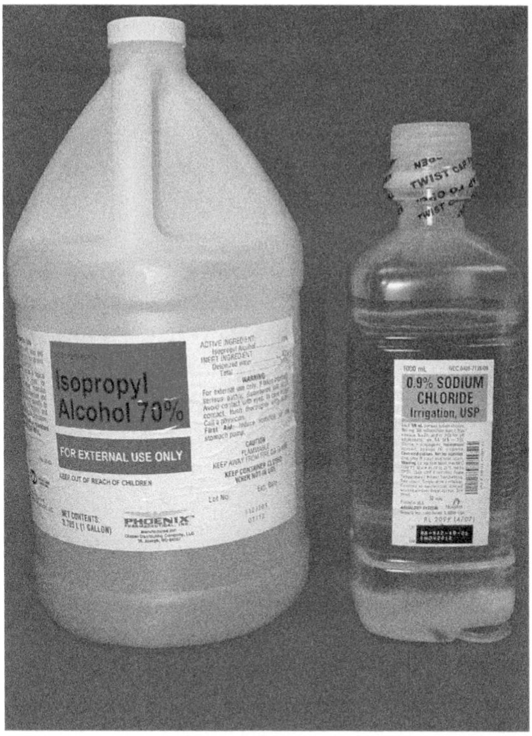

Figure 3.15 Rinsing products available for patient prep.

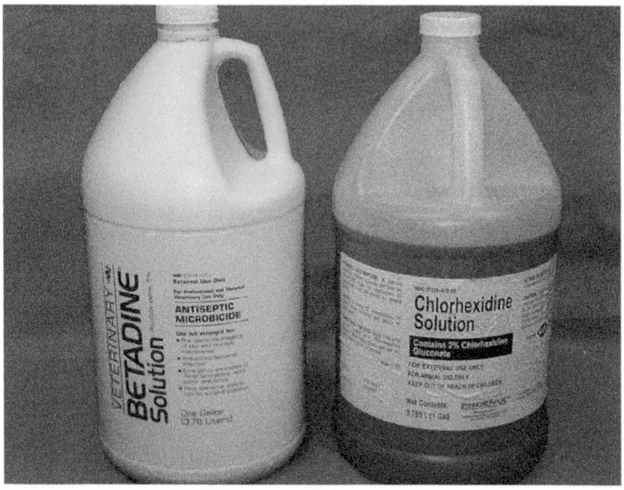

Figure 3.16 Final solution products available for patient prep.

have different molecular charges (cationic vs. anionic), it is recommended that the two products not be used together as the povidone-iodine may decrease the efficacy of the chlorhexidine. Povidone-iodine is used at full strength as it comes from the manufacturer. Chlorhexidine, however, is diluted according to the manufacturer's directions, which are generally 1 oz. chlorhexidine solution in 1 gallon of tap water.

Patient Prep Patterns

Target Pattern

Depending on the proposed incision site, there are various methods or patterns for cleansing the skin that can be utilized. For abdominal, thoracic, neurologic, or lump/mass removals, a target pattern should be used. It is aptly named the target pattern because when properly executed, it resembles a target or bull's eye. Starting at the center of the clipped area (which should be the proposed incision site), the skin is cleansed with surgical scrub applied in a linear, back-and-forth movement. When using a sponge, it is advantageous to fold the corners of the sponge to the center to better control the surface area of the sponge touching the patient. There need not be excessive pressure placed on the skin. In fact, too much pressure can result in abrading the skin which can create a breeding ground for bacteria and compromise the incision. If redness or capillary oozing appears, the amount of pressure being exerted by the person prepping must be greatly reduced to the point of barely touching the skin. Contact time with the surgical scrub is what affects the effectiveness, not the amount of pressure used to apply the product. After constant contact with the proposed incision site (about 15 s), the sponge continues to be moved in a small back-and-forth motion while moving outward from the center to the periphery of the clipped area (Figure 3.17). If the sponge becomes contaminated (by hair or other organic material), it should be discarded and a new sponge obtained. The new sponge should begin where the old one ended and continue moving in an outward motion toward the hairline. Once the sponge touches the hair, it may continue to be used if only touching hair. The entire area that is clipped should be scrubbed. After the initial scrub is completed, a decision needs to be made. Some surgeons prefer to have the site scrubbed two more times with the surgical scrub before rinsing with a rinsing agent. This approach provides a constant contact time. Other surgeons prefer to have the site scrubbed once, rinse with either 70% isopropyl alcohol or sterile water/saline, then scrub again, then rinse, then repeat the cycle one more time. This approach has interrupted contact time, but it is easier to remove all the scrub detergent from the skin. The critical point is that as long as the recommended contact time is achieved, either method can be used. Some clinics find setting a timer for the patient prep ensures appropriate contact time.

The rinsing agent should be applied to the shaven area using the same target pattern. If using sterile water/saline to rinse, a good squeeze of the sponge, to remove excess fluid, will be helpful. This will help decrease excessive sudsing as mentioned previously, which can hinder complete removal of the scrub agent. It is important that all detergent be removed from the skin as it can cause tissue irritation if transferred to internal tissues. The clipped area needs to be cleansed at

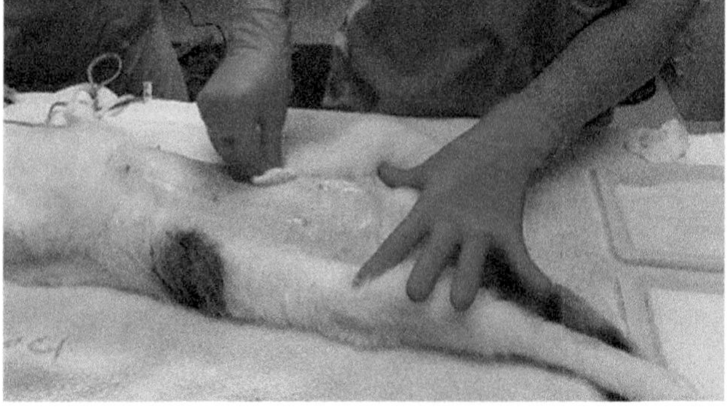

Figure 3.17 Abdominal prep.

least three times to meet the essential contact time without excessive drying or abrading of the skin. If, however, after checking the rinse sponge of the third cycle of cleansing, there is still dirt being removed, cleansing should continue until the rinse sponge is clean. Most small animals will be clean after the three cycles, but animals that live in an area where they are exposed to more dirt (outside kennel or farm) or those involved in a trauma (hit by car or penetrating wound) may need the additional cleansing. In an ideal situation, at this point, the patient would be transported to the surgery room, positioned on the surgery table, and then have a sterile prep performed. However, quite frequently this does not occur. If no sterile prep is performed, a final application of paint solution is applied, using the same target pattern. Paint solution may be applied with a spray bottle instead of with a sponge, although the disadvantages outweigh the advantages. Application with a spray bottle results in the solution falling on surfaces not intended to be sprayed (patient's fur, tabletop, and floor) and causes a mess. In addition, application with a spray bottle may mean the solution is sprayed in uneven amounts on the animal's skin which may mean not all solution is dry before surgery begins. Although spray application is accomplished quickly, this is the only advantage. Application of the final solution with a sponge allows for a controlled, even application of solution. However applied, the solution must be allowed to fully dry prior to draping and the incision is made to allow the product to perform to its full potential. The patient can then be moved into the surgery room, taking special care to not contaminate the prepped area. At a minimum, another final paint solution application should occur after final positioning on the surgery table.

Orthopedic Prep

Patients having surgery on any limb will most likely need an orthopedic prep. This method of skin preparation offers the surgeon the ability to have full circumferential access to the limb as well as the ability to handle and maneuver the limb as needed during the procedure.

First, the distal end of the surgical limb, if available, must be covered to the carpus/tarsus with an exam glove or a non-adhesive elastic-type bandage material (Figure 3.18). Once the distal limb is covered, a stirrup (for suspending the limb) must be made. Using 1″ or 2″ tape, rip a piece approximately 30″ long to be used to create the stirrup that will elevate the limb. Large breed dogs or dogs with long legs may need a slightly shorter piece, while small dogs or shorter legs will need a longer piece of tape. Regardless of the length, leave the last 1–2″ on either end as regular-width tape. The length in between needs to be folded on itself, lengthwise with the sticky side to sticky side, to form a non-sticky surface. The ends are then adhered to the covered paw, on either the medial and lateral surfaces or the anterior/palmar or plantar surfaces, leaving the loop visible. Tape is then used to cover the tape ends on the paw to secure the stirrup so it does not slip (Figure 3.19). If the distal portion of the limb is the surgical site, a Backhaus penetrating towel clamp can be clamped onto the web between two toes for limb suspension. A puncture wound to the web is considered less traumatic than a puncture to a toenail. The tape stirrup is then passed through the ring handles of the towel clamp, the free

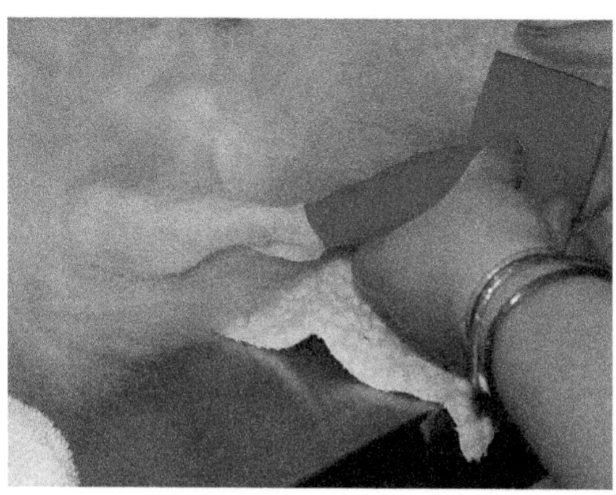

Figure 3.18 Covering the distal end of the limb.

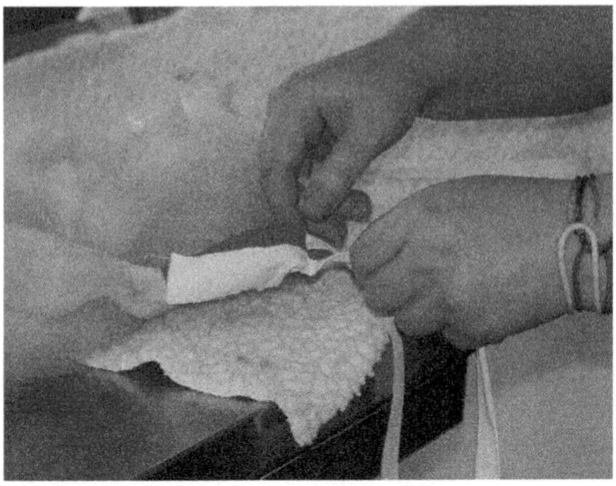

Figure 3.19 Applying a hanging stirrup.

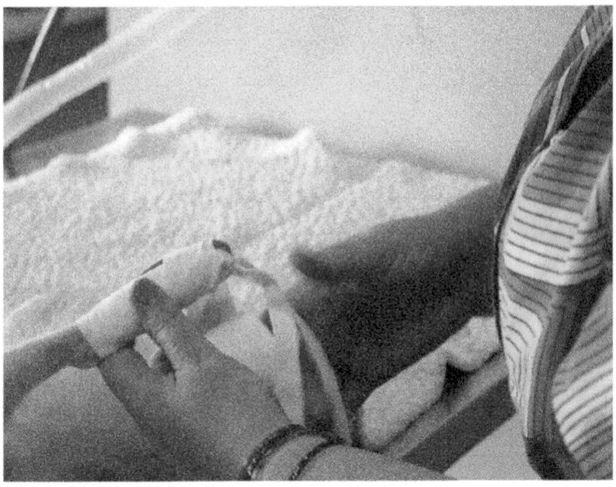

Figure 3.20 Securing the stirrup with tape.

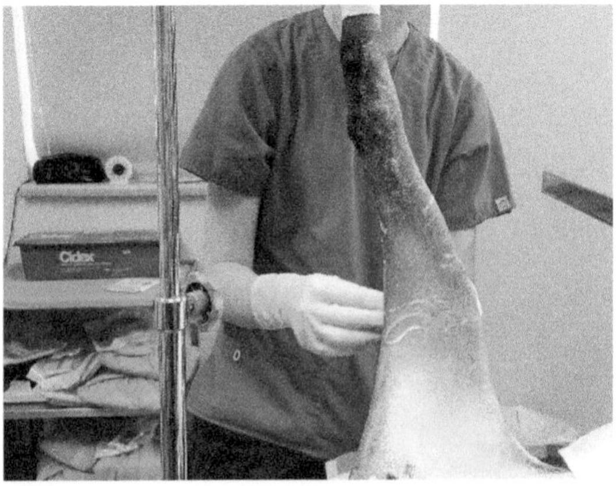

Figure 3.21 Orthopedic prep.

ends of the stirrup are secured to one another, and the limb is ready for suspension (Figure 3.20). Providing support to the limb, lift the leg and place the loop over an IV pole hook. Elevate the pole so the leg is straight, but not lifting the animal off the table. In the case of a fracture, providing support to the limb is imperative to avoid bone fragment ends from causing more trauma to the tissues. Once elevated, the traction on the tissues may in fact assist the surgeon with distraction and reduction of the fracture, as the muscles will be stretched and fatigued.

The orthopedic prep begins at the distal end of the limb by the taped foot. Fold the corners of the prep sponge into the middle and hold all four corners to better control the sponge. Without touching the tape, begin scrubbing the skin, moving the hand in short vertical strokes, circumferentially (all the way around) on the limb (Figure 3.21). Once one complete circling of the limb has been completed, the sponge is moved just proximally on the limb and the pattern is continued. Due to the larger surface that needs to be covered with this prep, subsequent sponges may be needed as the pattern moves proximally on the limb. When starting with another sponge, the prep should begin where the previous sponge ended. As with the target pattern, once the sponge touches hair, it can only continue to touch hair and may never return to the clipped skin. After scrubbing the entire clipped area, the pattern can either be repeated with another scrub sponge or a with a rinse sponge, as previously discussed. After the limb is sufficiently cleansed (at least three scrubs/rinses or until the rinse sponge is free of dirt and minimal contact time has occurred), a clean (not sterile) towel needs to be laid over the down limb. The surgical limb is then carefully lowered and laid on the towel. The patient is transported to the surgical suite and positioned on the surgery table. The leg is then carefully resuspended, and the towel is removed in preparation for the final prep. All orthopedic procedures should always have a sterile prep performed following final positioning of the patient on the surgery table.

Perineal

Perianal/perineal procedures are generally prepped utilizing a modified target pattern. Once the clipping and vacuuming are complete, the next step is the placement of a purse string suture in the anus. This is done to help eliminate the leakage of fecal material onto the surgical field. Unless the surgeon requests this not be done, it is a standard inclusion in the patient preparation. It is easiest to place this suture with a straight needle on any type of suture that is 2–0 or 3–0 in size. Since it is a limited-term suture, whether the suture is absorbable or non-absorbable is not an issue, but a monofilament is preferred. In this situation, placement of this stitch is not a primary wound closure, nor a curative measure, so it should be allowed by most jurisdiction's Practice Acts. If any doubt arises regarding the legality of a credentialed veterinary technician performing this procedure, the Practice Act should be consulted. To place the suture pattern, start first by looking at the anus and imagining it as a clock face. With the needle at the 11 o'clock position, take a superficial bite and have the needle exit at the 1 o'clock position. Starting the next bite where the previous one exited the skin, drive the needle superficially and exit at the 5 o'clock position. For the ventral placement, enter the skin at 5 o'clock, drive the needle superficially, and exit at the 7 o'clock point. The final bite begins at 7 o'clock and moves in a dorsal direction, superficially, and exits at the 11 o'clock point. Superficial placement is imperative for all the bites, but especially for the lateral stitches to avoid inadvertently penetrating the anal glands. In essence, a "box" has been placed around the anus (Figure 3.22). Pull the suture tight to cinch down the anal opening and tie the suture. A simple one-throw knot or square knot is sufficient. Cut the suture tails long enough to be able to find them, but not so long that they interfere with the procedure. A bold note should be made on the anesthesia sheet or the surgical report indicating the placement of the purse string. Some clinics have found that placing a piece of tape on the patient's head with "Purse String" written on it is an equally

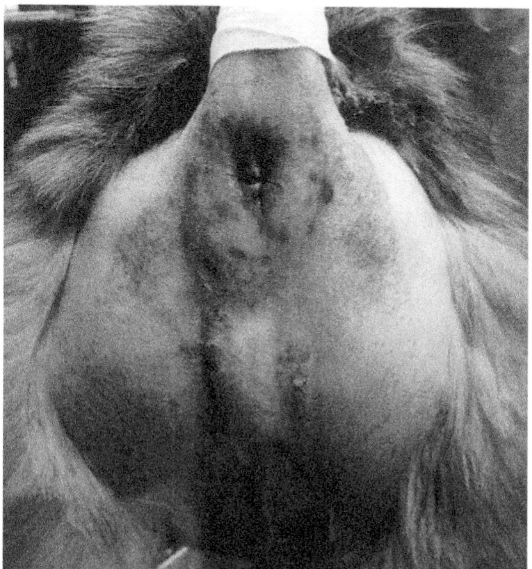

Figure 3.22 Purse string suture in anus – irritation from fecal matter. *Source:* Courtesy of Cassandra Simmons.

effective bold reminder. Whichever method is utilized, it will act as a reminder to remove the suture postprocedure, but before recovery.

After the purse string stitch has been completed, the prep can begin. Working from clean to dirty areas, the clipped area lateral to the anus should be scrubbed with the target pattern. Using a new sponge for each side, perform the target pattern until hair is touched. Use a new sponge and scrub just the anus, then discard that sponge. This modified pattern is repeated until the rinse sponge is free of dirt, with a minimum of three repetitions. The final solution is applied using the same pattern.

Patient Positioning

Once the patient has received the initial prep, they are ready to be transported to the operating room. There are many devices available for assisting with positioning the patient on the surgery table. Proper positioning of the patient is a critical step in the patient prep process. Surgeons require the patient to be positioned in a straight and anatomically correct fashion. Once a patient is positioned to the surgeon's liking, they must not shift to move from that position until the end of the surgery. Some surgery tables have a split top that allows either one or both sides of the tabletop to be adjusted. Options from a flat surface to a full "V" position are available. For patients in dorsal recumbency, this may be all that is required to maintain the patient in the surgical position required. For deep-chested dogs, long sandbags will be an effective method for maintaining dorsal recumbency in addition to the table "V." Foam wedges may also be used but may slip and if contaminated by blood or other fluids may be difficult to clean. Also available for use, if the tabletop is solid and cannot be adapted to the animal's shape, is a thoracic positioner (Figure 3.23). Additionally, patients in dorsal recumbency will need to have their limbs restrained away from the surgical field. Soft ropes or "leg ties" are available and work well. Roll gauze, IV tubing, or elastic bands are not recommended as they may apply too much pressure to the soft tissue and impede distal limb circulation. Leg ties should be placed just proximal to the carpus and tarsus, with a half hitch placed just distal to those joints (Figure 3.24). Double placement aids in better distribution of pressure to reduce circulation issues. Most surgery tables have either brackets or rubber rollers on the sides of the table near each corner. Brackets require a figure 8 method of securing the leg tie with a half hitch on the last loop to hold the rope (Figure 3.25). Rubber rollers are easier to use and simply require the leg tie to be passed between the two rubber rollers to securely hold the rope (Figure 3.26).

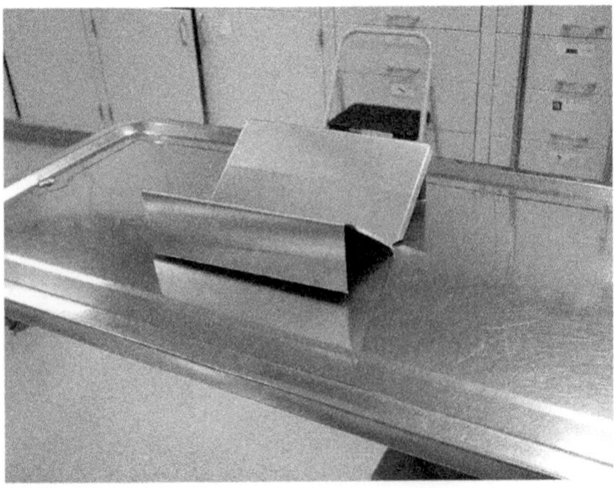

Figure 3.23 Thoracic positioner for maintaining dorsal recumbency.

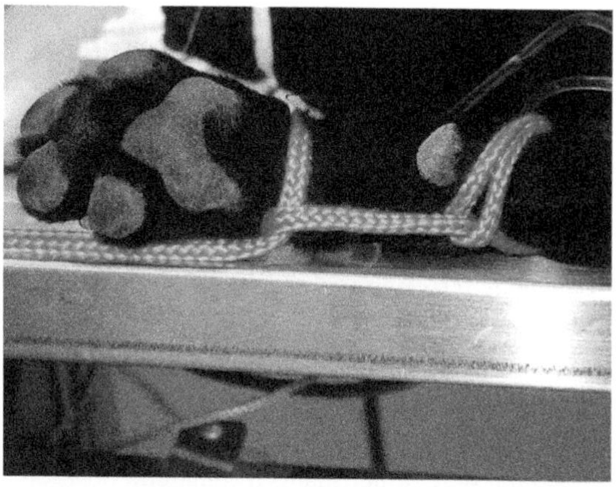

Figure 3.24 Leg tie with half hitch on limb.

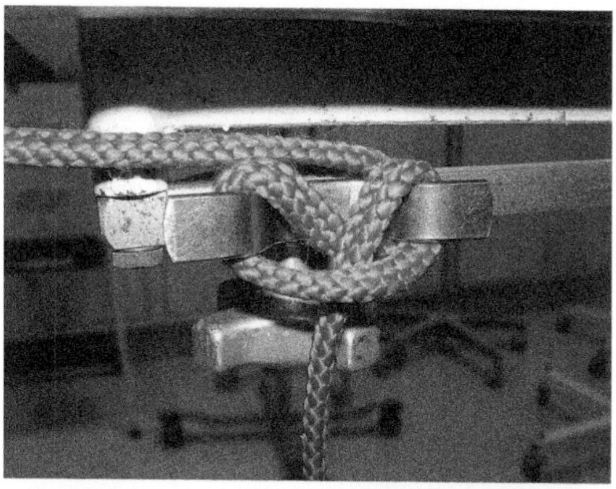

Figure 3.25 Table bracket with figure 8 leg tie.

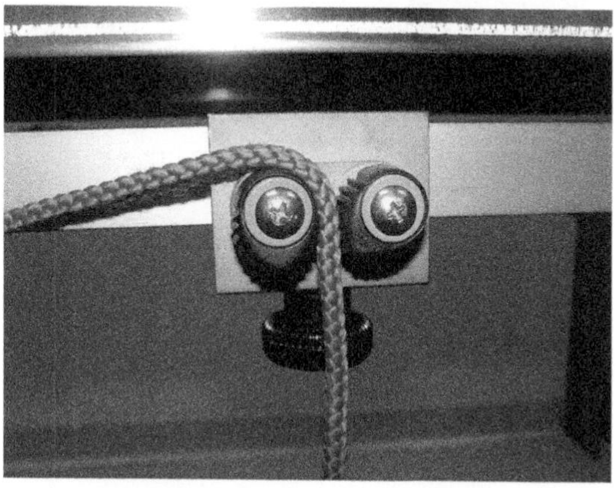

Figure 3.26 Table roller for securing leg tie.

Care should be taken to avoid excessively extending the limbs. The forelimbs should have the leg ties brought over the head of the table, not the sides, to help maintain normal joint anatomy. Hind limbs should be extended to full range of motion, although not excessively stretched, and the ropes should be brought over the end of the table, not the sides. Normal anatomy of the hind leg joints can be maintained with this approach. Rear limb leg ties brought over the side of the table force the hips into a "frog leg" position, and for lengthy procedures, this is not recommended. Additionally, the limbs will be closer to the animal's body and not impede the surgeon's work. There is a special type of positioning aid for dogs having arthroscopic surgery on the stifle. The brace holds the limb in a flexed position to assist the surgeon. The brace must be covered by a sterile drape before the limb can be placed on it. If an additional procedure will be done after the arthroscopy (i.e. Tibial Plateau Leveling Osteotomy [TPLO]), then the brace will not be used.

Patients in lateral recumbency may be maintained in the desired position by the use of sandbags or vacuum positioning aids. Hug-U-Vac® and Vac-Pac® are both positioning devices that conform to the patient to maintain the position, and then a vacuum process is used to evacuate the air from the device. As the positioning aid hardens as the air is removed, the patient is held in the desired position. These devices help with thermostasis as well as they are insulated and protect the patient from the cold surface of the surgery table. Vacuum aids are especially helpful when positioning patients for ophthalmic procedures or thoracic cases that necessitate the patient be positioned in an oblique state rather than a level lateral position. Patients in lateral recumbency will also require the limbs to be restrained by leg ties. Larger breed dogs may have sandbags, foam, or some other type of "spacer" placed between the upper and lower limbs to help alleviate stress on the upper limb joints.

Patients undergoing spinal surgery are generally placed in ventral recumbency. The use of sandbags and/or vacuum aids is required in order to achieve and maintain proper positioning of the patient. Patients in this position must be monitored for adequate respiratory capability. The vacuum position aids are quite stiff and hard following evacuation of the air and are therefore not very good at allowing expansion of the chest wall if conformed too tightly to the patient. Positioning aids should not be "wrapped around" the chest of the patient, but rather gathered or formed along the sides of the chest (Figure 3.27).

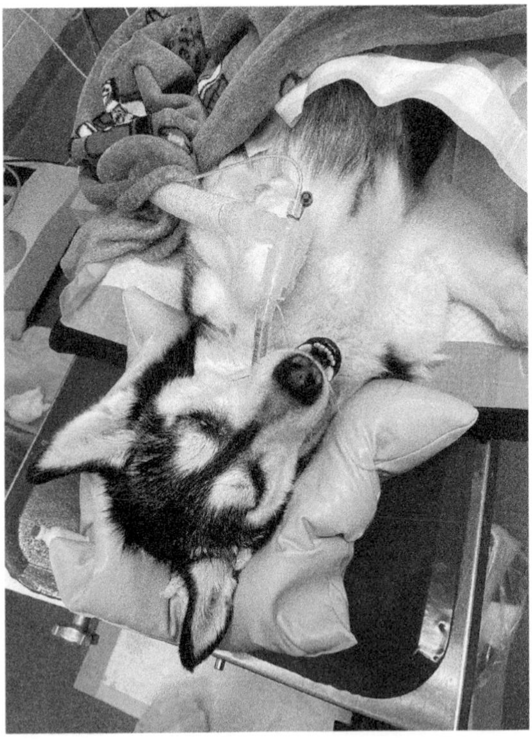

Figure 3.27 Vacuum positioning device. *Source:* Courtesy of Charlotte LeMieux.

Patient Warming

Normal body thermoregulatory systems are compromised by anesthesia, so maintaining an appropriate body temperature for the patient is very challenging. Surgical complications can often be linked to patient surgical/postsurgical hypothermia, so external supplementary means must be used. In addition to peripheral vasoconstriction, hypothermia can compromise the immune system and elevate both blood pressure and heart rate, thus affecting wound healing.

Heated Surgery Tables

One method of supplemental heat is the use of a heated surgery tabletop. Some surgery tables are constructed with heating elements enclosed within the tabletop (Figure 3.28). As a constant source of heat there is the potential for a thermal burn, so placing a thick towel between the table and the patient is advised.

Circulating Water Blankets

Other types of supplemental heating generally revolve around the use of a pad of some sort and a control unit or box. Circulating water blankets have been employed for a long time and are now available with hard Plexiglas pads as well as the traditional softer vinyl pads. Softer vinyl pads are appropriate for use on a surgery table. Placing a towel both under the pad as well as between the patient and the pad is required. A towel between the tabletop and the pad will help avoid the loss

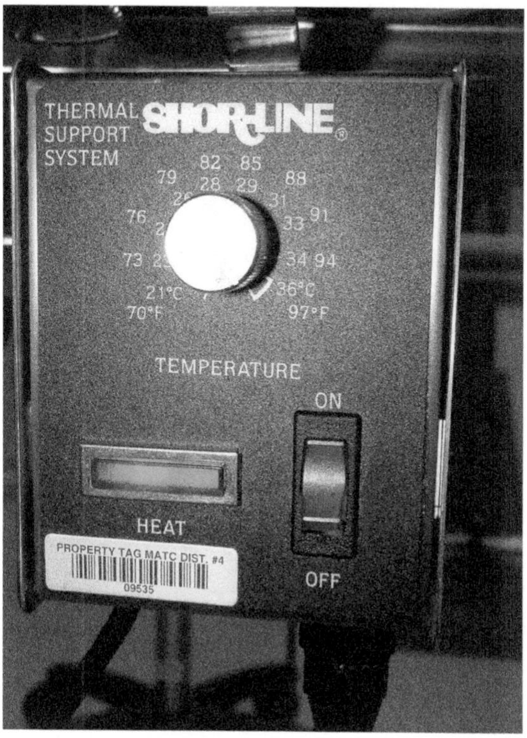

Figure 3.28 Control box for heated surgery table.

of heat to the cold stainless tabletop. A towel between the patient and the pad is necessary to guard against thermal burns from extended direct contact with the skin. Although perhaps not as comfortable as the pliable pad, the increased security of knowing a claw or a tooth will not puncture the pad makes the Plexiglas pads appealing for use postoperatively. Returning to the recovery area to check on a patient only to find a flood and a soaking-wet patient is very frustrating.

Convection Warming Systems

The use of forced warm air enveloping the patient has become a standard in recent years. A lightweight disposable paper pad with many small holes or a cloth reusable pad is positioned to cover as much of the patient as possible (Figure 3.30). A towel should be placed over the pad to contain the generated heat around the patient. Once the patient is positioned on the surgical table, and after the surgical drapes have been placed, the unit is turned on. While the drapes do assist in keeping the warm air close to the patient, there is some concern with increased air particles and potentially compromising aseptic technique with the addition of the warm forced air.

Solid Warming Pads

Multiple styles of solid warming pads that can be used are also available. Many of the pads deliver a low-voltage current to the solid pad. Internal sensors regulate the temperature of the pad and greatly reduce the risk of hot spots or uneven heating. Some models have an automatic shut off which inhibits thermal burns as well. Some of the styles of solid pads can be wrapped around (envelope) the patient, which in turn results in less hypothermia (Figure 3.29).

Alternative Methods

Alternative methods of supplementary heat include warmed bags of fluids, rice socks, warming discs, and hot water gloves (Figure 3.31). These devices, while warm, can certainly provide external heat for the patient. They are readily available, relatively inexpensive, and reusable, but the disadvantages must be considered. First, smaller warming devices will provide supplemental heat to only an isolated area of the body. Other methods previously discussed have a much greater body surface contact area, thus increasing heat absorption. Second, the warmed devices only provided warmth for a limited period of time and then they start to cool. As the rice socks or any other such

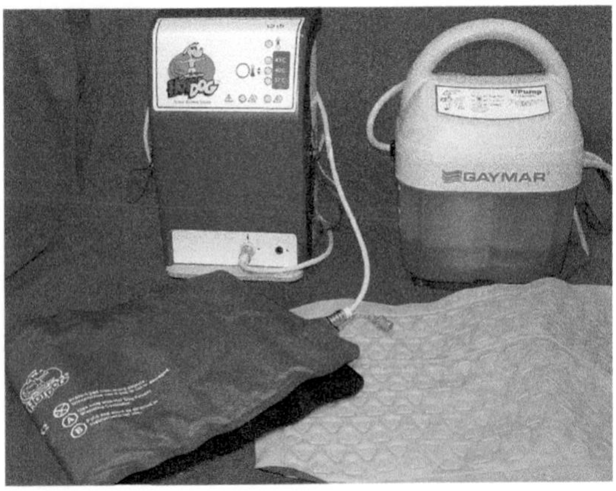

Figure 3.29 Supplemental heating devices.

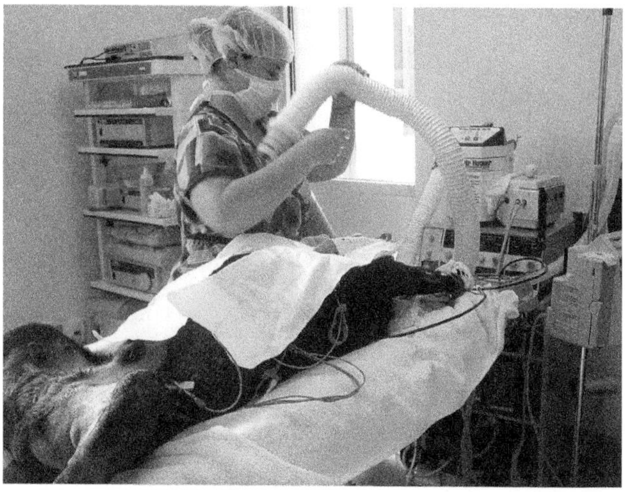

Figure 3.30 Hot-air warming system.

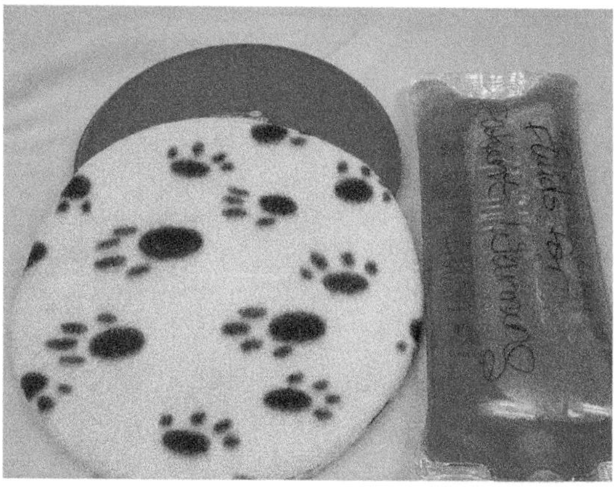

Figure 3.31 Alternative warming devices.

device cools, it will also cool the patient, therefore making these choices contraindicated for procedures longer than 30 minutes. Heating these types of devices requires the use of a microwave. Uneven heating from the microwave may put the patient at additional risk with prolonged contact. Strict instructions for times and power levels to use with the microwave must be posted to ensure all staff warm the devices in the same manner.

Patient Sterile Prep

Following positioning of the patient, the sterile prep may begin. A sterile patient prep is done the same as the initial prep, with the major difference being the use of sterile products. Prep sets can be made a couple of ways, depending on clinic choice. A small instrument pan (3″ × 8″) or a kidney basin (emesis basin) can be used as the pan. Two stacks of ten 4″ × 4″ gauze sponges are placed side by side in the pan. An indicator strip should be placed in the middle of the sponges. A right-hand glove (size 7–7 1/2) can then be laid on top of the sponges. The pan is double wrapped using the envelope style of wrapping and is steam sterilized (Figure 3.32). Some clinics prefer to use sterile packaged gauze and a fresh pair of sterile gloves, which is an acceptable adaptation.

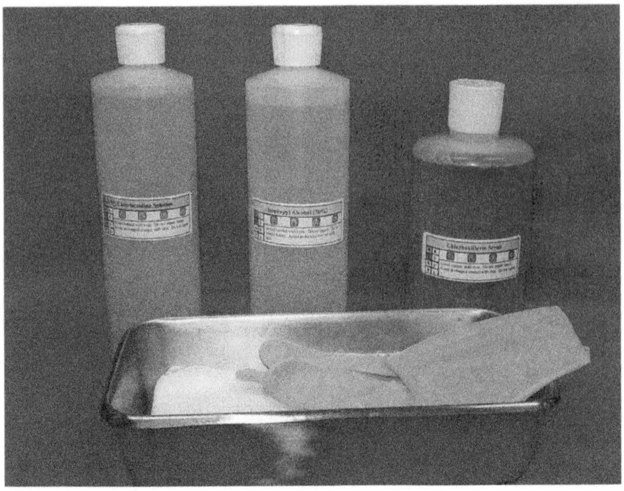

Figure 3.32 Sterile prep set with squeeze bottles of solutions.

In addition to the prep set, squeeze bottles of the prep solutions are needed. The solutions and prep set should be set up in the surgery room when the rest of the packs and equipment are placed in the room. Once the patient is placed on the table and positioned, the prep set can be opened. Both wraps are aseptically opened to reveal the sterile contents. Before proceeding, the caps of the solution bottles should be opened. If a glove was not included in the sterile prep set, a pair of gloves should now be aseptically opened, and using the open gloving technique, put on one glove on the dominant hand. If a glove was included, it is now aseptically placed on the dominant hand. Having one sterile and one non-sterile hand allows the technician the versatility to perform the sterile prep without assistance. The non-sterile hand is available to pick up the solution bottles to apply product as well as to stabilize the suspended limb in the event of an orthopedic case.

With the sterile gloved hand, a sponge is picked up. The non-sterile hand picks up the surgical scrub bottle and aseptically applies some scrub solution to the sterile sponges. Care must be taken to ensure the cap of the bottle does not touch the sponges. The prep now continues using the same pattern as was used with the initial prep. New prep sponges should be retrieved as needed. The rinsing agent is aseptically applied to the sponges as needed. Be sure to save a few dry sponges to be used for the application of the final paint solution. An alternative to this type of final prep is a One-Step Prep of chlorhexidine and alcohol (Chloraprep®) or povidone-iodine and alcohol (Duraprep®) in 1.0, 1.5, 3.0, 10.5 and 26.0 ml wands (Figure 3.33). Chlorhexidine One-Step Preps are sold in clear, orange, or teal solution. A One-Step Prep is painted on as a final sterile prep. One should don a sterile surgical glove using the open gloving technique, then break the inner tube of the One-Step Prep wand by compressing the wand tabs and shaking the chlorhexidine or povidone-iodine with the alcohol. Once the pad is saturated with the solution, the intended surgical site can be painted in the chosen pattern. Proper application is to overlap each pass of the wand by 50% and to discard the wand once hair is touched. The prep solution must be dry for 2–3 minutes before the patient is draped. This method of patient prep has been shown to be as effective in preventing bacterial growth as a full scrub.

Once the final paint is applied, the draping may begin. Every effort should be made to allow the final solution to dry prior to draping to encourage optimal efficacy.

Figure 3.33 Chloraprep™ final prep applicator.
Source: Courtesy of Heidi Reuss-Lamky.

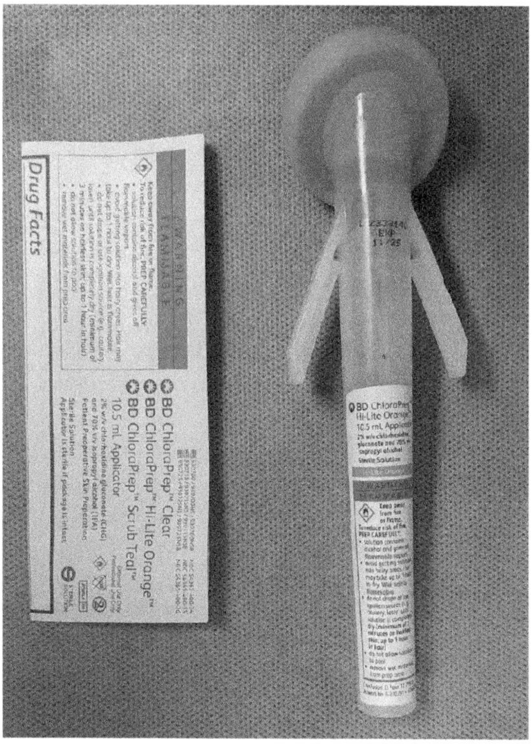

Personnel Preparation

Attire

Any person entering the surgery room must have on the appropriate attire. Clean scrubs, with the top tucked into the pants, an appropriate head covering, and shoe covers or facility-dictated footwear should be a minimal dress code. Personnel in the operating room, whether they are scrubbed in or not, must also adhere to several personal hygiene rules. Bathing or showering should occur every day. The use of fragrance or cologne should be minimal if at all. With increased sensitivity to fragrance by many people, it is simple consideration to not heavily apply a fragrance. More importantly, if the room or area is filled with the odor of cologne, the anesthetist will have a difficult time detecting any odor of inhalant gas that may indicate a leak in the anesthetic system. Finally, due to the increased sensitivity of the smelling sense of animals, heavy odors may be irritating to the patients.

Jewelry worn should be minimal and simple. If acting as the surgical assistant, no rings, watches, or bracelets can be worn. Even necklaces such as simple chain are discouraged. Some facilities allow small poststyle earrings to be left in the ear lobes, but never should hoops or large dangling earrings be worn. Ideally, earrings should be removed or not worn at all. Circulating technicians may have simple band-style rings and watches left on. Rings with large precious gemstones risk damage from chemicals or getting caught on equipment and would best be left at home. Earrings may be left in and should be a small poststyle earring. Simple single-chain necklaces may be left on.

Fingernails of all surgical team members should be short, well-groomed, and clean. Nails should not be longer than passed the pad of the finger. Current literature suggests the maximum length of nails that should be allowed for surgical personnel is 2 mm. Long fingernails can cause pain to feline patients while scruffing them and can puncture surgical gloves. Artificial nails and/or nail polish are strictly prohibited. Chipped or flaking nail polish may contaminate the field or worse, harbor bacteria that may infect the patient. Additionally, nail polish may mask the number of contaminants under the nail.

Surgeons Hand Scrub

Members of the surgical team who are scrubbing in need to perform a surgeon's hand scrub or rub. The hand scrub is a specific method of cleansing the hands, wrists, and forearms of a person that will be wearing a sterile gown and gloves. A surgical scrub, or cleansing, is performed in addition to the use of the sterile gown and gloves. It has been reported that the overall incidence of glove defects is 23% and glove defects increase as the duration of the procedure increases. Since the presence of glove defects can often be undetected, the surgical hand scrub is an essential step. Products used for a hand scrub must be rapid acting, should be effective against broad spectrum of bacteria, and should be non-irritating as well as effective at inhibiting bacterial growth. There are three products available that may be used for this procedure – povidone-iodine, chlorhexidine, and chloroxylenol (PCMX). Other newer products are available but will be discussed under the hand rub (brushless scrub) section. Povidone-iodine has a broad spectrum of activity but it is inactivated by organic material. Additionally, it requires a minimum of 2-minute contact time, which can easily be achieved using either method of surgical hand scrub patterns. Chlorhexidine also has a broad spectrum of activity and has the best residual effect due to its binding to keratin. It is not inactivated by organic material and causes less skin irritation than povidone-iodine. Chloroxylenol is available as scrub-impregnated sponges and traditionally has been outperformed by chlorhexidine.

Before a surgical scrub can begin, all jewelry must be removed from the hands and arms. Nails should be inspected and if too long, they must be trimmed. Neither nail polish nor artificial nails are allowed. Appropriate head and face attire must be put on and the surgical scrub top must be tucked into the scrub pants. If shoe covers are used, they must be placed on the footwear prior to the scrub beginning. The next step is to thoroughly wash the hands and arms with an antimicrobial product. Leaving the lather on the hands and arms, the nails must be cleaned. Nail cleaners can either be found in the package of a disposable scrub brush or purchased commercially and left in a receptacle near the scrub sink. In either case, the nail cleaner is disposable and should only be used once and then thrown away (Figure 3.34). After cleaning under the nails, the hands and arms can be rinsed. If an antiseptic-impregnated disposable sponge is used, it can be saturated with

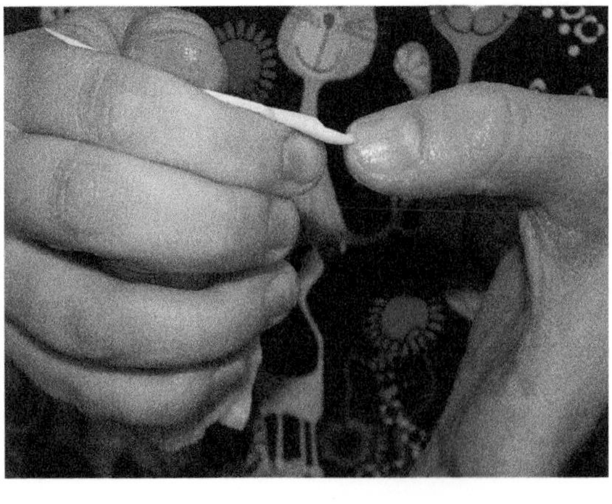

Figure 3.34 Cleaning nails.

water and squeezed to produce a lather. If a re-useable brush is used, it is aseptically removed from the sterilized brush dispenser. The foot-operated pedal for dispensing the soap is then depressed and the scrub brush is saturated with scrub product. The surgical scrub should be approached systematically and always performed the same way to avoid missing any of the steps. As the scrub begins, the elbows must remain bent, with the fingers pointing toward the ceiling. Not only does this allow the water to run from the fingertips to the elbows (clean to dirty) but it also ensures the hands and arms do not touch the scrub top.

Starting with either hand, the scrub brush is moved back and forth (which equals 1 stroke) on the nails for 30 strokes (Figure 3.35). Care should be taken to ensure the brush reaches under the nails as well as the nails themselves. Once the nails are done, the fingers are scrubbed next. It really does not matter if the scrub starts with the thumb or the little finger, as long as the same process is always used to avoid mistakes. The little finger is divided into four sides. Start the scrub on the lateral side moving from the tip of the finger to the base of the finger, counting as one stroke (Figure 3.36). Scrub the lateral side of the finger for 20 strokes. Move onto the palmar side of the finger for 20 strokes. The medial surface is scrubbed for 20 strokes next, and finally, the dorsal surface of the little finger is scrubbed for 20 strokes. That completes the scrub for one finger, so now the ring finger can be scrubbed using the same approach. Be sure to cleanse and scrub the webbing between each finger as well. After the ring finger is completed, the scrub follows the same pattern on the middle finger, index finger, and finally, the thumb. Following the scrub of the

Figure 3.35 Scrubbing the nails.

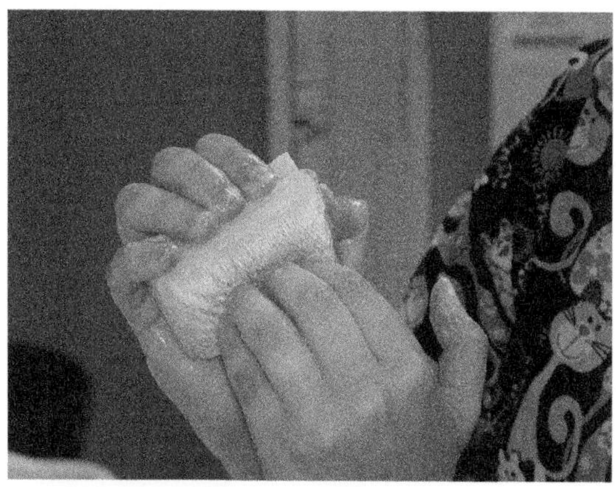

Figure 3.36 Scrubbing fingers: start at the little finger and divide each finger into four sides.

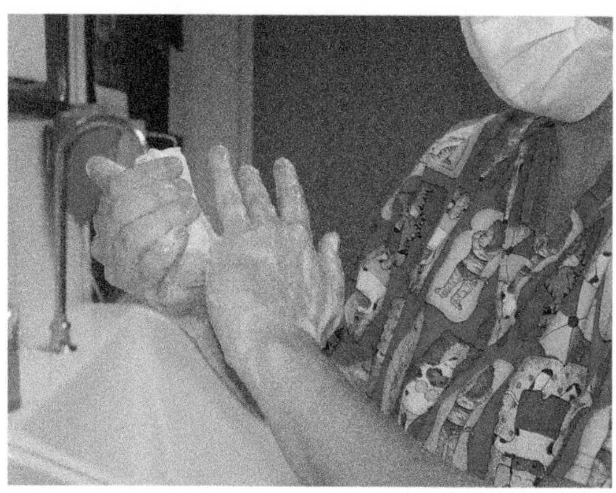

fingers, the entire palmar surface of the hand is scrubbed for 20 strokes (Figure 3.37). Following the palm, the dorsal surface of the hand is also scrubbed for 20 strokes (Figure 3.38). Completing the scrub of the hand allows progression to the arm. Dividing the arm into four equal sides, each side is scrubbed for 15 strokes, from the wrist to 2 in distal to the elbow (Figure 3.39). Leaving the antimicrobial detergent on the first arm, the sponge is transferred to the scrubbed hand, and the same process is followed to scrub the second hand and arm. At any time, more water may be added

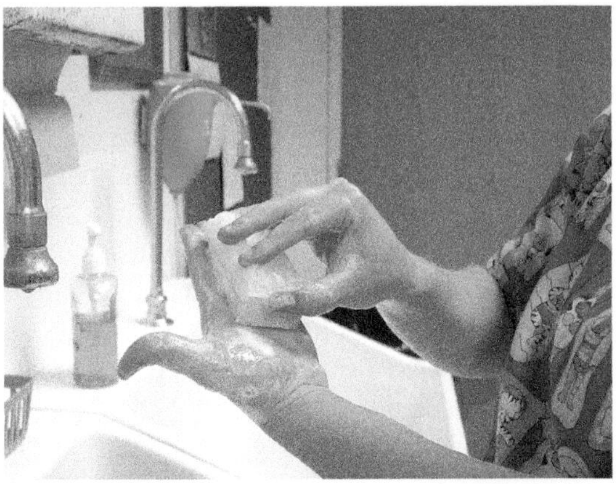

Figure 3.37 Scrubbing the palmar surface.

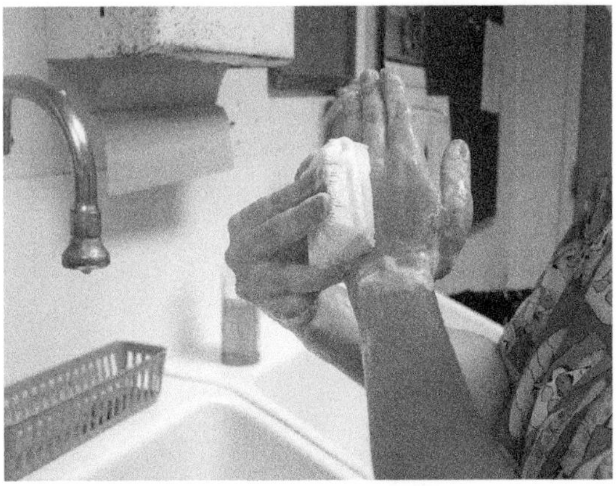

Figure 3.38 Scrubbing the back of the hand.

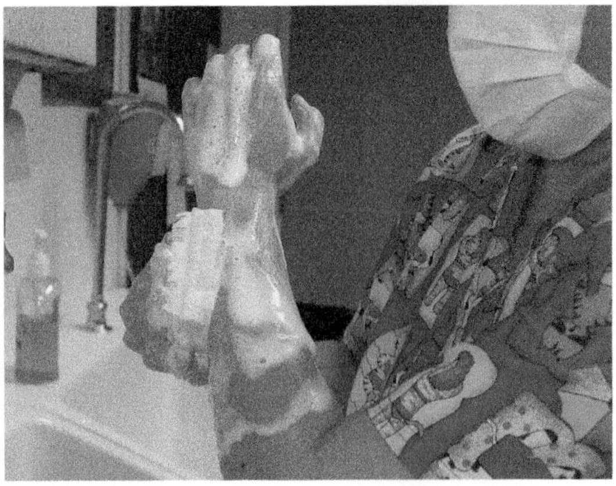

Figure 3.39 Scrubbing the arm: divide the arm into four sides.

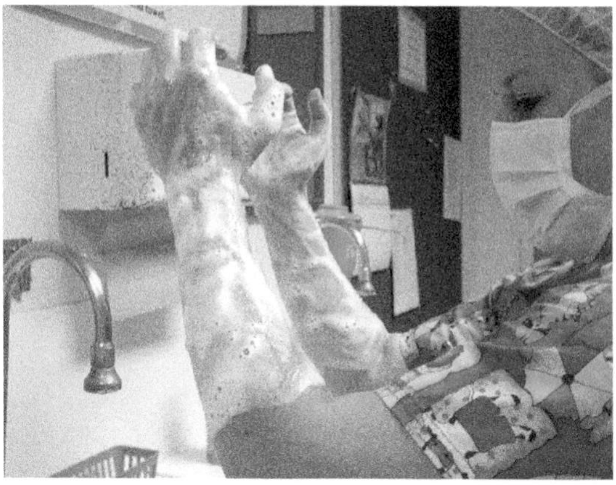

Figure 3.40 Both arms and hands scrubbed.

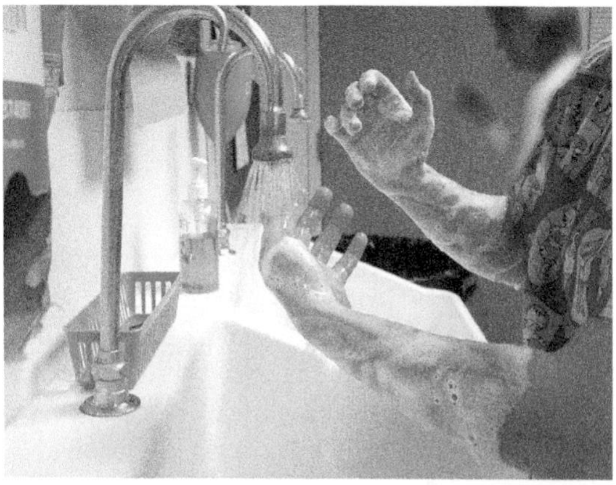

Figure 3.41 Rinsing first arm.

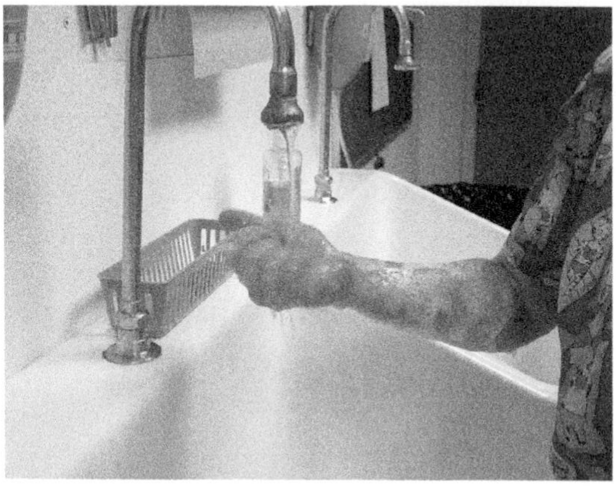

Figure 3.42 Rinsing second arm.

to the sponge to generate more lather or more soap may be added as needed. When the second hand and arm are completed, the first hand and arm are then rinsed (Figure 3.40). Being careful to not touch the faucet, the rinsing begins at the fingertips (Figure 3.41). With the elbows bent and the fingers pointing toward the ceiling, the rinse is continued down the hand, wrist, and arm. Care needs to be taken to keep the elbow bent so the water always runs from the fingers to the elbow. After completely rinsing the first arm, the second arm is rinsed in the same fashion (Figure 3.42).

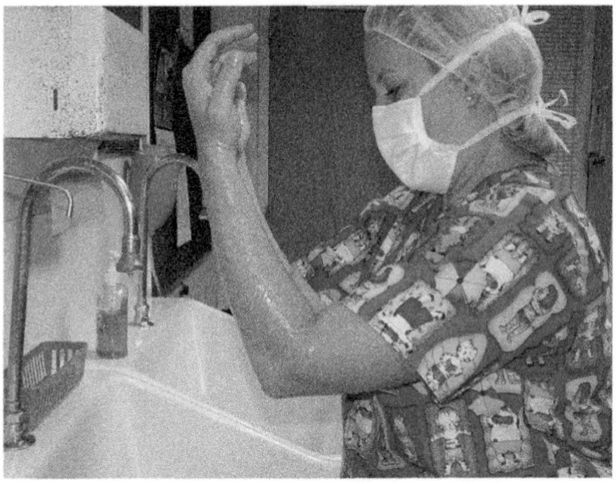

Figure 3.43 Letting arms drip at sink.

A slight end forward at the waist will help avoid splashing water onto the scrubs. After rinsing both arms, 15–30 seconds should be spent at the scrub sink allowing the water to run off the arms (Figure 3.43 and Video 3.1).

Surgical Hand Rub

One of the most recent advances in veterinary surgery is the introduction of the hand rub or surgical hand antisepsis. This procedure, performed with designated products, is intended to replace the surgical scrub. For surgeons and assistants who regularly scrub for multiple procedures in a day, this is a welcome alternative. There are various products available (Avagard®, Sterillium®, Surgicept®), but the base chemical in most of the options is ethyl alcohol. Current literature recommends a combination of chlorhexidine gluconate and ethyl alcohol as the ideal mixture for optimal effectiveness. It is imperative that manufacturer's recommendations be followed. Product should be applied to clean dry hands, so routine handwashing should be performed with the hands and arms being dried with a paper towel. It is advised for the first procedure of the day to use a nail pick to clean under nails. After rinsing the hands and forearms, they are dried with a paper towel. The recommended amount of product (usually one pump from an automatic delivery system) is dispensed into one hand. The nails and fingertips of the opposite hand are submerged in the solution. The remaining product is then rubbed into the hand and forearm to the elbow. Another dose of product is dispensed into the other hand and the procedure is repeated. A third dose of product is dispensed into either hand and reapplied to both hands and arms. Continuous rubbing will thoroughly dry the arms and hands prior to gloving. Proper exposure time to the product, as recommended by the manufacturer, must be adhered to (Video 3.2).

Drying the Hands and Arms

While the surgeon or assistant is performing the hand scrub, the circulating nurse should be opening the sterile gown pack. Both wrappers need to be opened in an aseptic fashion to permit access to the sterile hand towel. After performing a traditional hand scrub, the hands and arms need to be dried before gowning and gloving. The sterile hand towel must be picked up with either hand, by one corner (Figure 3.44). The hand that picked up the towel holds the towel as it is allowed to fully unfold. The hand holding the towel then gathers the towel into that hand. Starting with the little finger of the opposite hand, dry all surfaces of that finger (Figure 3.45). Move sequentially through the rest of the fingers and thumb, drying all surfaces as well as in between the fingers. It is

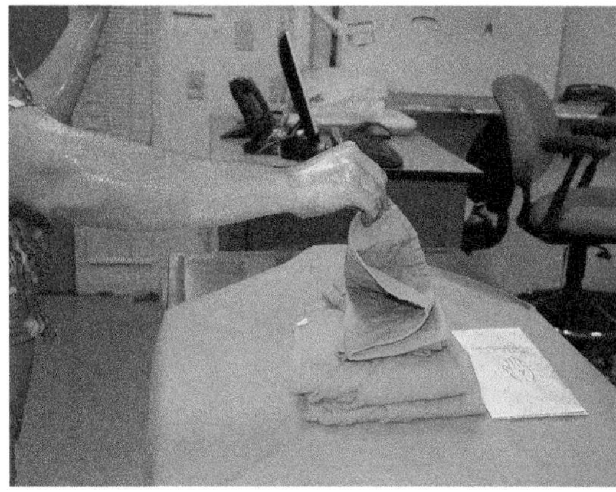

Figure 3.44 Picking up the towel by just one corner.

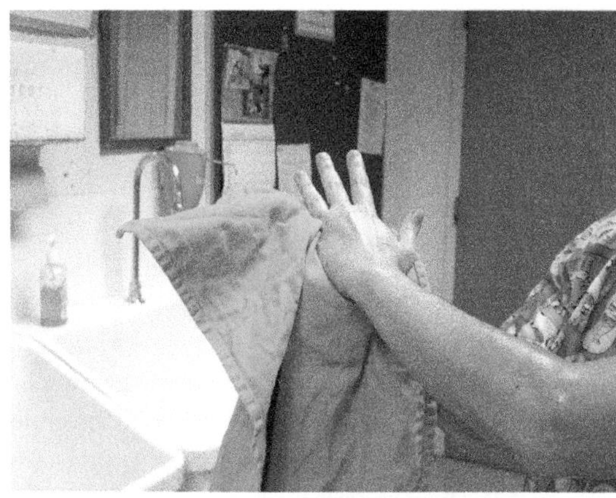

Figure 3.45 Drying the hand starting at the little finger and working through all the fingers.

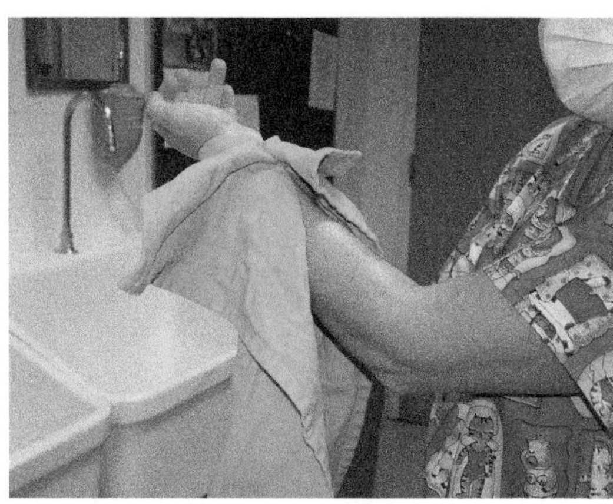

Figure 3.46 Drying the arm by pushing the arm through the towel.

important to remember that once an area has been dried, it *cannot* be re-visited. Upon completion of drying the fingers, the palm of the hand and then the back of the hand are dried. Extending arms in front as well as slightly bending forward at the waist will assist with keeping the sterile towel from touching the non-sterile scrub suit. To dry the arms, the hand holding the towel is wrapped around the wrist to be dried. Push the wrist and arm *away* from the body while the towel twists around the arm until the elbow is reached (Figure 3.46). Never dry the arm using a

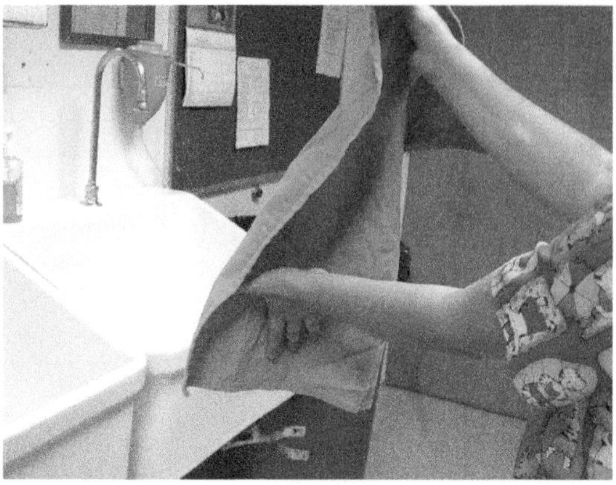

Figure 3.47 Place the dry hand on the underside of the towel. Drop the wet side to reveal the dry side for use on the other hand of the arm.

back-and-forth motion from the wrist to the elbow. Once the elbow has been reached, the dry hand is placed on the opposite end of the towel, on the underside (Figure 3.47). The wet end of the towel is dropped, leaving a clean dry surface with which to dry the second arm and hand. Upon completion of drying the second hand and arm, the towel is dropped onto the floor without having either hand drop below waist level.

Gowning

It is important to be familiar with how the gown is folded in order to aseptically pick up the gown and properly put it on. Whether a paper (disposable) gown or a cloth gown is used, proper donning of the gown is critical. Often the gown is folded with the seams of the sleeves on the top of the pack, so if the arm sleeves seams are visible, the person putting on the gown should use one hand to grasp the seams. The other hand is slid under the folded gown. The gown is then lifted off the wrapper and a step is taken back from the table (Figure 3.48). The hand under the gown is removed and the gown is allowed to unfold (Figure 3.49). At this point, it should be possible to identify both sleeves. One arm is advanced into the corresponding sleeve but stopped before the fingers come out of the sleeve cuff (Figure 3.50). As the gown is put on, it is important to permit the arms to move to the side only – never up above the shoulders or down below the waist. After one arm is in

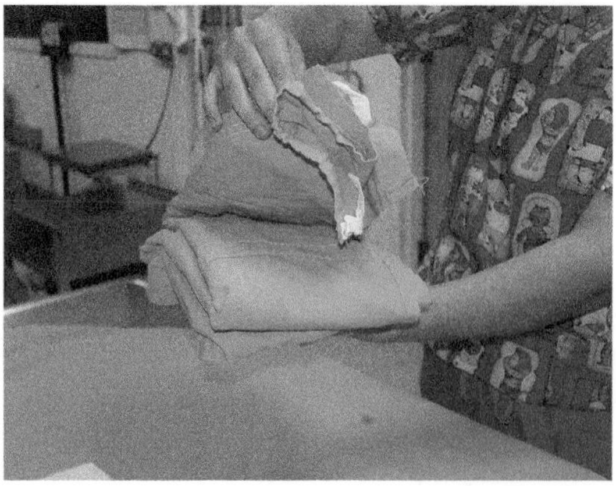

Figure 3.48 Picking up the gown holding the arm sleeve seams, just down from the neck. The other hand is slid under the gown.

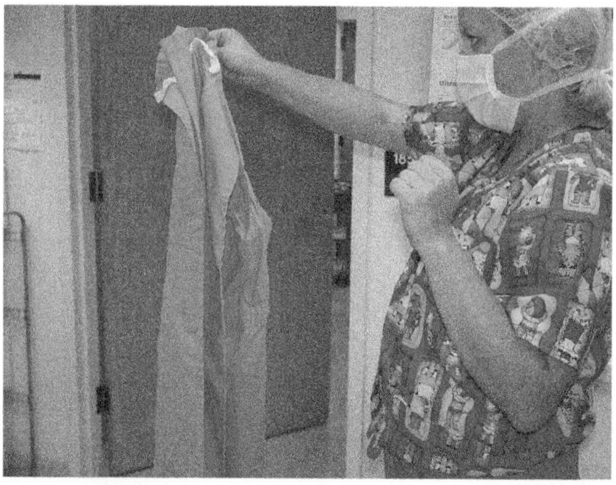

Figure 3.49 Let the gown unfold.

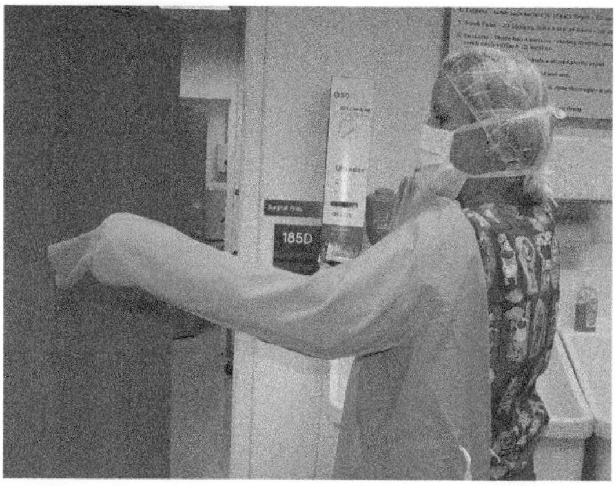

Figure 3.50 Slide one arm into the sleeve.

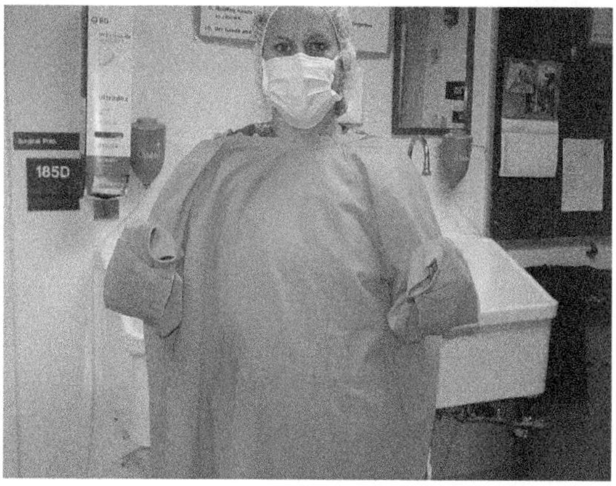

Figure 3.51 Slide the other arm into the other sleeve, keeping both hands inside the sleeve.

the sleeve, the other arm is advanced into its corresponding sleeve. Again, care must be taken to not allow the gown to fall down or touch the floor as the second arm is advanced into the sleeve (Figure 3.51). At this point, the non-sterile circulating nurse needs to "tie in" the sterile person. Without touching any area of the gown that is considered sterile, the circulating nurse must get access to the neckties. Placing the hands on the underside of the gown (that which is touching the

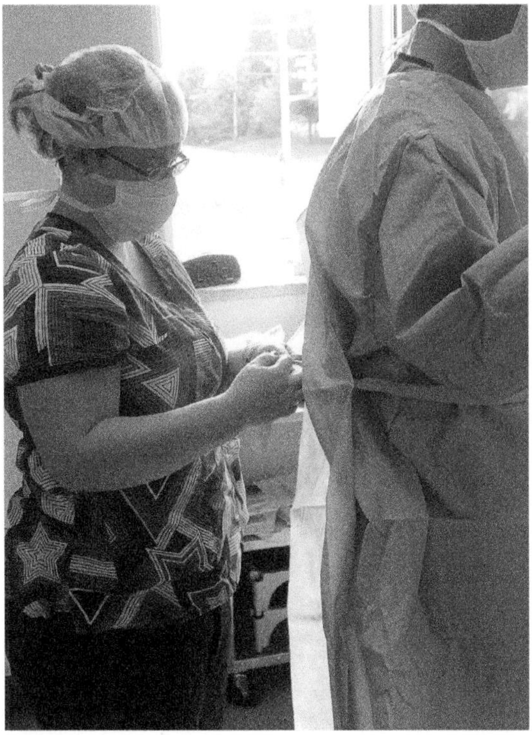

Figure 3.52 Tying the waist of the gown.

person) allows the circulating nurse to "flip" back the neckties to the back of the person. A simple bow is made to secure the ties at the neck. Depending on the type of gown that is used, the next step can be accomplished in one of two ways. Since the back of the gown is not considered sterile, the circulating nurse may touch anywhere on the backside to retrieve the ties. If the gown is a non-sterile back style, then the two waist ties are tied in a bow at the waist. If the gown is a wraparound or sterile back style, the circulating nurse must be careful to touch only those ties which are considered non-sterile. One tie will be on the edge of the left flap of the back of the gown. The other ties will be on the inside of the gown on the right-side seam. These two ties are tied into a snug bow (Figure 3.52). The ties on the edge of the right side, which may be tied to a front tie, are not touched. Standing behind the gowned person, the circulating nurse bends his/her knees to get to floor level. Reaching around to the front of the gown, a gentle tug is given to the bottom edge of the gown to alleviate any bunching of the gown. If the gown is a sterile back/wraparound style, the tying process of the front ties will need to be completed once the gloves have been put on. Once gloved, the sterile person detaches the tie attached to the gown from the card. The card is handed to the circulating nurse and the sterile person slowly spins in a circle to wrap the gown around them. The sterile person then grabs the tie from the card without touching the card and pulls the tie off the card (Video 3.2). Once the gown is completely secured, there are sterile areas of the gown that must be protected during the procedure. The front of the gown from the chest to the level of the surgical field is considered sterile. Gloved hands must remain within this area throughout the procedure. Areas of the gown below the surgical field and out of sight of the sterile person are considered non-sterile. Non-sterile areas include the back of the gown (even if it is a wraparound gown), neckline, shoulders, and area under the arms that may be contaminated by perspiration or

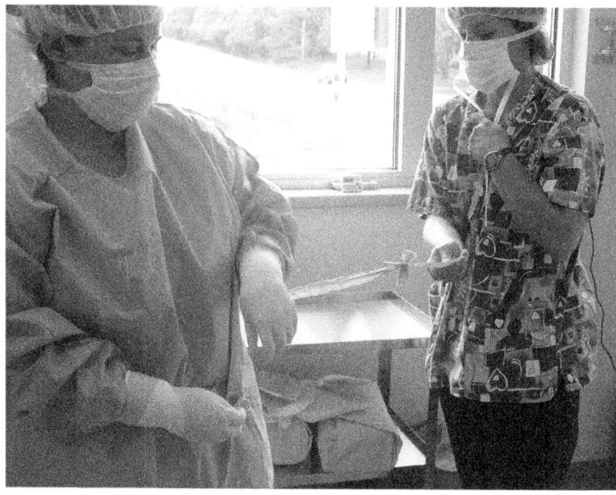

Figure 3.53 The sterile person spins slowly to wrap the gown around them while the circulating nurse holds the card.

contact with non-sterile items (i.e. mask) during normal head and neck movements. The sleeves of the gown are only considered sterile from 2″ (5 cm) above the elbow to the stockinette cuff at the wrist. The cuff of the gown must be covered by sterile gloves at all times (Figure 3.53).

Gloving

Closed Gloving

The preferred method of donning sterile gloves when a sterile surgical gown has been put on is by a technique called closed gloving. The intention of closed gloving is that by keeping the hands within the sterile sleeves there is little risk of contaminating the sterile gloves during application. Closed gloving can *only* be performed while wearing a sterile gown. After the ties of the neck and waist of the gown have been secured, gloving may begin. Sterile gloves should have been opened onto a sterile field by the circulating nurse. With hands and fingers staying within the gown sleeves, open the glove wrapper so the gloves appear with the palms up, fingers pointing away. Fold the bottom edge of the wrapper under to avoid the paper wrapper from springing back to original shape (Figure 3.54). The folded cuff of each glove should be closest to the person putting the gloves on. Remember, before touching the gloves, all areas of the gloves are considered sterile, but once the

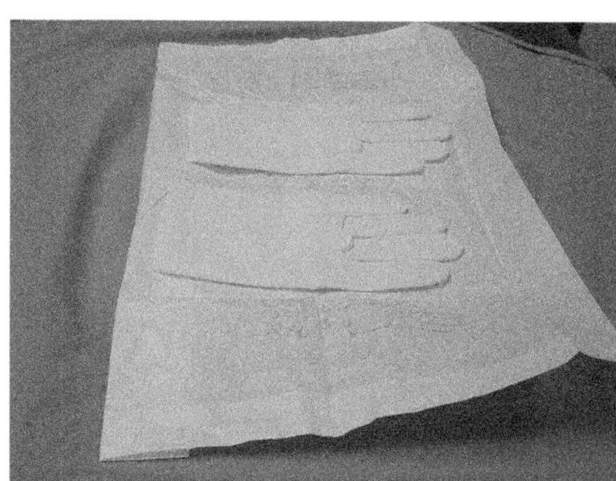

Figure 3.54 Glove wrapper edge folded under.

gloving process begins, the inside of the glove is considered non-sterile because it will eventually touch the non-sterile hands. Use the following technique to aseptically perform closed gloving:

1) Until one glove is successfully and correctly placed on the hand, all contact with the gloves and glove wrapper is done with the hands inside the gown sleeves.
2) Keeping the hands within the sleeves, turn the left hand so the palm is facing up. The right hand grabs the left glove on the top folded edge of the cuff (Figure 3.55).
3) Pick up the left glove and hold it vertically so the fingers are facing the floor (Figure 3.56).
4) Gently flip the glove and place it on the waiting left hand. The thumb of the glove should be facing the thumb of the hand and the fingers of the glove should be facing the forearm and elbow of the left arm (Figure 3.57).
5) Working through the sleeve, the fingers of the left hand grab the bottom folded edge of the glove while the right hand (through the right sleeve) grabs the upper fold of the glove cuff (Figure 3.58).
6) With each hand securely holding the folded edge of the glove, stretch the glove to create a larger opening (Figure 3.59).
7) Pull the glove over the left hand. The entire knit cuff of the gown sleeve must be covered at this point (Figure 3.60).
8) Unroll the cuff of the glove completely to keep the gown sleeve secure (Figure 3.61).
9) Pull on the left-hand fingers (with the right hand still inside the gown sleeve) to match up with the finger holes on the glove.

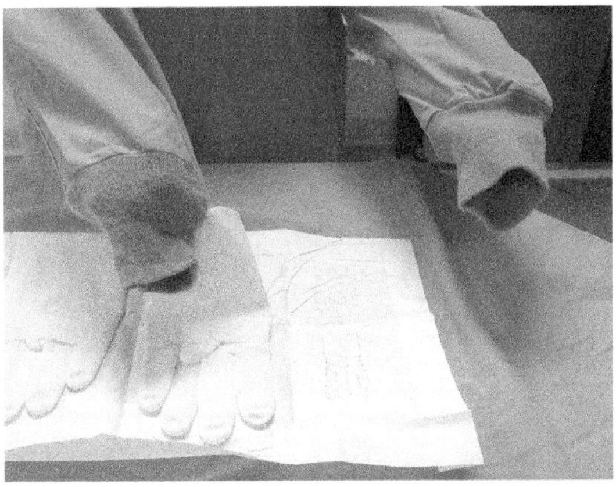

Figure 3.55 Right hand grabs the folded edge of the cuff.

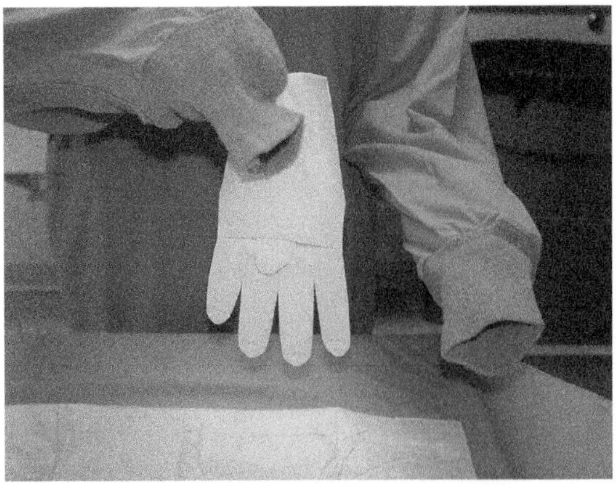

Figure 3.56 Hold the glove vertically.

Figure 3.57 Flip the glove onto the hand, thumb to thumb, fingers pointing toward the operator.

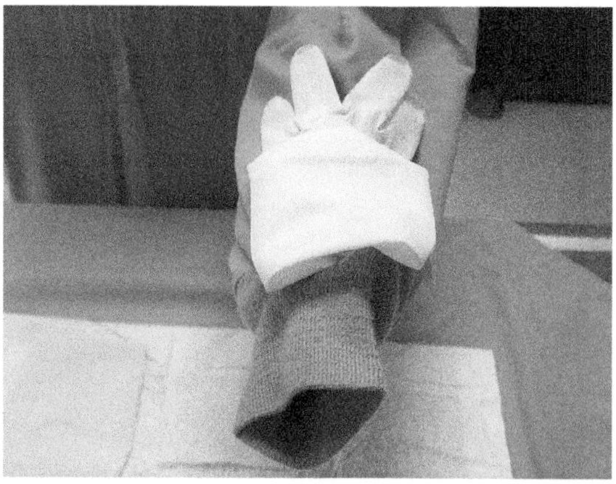

Figure 3.58 Each hand grabs a folded edge of the cuff – through the gown sleeve.

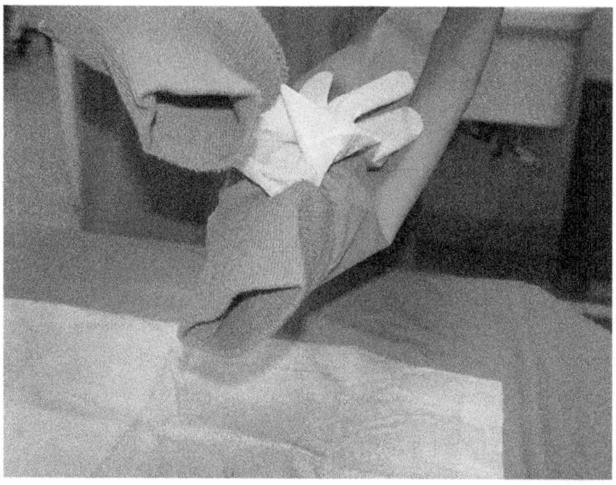

Figure 3.59 Stretch the glove to insert the hand.

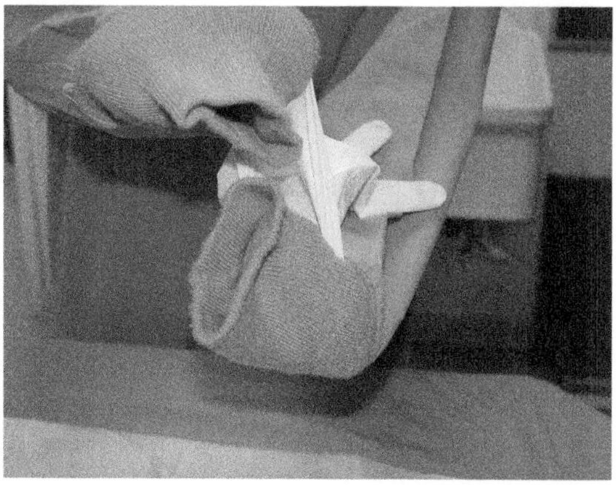

Figure 3.60 Pull the glove over the hand and completely cover the cuff of the sleeve.

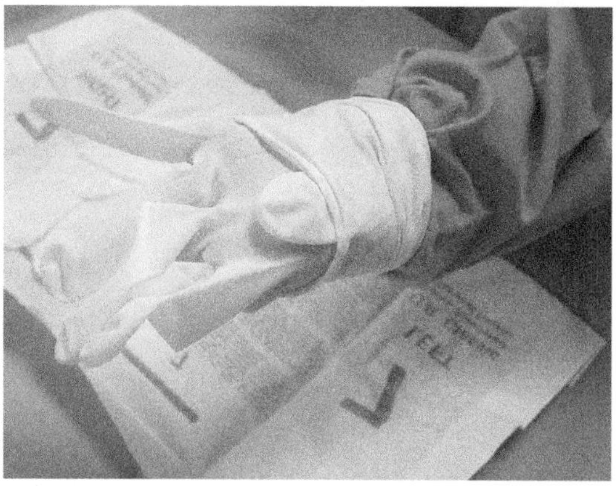

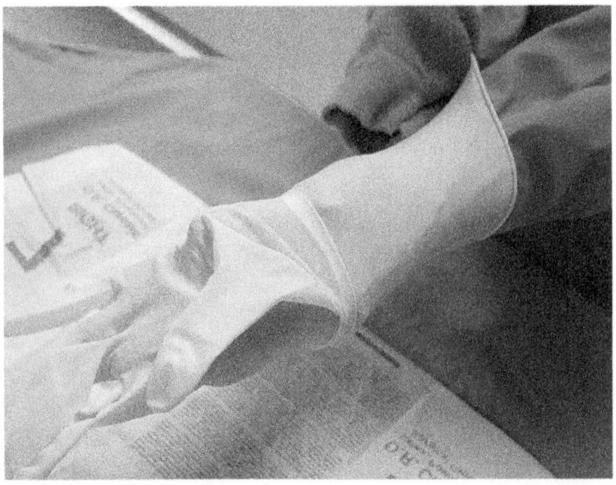

Figure 3.61 Unroll the cuff of the glove.

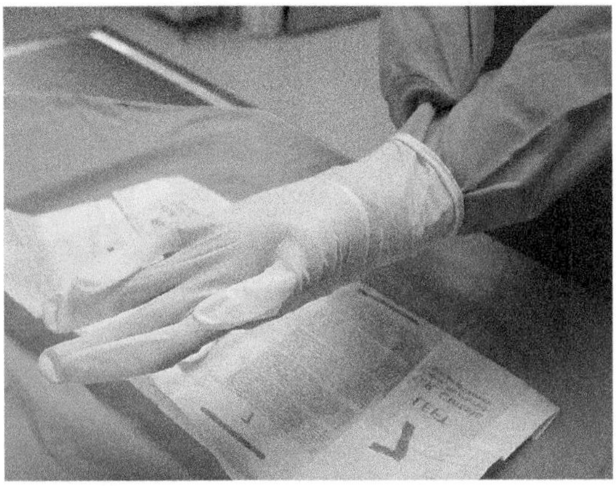

Figure 3.62 Pull sleeve to get fingers into finger holes.

10) Any adjustment of the glove fingers must be done with the right hand still within the right gown sleeve.
11) The sleeve of the gown may be pulled to get the cuff of the sleeve off the hand (Figure 3.62). The knit cuff of the gown sleeve must never extend beyond the glove cuff so excessive pulling of the sleeve is not recommended. Care should be taken to avoid wrinkles on the gown sleeve cuff to avoid compromising circulation to the hand.
12) The process is repeated with the right hand. After both gloves are in place, final adjustments to the gloves may be made to ensure the best possible fit (Video 3.4).

Open Gloving

The open gloving technique is used when a sterile gown has not been put on, but sterile gloves are still required (i.e. urinary catheterization, jugular catheter placement, etc.). Open gloving may also be performed if a glove was contaminated during surgery and a replacement glove must be put on. Use the following technique to properly perform open gloving.

1) One of the most important things to remember when open gloving is being aware of what is considered sterile vs. non-sterile. Even though all surfaces of the gloves have been sterilized, some surfaces are considered non-sterile once open gloving begins.

2) The glove wrapper is carefully opened revealing the gloves in a palm-up position in the wrapper. Fold the long edge of the wrapper under to keep it from springing closed (Figure 3.63). The folded cuff of the gloves should be closest to the person putting on the gloves.
3) The entire inner surface of the glove wrapper is considered sterile but can only be touched from the edge to within 1″ of the edge of the wrapper.
4) The right hand picks up the top folded edge of the cuff of the left glove. Do not touch the wrapper underneath or any other part of the glove (Figure 3.64).
5) The left-hand fingers are cupped together, and the hand is slid into the glove, palm up. Fingers should be aligned with the glove fingers (Figure 3.65).
6) Leave the cuff of the glove folded until the other hand is gloved (Figure 3.66).
7) The sterile left hand is slid between the cuff and the sterile glove of the right hand. This position allows the sterile left hand to contact the outside of the sterile right glove (Figure 3.67).
8) Bring the thumb of the left hand down to hold the cuff against the left hand.
9) Keeping the palm of the right hand up, cup the fingers and slide that hand into the glove. DO NOT allow the sterile left thumb to touch any part of the non-sterile right hand (Figure 3.68).
10) The cuff of the right glove may be carefully unrolled if the sterile left hand does not touch anything non-sterile (Figure 3.69).
11) The now sterile right hand may slide under the cuff of the sterile left glove and carefully unfold the cuff (Figure 3.70). No part of the sterile right hand may touch a non-sterile surface (Video 3.5).

Figure 3.63 Glove wrapper edge folded under.

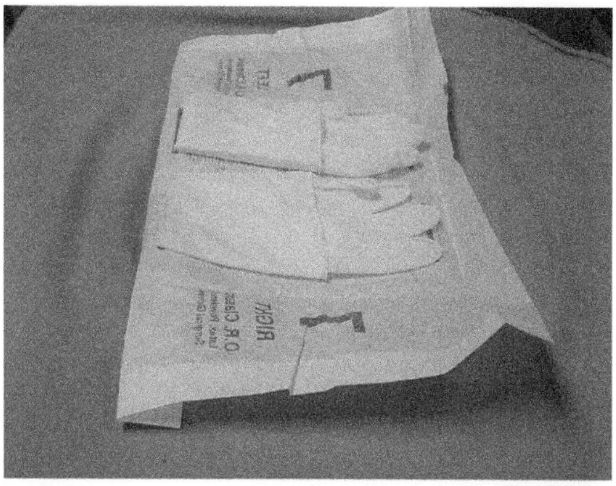

Figure 3.64 Right hand picks up the top fold of the cuff.

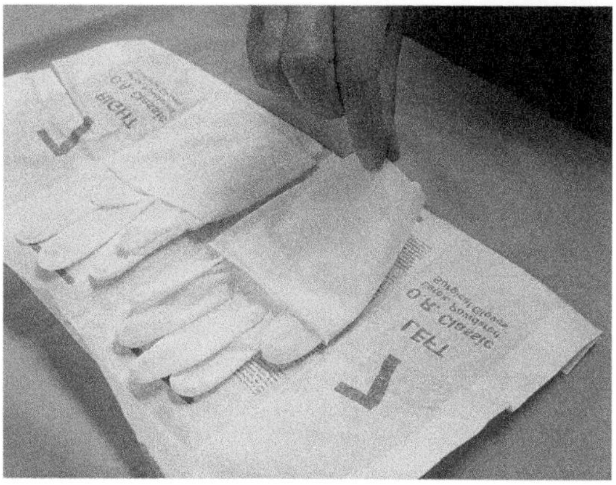

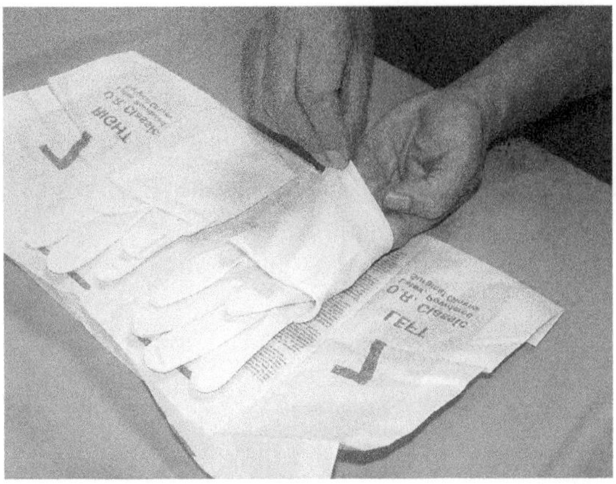

Figure 3.65 The left hand is cupped and slid into the glove.

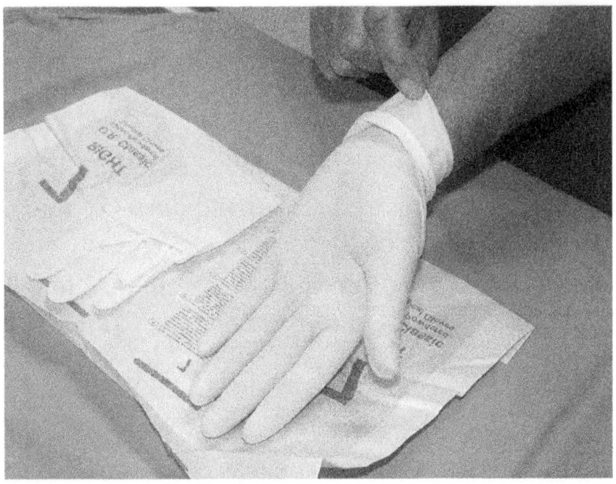

Figure 3.66 The cuff is left folded.

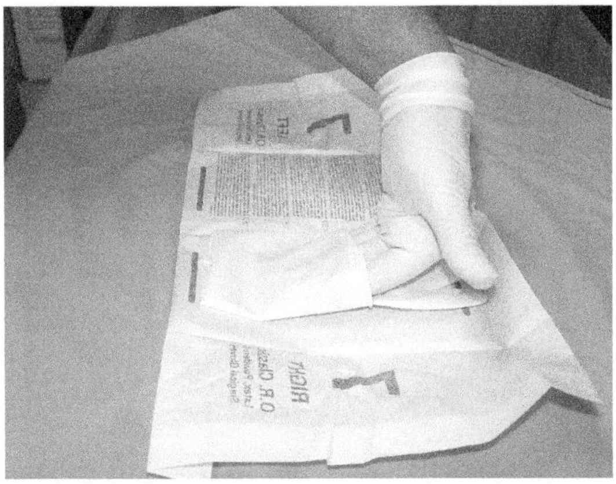

Figure 3.67 The left hand is slid under the cuff of the right-hand glove.

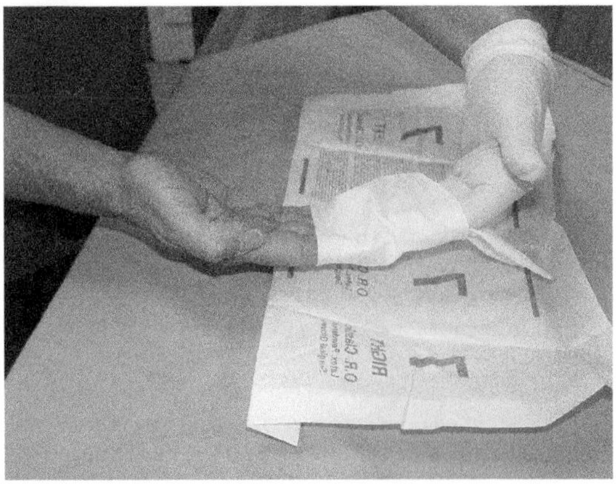

Figure 3.68 The right-hand is cupped and slid into the glove.

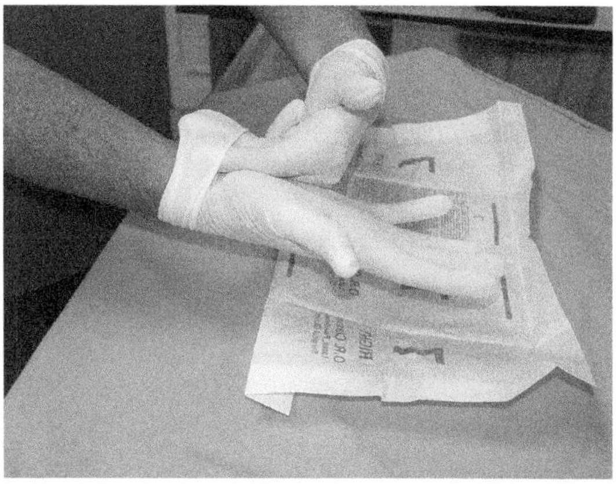

Figure 3.69 The cuff is unrolled.

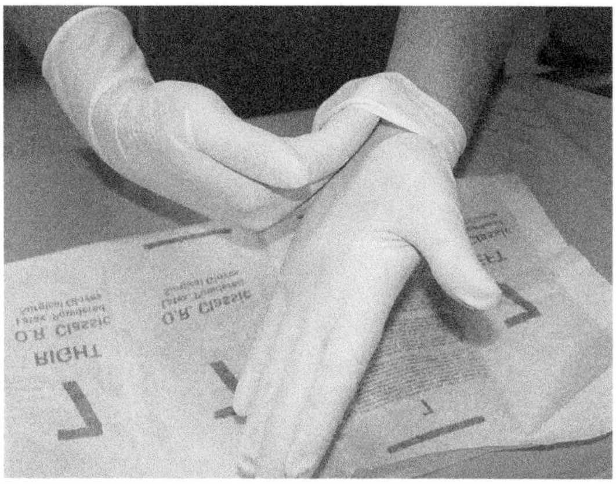

Figure 3.70 The right-hand returns to the left glove and unrolls the cuff.

Assisted Gloving

Although infrequently used in veterinary surgery, this is the preferred method of re-gloving once a sterile gown has been put on. This method does require at least two sterile members of the surgical team, hence its limited use in veterinary surgery. To appropriately perform the assisted gloving technique, the following steps must be done.

1) A non-sterile person aseptically removes the contaminated glove (see following section).
2) The sterile person who will be assisting with the gloving receives the gloves from the circulating nurse and opens the glove wrapper on a sterile surface.
3) The assisting sterile person picks up the glove that will be put on and places both hands under the cuff of the glove.
4) They then pull the opening of the glove wide to accept the hand needing the glove. The person receiving the glove may also place their remaining sterile hand under the cuff to assist with stretching the glove.
5) Orient the glove so the palm of the glove is facing the person receiving the glove.
6) The team member needing the glove then inserts his/her hand into the glove. Be sure the fingers of the accepting hand are pointing downwards prior to insertion.
7) Pull the cuff of the glove over as much of the gown cuff as possible.
8) The person who received the glove may now make minor adjustments to the fit of the new glove.

Removing a Contaminate Glove

For multiple reasons, a glove may become contaminated during a procedure. The glove must be changed immediately to avoid further contamination of the surgical field. The following is the procedure for removing a contaminated glove during a procedure.

1) A non-sterile person must remove the contaminated glove.
2) The person having the glove removed presents the contaminated hand in a sideways orientation as if shaking hands (Figure 3.71).
3) Care should be taken to ensure that the non-sterile person does not touch any part of the gown sleeve.
4) The non-sterile person grasps the glove at the level of the hand and pulls the glove off inside out (Figure 3.72). The cuff of the gown should not be pulled over the hand as the inside of the gown has touched skin and would therefore contaminate the hand if they came in contact with one another (Figure 3.73).
5) The sterile member must now either open glove to replace the contaminated glove (if working alone) or be re-gloved using the assisted gloving technique if another sterile member is available.

Double Gloving

Some surgeons will elect to double glove when draping a patient, then remove the outer gloves once draping is completed. This will greatly reduce the risk of introducing any contaminants from

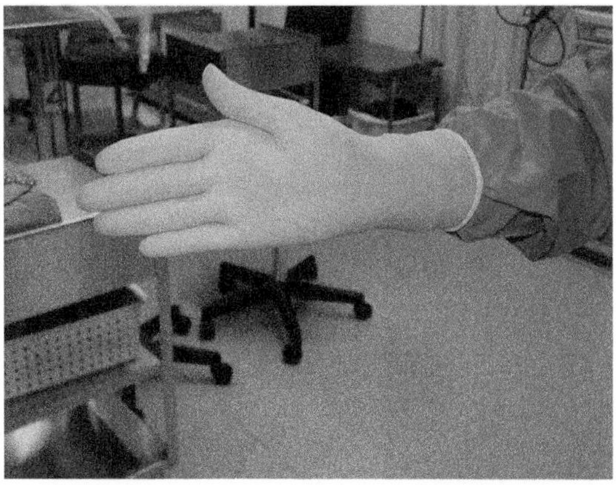

Figure 3.71 Presenting contaminated gloved hand for glove removal.

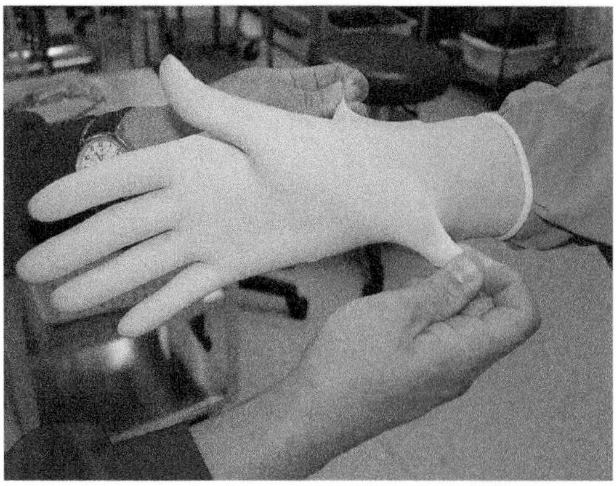

Figure 3.72 The circulating nurse grabs *only the glove* and pulls the glove off inside out.

Figure 3.73 The open hand is left to re-glove.

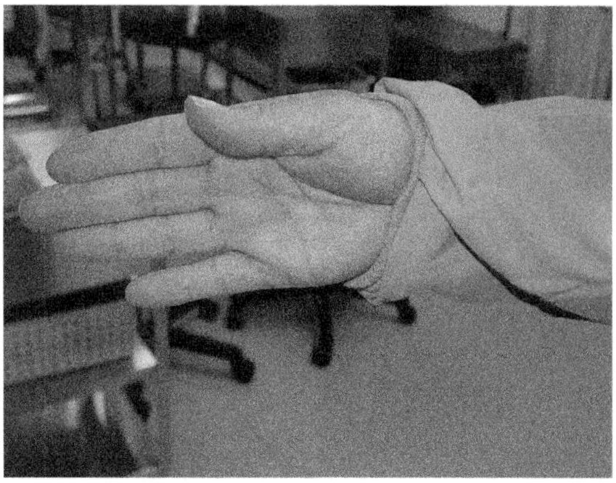

draping into the surgical field. Some surgeons, especially those performing a joint replacement procedure, will require all team members to wear double gloves for the entire procedure. Glove integrity has been shown to fail as often as 51% of the time. Double gloving can reduce that failure rate to 7%. When double gloving, the second (outer) pair of gloves is generally half size large than the first pair of gloves. Specifically, manufactured "orthopedic" gloves are thick than regular gloves and have improved durability for use during orthopedic procedures. Double gloving may still take place during the draping, but double gloving for the entire procedure can be eliminated if ortho gloves are used.

Stress Mats

Once properly gowned and gloved, the surgeon and/or assistant should proceed immediately to the surgery room, if they are not already there. Gaining interest in the surgery room is the use of stress mats for people standing still for long periods of time. Designed to help relieve stress and fatigue of legs and feet, stress mats can be positioned on the floor so the surgeon and assistant will stand on them during the procedure. When purchasing the mats, it must be noted that mats with a protective covering on all sides are desired. Mats that only have a vinyl top may have blood, solutions, or other fluids soak into the bottom of the mat and potentially harbor harmful bacteria. Mats are available commercially from many veterinary product distributors (Figure 3.74).

Figure 3.74 Stress mat in surgical suite.

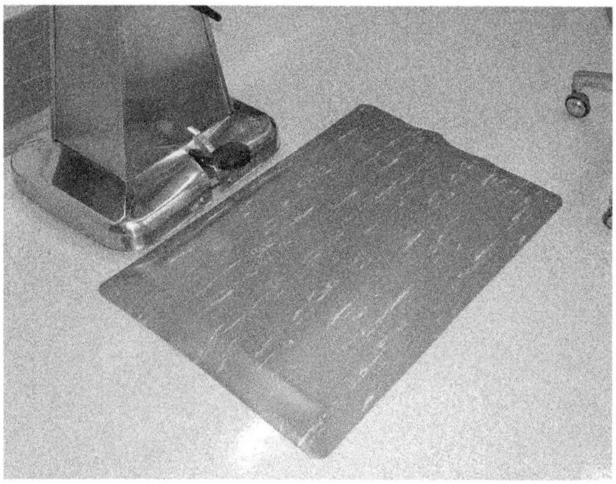

Instrumentation

Surgical instrumentation is an expensive and valuable asset of any hospital. Access to the correct, functioning instrument may determine the outcome of a surgical procedure. There may be one best instrument needed for a case and if it is not available something of lesser quality and unequaled function will have to be substituted. Efficient use of specialized veterinary surgical instrumentation requires those using it to understand proper application, handling, care, and troubleshooting. Often the surgeon relies on the veterinary technician for such knowledge.

Instrument Manufacturing

The production of surgical instruments is a fine art with the end product being depended upon for proper function and longevity. Surgical-grade instruments are generally made from stainless steel and other metal alloys such as carbon and chromium. These metals are chosen due to their resistance to marring, pitting, scratching, and dulling. Floor-grade instruments, while less expensive, are made from inferior-quality metals and will rust within two to three steam sterilization cycles. Floor-grade instruments are generally referred to as single-use items such as suture removal scissors and disposable suture kits.

Finishes on surgical-grade instruments can be a bright/mirror finish, a satin/dull finish, or an ebony finish. The bright/mirror finish is a highly polished shine that reflects light. Due to the reflection, it may cause a glare and be annoying or interfering to some surgeons. The dull/satin finish is as the name implies a non-reflective finish that does not glare, which is often preferred by many surgeons. The ebony finish is a black chromium finish for instruments used in laser surgery. The black finish deters the laser from bouncing off a shiny finish and damaging nearby tissues.

The instrument composition is either a martensitic stainless steel or an austenitic stainless steel. Martensitic stainless steel has higher carbon content and is used more often in cutting instruments for increased hardness and increased sharpness on the cutting edges. Austenitic stainless steel has higher chromium content and is usually used for hemostats and needle holders. Needle holders can also have tungsten carbide inserts in the tips of the instrument (Figure 3.75). The inserts are used to increase the durability of the needle holder. Although initially more expensive, the inserts can be replaced as they wear out. Needle holders that wear out, but do not have a tungsten carbide insert must have the entire instrument thrown away, because repair is not possible. In the long term this would be more costly for the clinic. Tungsten carbide

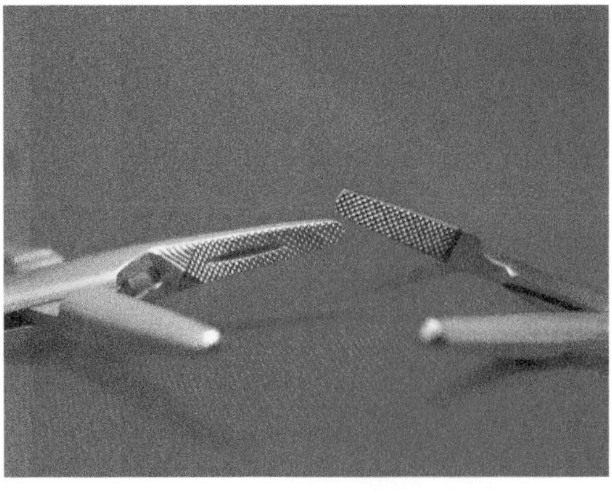

Figure 3.75 Tungsten carbide insert (right) in a needleholder jaw.

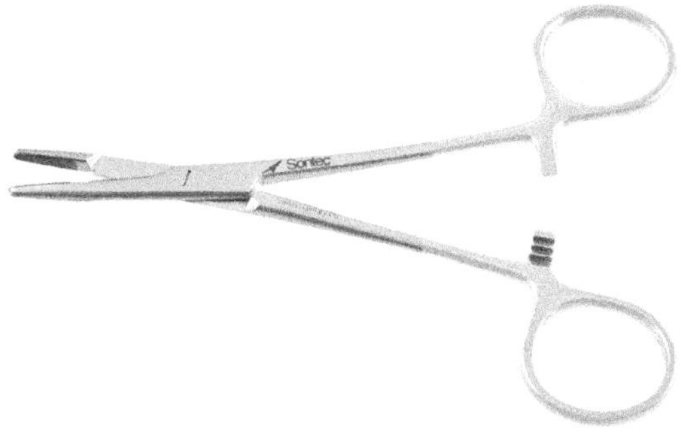

Figure 3.76 Gold ring handles indicating tungsten carbide inserts. *Source:* Courtesy of Sontec Instruments, Inc. (Cat. # 1100-108).

inserts can also be used on the cutting edges of scissors. As with the needle holder, the insert edges can be replaced when worn out, instead of replacing the entire instrument. Any instrument having a tungsten insert will have gold ring handles as the industry standard for quick identification of those instruments (Figure 3.76).

A five-step process is used in the creation of any surgical instrument. The first step is forging. Forging is the shaping or forming of the instrument through hammering and the use of heat. Second, the instrument undergoes a milling process. Milling is the cutting of a forged piece to create the final instrument. Tempering is the third step. Slowly heating the instrument in a salt bath and then immersing it in oil completes the tempering stage. Tempering may also be referenced as quenching. The fourth step is that of passivation. A chemical bath to remove any particles from the grinding process as well as strengthen the instrument is the passivation stage. This step also helps in rust prevention. The final step is polishing. Either a shiny or matte finish is the end result of the polishing step.

There are several basic components of surgical instruments that must be understood by all who use and care for the instruments. The working parts may vary slightly between ring-handled instruments and non-ring handled, but some similarities do exist. For ring-handled instruments, the area of the instrument used on or near tissue is the jaw. The jaw may have horizontal, vertical, or cross-hatched serrations on the tip. The serrations can vary in depth, length, and closeness to one another depending on the intended function of the instrument. Occasionally, a ring-handled instrument will have teeth on the tip, as with the Rochester Kocher, but those instruments are infrequently used. The shape of the jaw will be straight or curved depending on the intended use of the instrument. Non-ring-handled instruments (thumb tissue forceps and hand-held retractors) may have varying styles of tips or ends. Thumb tissue forceps that have teeth on either side of the jaw are named to identify the number of teeth on each side. For example, a thumb tissue forceps may be a 1×2, 2×3, or 3×4 style. Teeth can also be construed in rows that are recessed or projected from the tip (i.e. Adson Brown).

The next part of the ring-handled instrument is the box lock. The box lock is the hinged portion of the instrument. Excessive force on the jaw can cause misalignment of the box lock, resulting in rubbing of the metal when the instrument is opened or closed. Another trauma to the box lock is cracking of the metal, making the instrument useless. Even when the instrument is used for its intended purpose, this area of the instrument absorbs a lot of stress. Box locks must be carefully inspected following each use for any resulting damage. Some instruments, especially scissors, have a screw hinge instead of a box lock. This area of the instrument continually is exposed to large amounts of stress so evaluating the integrity of the hinge as well as the presence of any cracks is very important.

The longest part of the instrument is known as the shank. When an instrument is available in varying lengths, the shank is the variable. Some instruments (i.e. needle holders) may be available in size from 3″ to 12″ in length depending on the shank length. When identifying instruments with instrument tape, the tape should be placed on the shank of the instrument. The next component is the ratchet. The ratchet is the locking portion of the ring-handled instrument. Few non-ring-handled instruments have ratchets (i.e. Mathieu needle holders). Ratchets have interlocking teeth that lock the jaws of the instrument closed. The more the ratchet teeth lock, the tighter the closure of the jaw. The interlocking teeth will wear down after time and the inability of the instrument to remain locked is a first indicator that the instrument is not functioning optimally. Finally, as previously mentioned, ring-handled instruments that have tungsten carbide inserts in the tip will have gold ring handles for easy identification within the pack. Instruments with diamond inserts will have black-colored ring handles.

Non-ring-handled instruments will have no box lock or ratchet. The tips and shaft are still there, but the two separate sides are joined at the end. This type of instrument that has a tungsten carbide insert in the tip will have a gold identifier at the joined end.

General Surgery Instruments

Many resources are available for learning surgical instruments. While this text is intended to show the basic instruments, there are hundreds of additional instruments available. Most instrument companies offer photos on their website.

There are many standard or general instruments that will be used in all surgeries. Thumb tissue forceps, scissors, needle holders, and hemostats do have some case specificity, but some style will be used in every surgical procedure.

Scissors

There are many types of scissors available ranging from ophthalmic to orthopedic uses. As with all instruments, it is imperative that scissors be used only for their intended purpose (Figure 3.77).

Operating Scissors Operating scissors are generally used scissors for cutting inanimate objects such as sutures, paper drape material, sponges, and drains. The blade tips of the operating scissors can be blunt or sharp and the overall blade shape can be straight or curved. The style of scissors is usually included in the name of the scissors (i.e. sharp/blunt curved operating scissors). The length of the blade is about one-third of the overall length of the instrument (Figure 3.78).

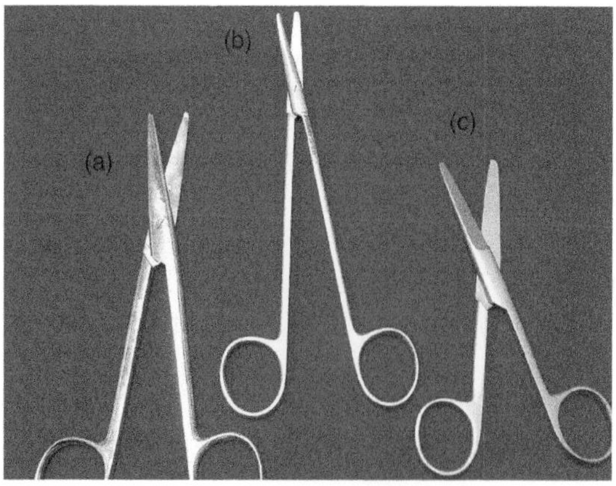

Figure 3.77 Scissors: (a) Mayo dissecting, (b) Metzenbaum dissecting, and (c) operating.

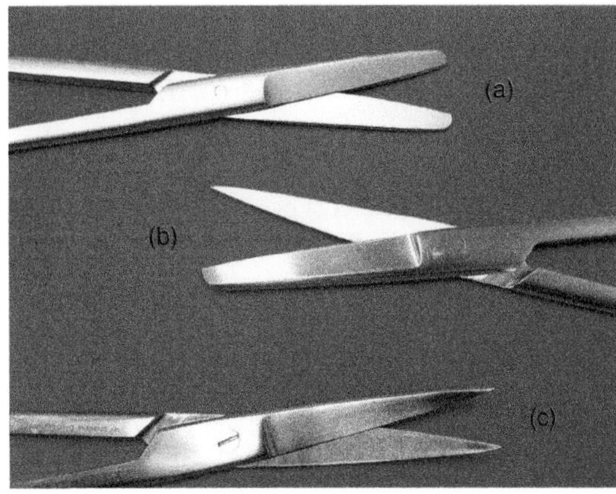

Figure 3.78 Operating scissors: (a) blunt/blunt, (b) sharp/blunt, and (c) sharp/sharp.

Mayo Dissecting Scissors Mayo dissecting scissors generally have a thicker, heavier blade than other scissors. The tips are rounded but are not classified as sharp or blunt. The blades may be curved or straight. Mayo dissecting scissors are used for cutting large muscle mass, dissecting non-delicate tissue, or cutting tougher tissue such as cartilage or tendons. The blade length is approximately one-third the length of the entire instrument.

Metzenbaum Dissecting Scissors Metzenbaum dissecting scissors are designed for the dissection of delicate tissue. The blades are fine, delicate, and only about one-fourth of the length of the entire instrument. Delicate tissue and vessels are often dissected with this type of scissors, so keeping the blade tips fully functionally and extremely sharp is very important.

Miscellaneous Scissors Ophthalmic scissors often have a spring-loaded handle instead of ring handles to permit cutting with less overall instrument movement (Figure 3.79). Intra-ocular scissors such as Castroviejo scissors are extremely delicate and usually have sharp-tipped blade. Extra-ocular scissors such as Stevens Tenotomy scissors or Iris scissors have ring handles as motion with cutting is not as much of an issue with extra-ocular procedures (Figure 3.80).

Bandage Scissors Bandage scissors are not considered a general surgery instrument but deserve comment. Bandage scissors are designed to be used to cut off bandages. The longer blade has a blunt probe at the tip of the blade to assist with cutting through the bandage material (Figure 3.81).

Orthopedic Scissors Orthopedic scissors such as wire-cutting scissors and cartilage scissors have a very specific function. As the name implies, wire-cutting scissors are used for cutting orthopedic wire. Wire can be very damaging to the cutting edge of scissors, but this instrument is designed with short sturdy blades to be used exclusively with wire. Cartilage scissors have a serrated cutting edge to grip cartilaginous type tissue while cutting, instead of having smooth cutting edges which would slide on the tissue and create a more uneven cut edge.

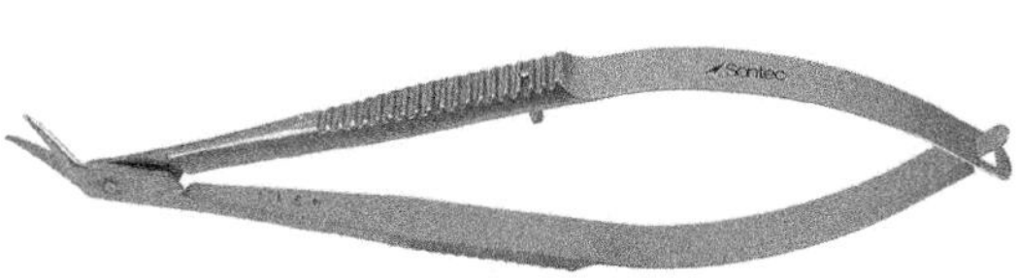

Figure 3.79 Castroviejo corneoscleral scissors. *Source:* Courtesy of Sontec Instruments, Inc. (Cat. # 13-1306).

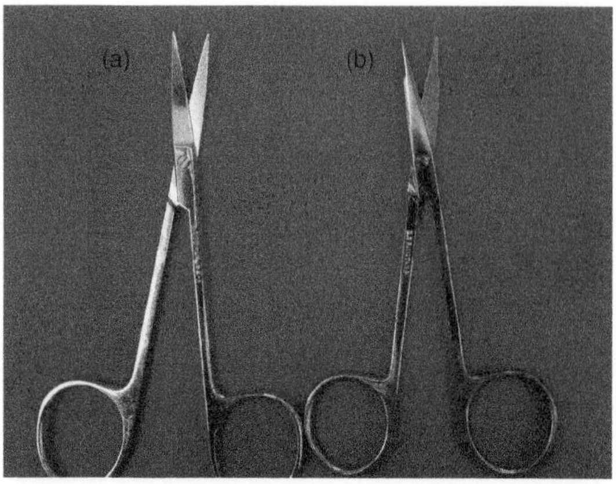

Figure 3.80 Ophthalmic scissors – Iris (a) and Stevens tenotomy (b).

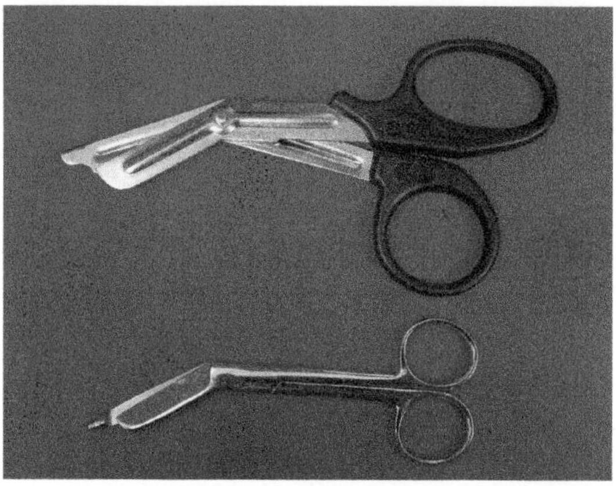

Figure 3.81 Bandage scissors.

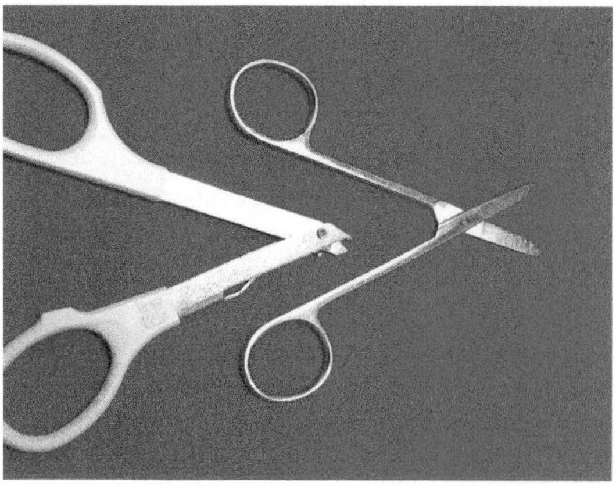

Figure 3.82 Suture removal scissors and staple remover.

Suture Removal Scissors Suture removal scissors have a short blunt tip blade on one side and the other blade has a hooked tip. By its name, it is designed to aid in the removal of skin sutures. The hooked blade is slid underneath the suture loop and then the suture is cut. The staple remover is not scissors, but a required piece of equipment for staple removal. The two-prong tip is placed under the staple and the handle is squeezed. The squeezing action closes the tip together which bends the staple, allowing removal (Figure 3.82).

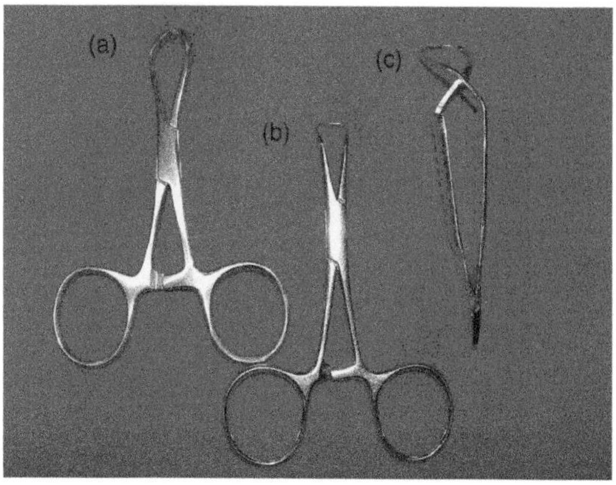

Figure 3.83 Towel clamps: (a) Lorna Non-Penetrating, (b) Backhaus Penetrating, (c) Jones.

Towel Clamps

Towel clamps are instruments designed to hold drapes in place when preparing a patient for surgery. Penetrating style towel clamps hold the sterile drapes to the patient by piercing the skin and holding the drape securely. Non-penetrating styles are designed to hold sterile drapes to other sterile drapes (Figure 3.83).

Backhaus Penetrating Towel Clamps Backhaus towel clamps are the most common penetrating clamp used and are available in 3 ½″ or 5″ sizes. When draping a patient, this type of towel clamp is used to secure the drapes to the patient.

Roeder Towel Clamps Roeder towel clamps are a penetrating style with balls about ½″ from the tip of the jaw. The balls are in place to avoid penetrating the skin too deeply. This type of towel clamp is often used in large animal surgery.

Jones Towel Clamps The Jones towel clamp is a spring-loaded, squeeze-handle type of clamp. It is smaller in size and more lightweight than other penetrating clamps. They are best suited for small drape placement in delicate tissue or with patients that are very small.

Lorna (Edna) Non-penetrating Towel Clamps Lorna towel clamps – sometimes called Edna towel clamps – are a non-penetrating style of towel clamp. They are used on a second layer of draping and attach the top layer of drape material to the underlying first layer of drapes. They are available in 3 ½″ and 5″ sizes.

Scalpel Handles and Scalpel Blades

Scalpel handles have the function of holding the scalpel blade to allow the surgeon to make a skin incision, or other types of incisions, in a safer manner (Figure 3.84). Number 3 scalpel handles are used with scalpel blades numbered 10–19. Number 4 scalpel blade handles are used with scalpel blades numbered 20–29. Number 7 scalpel handles are a slender, longer style that fits blades 10–19. A Beaver handle is a short cylindrical handle designed to work with Beaver blades. Beaver handles and blades are often used in ophthalmic surgery and arthroscopy. Scalpel blades are designed for very specific applications. Number 10 blades are the most common type of blade for skin incisions. With a full blade, it is great at creating a swift, clean incising of the skin. The number 11 blade has a very sharp point and a straight cutting edge. This blade is often used for stab incisions such as for

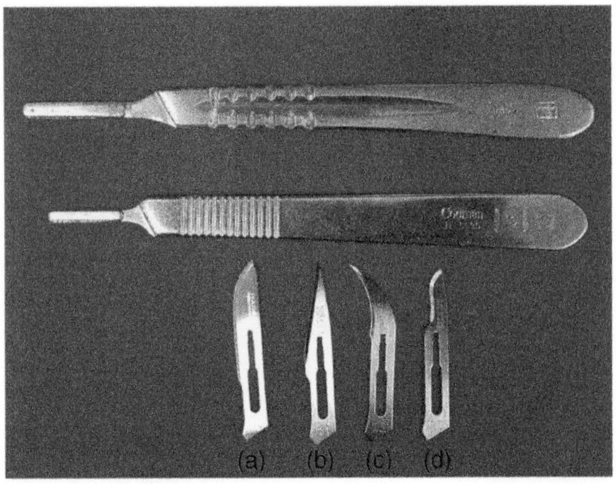

Figure 3.84 Scalpel handles (numbers 3 and 4); and Scalpel Blades (a–d) numbers 10, 11, 12, and 15.

an arthroscopy or abscess. A number 12 blade is in the shape of a hook with the cutting edge on the inside curve of the hook. A number 12 blade is often used for dissection around bone within a small joint. The final blade most frequently seen in veterinary surgery is the number 15 blade. This blade has a cutting surface the same shape as a number 10 blade, but it is only half as large as a number 10. The blade can be used where a small delicate blade is needed. A number 20 blade on a number 4 blade handle is sometimes used in large animal surgery. The initial skin incision is made with the number 20 blade, then a number 10 blade is used for deeper tissue. The number 4 handle and 20 series blades have limited use and application in small animal surgery.

Hemostatic Forceps

Hemostatic forceps are available in a variety of sizes and styles. As the name implies the function of a hemostatic forceps is to occlude flow from a vessel or tissue mass. The tips of a hemostat can be straight or curved, but the style used is often surgeon's preference. The serrations on the tips can be horizontal, vertical, or a combination of the two. When placing a hemostatic forceps on tissue, if a curved style, the curve should always be placed facing up. The smallest amount of tissue possible should be clamped to avoid excessive tissue damage (Figure 3.85).

Mosquito Hemostatic Forceps The mosquito hemostat is the smallest forceps of the most commonly used instruments. It is available in both 3 ½ and 5″ sizes with the shank length being the only

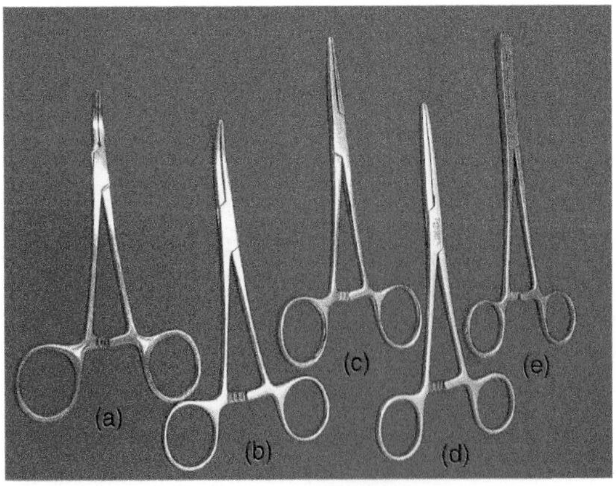

Figure 3.85 Hemostatic forceps: (a) Mosquito, (b) Kelly, (c) Crile, (d) Rochester-Carmalt, and (e) Ferguson-Angiotribe.

difference. The 3 ½″ version is called a Hartmann mosquito hemostatic forceps. The 5″ version is called a Halsted mosquito hemostatic forceps. Both styles are available with curved or straight tips. The fine, closely positioned, transverse serration extends from the tip of the jaw to the box lock. Mosquito hemostats are used to occlude flow from small vessels.

Kelly Hemostatic Forceps Kelly hemostats are a larger clamp usually 5 ½″ in size. The horizontal serrations are wider than the mosquito serrations and most significantly extend from the tip of the jaw to only halfway down. Kelly hemostats are used on larger vessels or tissue bundles that can be best accommodated by the larger jaw.

Crile Hemostatic Forceps Crile hemostats are very similar to Kelly hemostats in size, design, and intended function. The primary difference is that the transverse serrations on the Crile extend the entire length of the jaw, from the tip to the box lock. Like the Kelly hemostat, the Crile is used for larger vessels or tissue bundles (Figure 3.86).

Rochester-Carmalt Hemostatic Forceps The Rochester-Carmalt is a large instrument with a jaw length approximately twice as long as the Kelly or Crile. The Rochester Carmalt has longitudinal serrations the entire length of the jaw and horizontal cross serrations at the distal tip of the jaw. This larger instrument ranges in size from 7 ½″ to 9 ½″. The larger jaw enables this clamp to be used to occlude larger tissue bundles such as during an ovariohysterectomy.

Rochester-Ochsner Hemostatic Forceps A Rochester Ochsner forceps is a large clamp like the Carmalt. It has widely spaced horizontal serrations on the entire jaw and there is one large traumatic tooth at the tip of the jaw.

Rochester-Pean Hemostatic Forceps The Rochester-Pean is a forceps that is exactly the same in appearance as the Ochsner, without the toothed tip. Wide horizontal serrations on the entire jaw and a long instrument overall make it useful for large muscle or tissue masses.

Thumb Tissue Forceps

Thumb tissue forceps are tweezers-like instruments that are used as an extension of the surgeon's fingers. Many different styles are available for many situations (Figure 3.87).

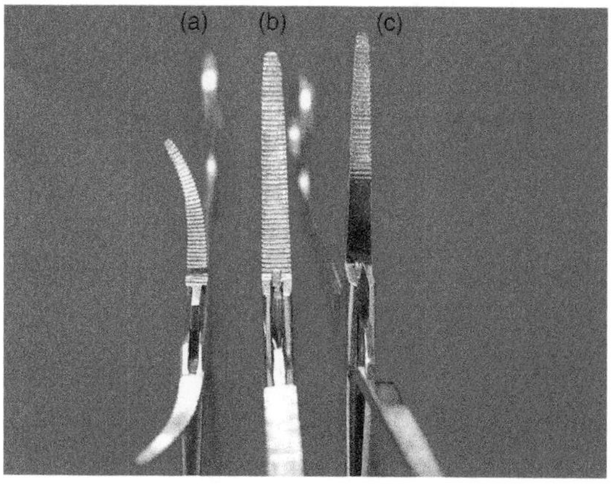

Figure 3.86 Hemostatic forcep tips: (a) Mosquito, (b) Crile, and (c) Kelly.

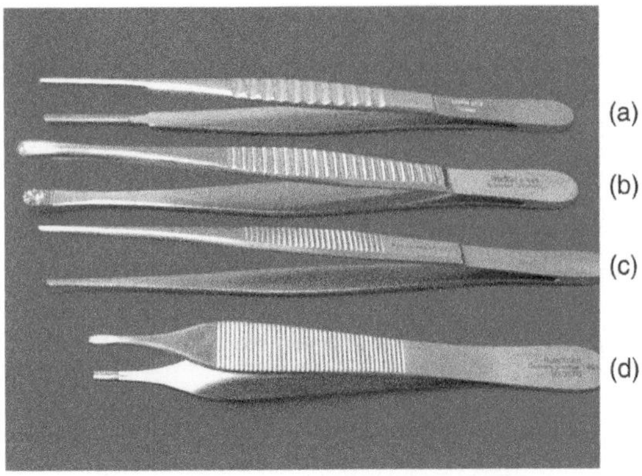

Figure 3.87 Thumb tissue forceps: (a) Debakey, (b) Russian, and (c) Rat Tooth, (d) Adson.

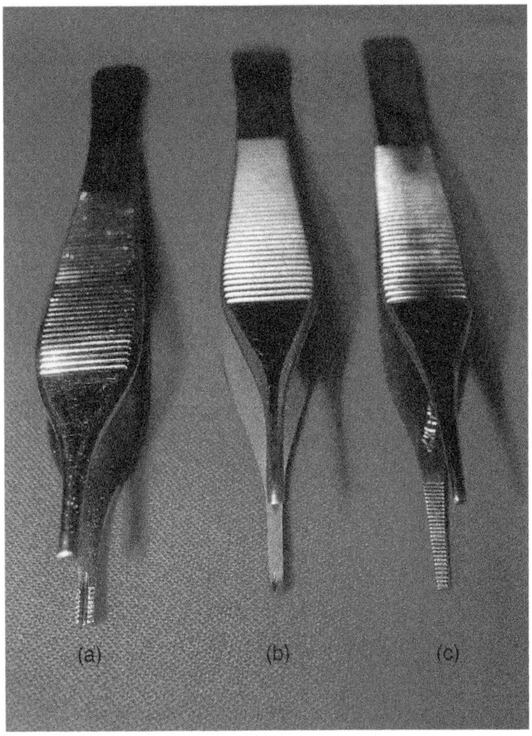

Figure 3.88 Adson tips: (a) brown, (b) 1 × 2, and (c) dressing.

Adson Adson forceps can be recognized by a very distinctive shape. A broad shank that narrows to a small tip describes its classic appearance. The Adson-Brown has two rows of teeth on either side of the tip. The Adson 1×2 has one tooth on one tip and two teeth on the opposite tip. The teeth interdigitate for secure grasping. There is also an Adson 2×3 style that has the same purpose. The Adson dressing forceps has the standard Adson shank, but the tips are smooth with horizontal serrations. This forceps is atraumatic but was designed for use with wound dressings (Figure 3.88).

Rat Tooth Rat-toothed thumb tissue forceps have toothed tips, and they have straight shanks. The 1×2 and the 2×3 styles are most frequently used.

Russian Russian thumb tissue forceps are broad-tipped, straight-shanked forceps. The tip is circular in shape with a very traumatic toothed end. This forceps is usually used on inanimate objects or tissue being removed from the patient.

Debakey The Debakey thumb tissue forceps was originally designed for vascular surgery. Its slender shank and fine tip make it easy to use. The tip has either a groove with two vertical rows of fine teeth or a ridge. This atraumatic instrument is used primarily for handling delicate tissue during general, thoracic, and neurologic surgical procedures (Figure 3.89).

Needle Holders

Needle holders were designed to hold suture needles when closing wounds. They are also the instrument of choice when placing a scalpel blade on a scalpel blade handle. They are not intended to handle tissue of any sort. Sometimes after a needle holder is no longer useful for the intended purpose due to worn tips, it will be "converted" to use as a wire twister. If this happens, the instrument must be very clearly marked as a wire twister rather than a needle holder to avoid any accidental misuse.

Needle holders have very short tips that can either be stainless or have carbide tungsten inserts. As previously discussed, the carbide tungsten inserts can be replaced when they get worn. Regardless of the type of tip, the instrument will have serrations or cross-hatching to better grip the suture needle. It also helps grip the scalpel blade as it is placed on the scalpel blade handle. Needle holders are available in lengths from 4″ to 12″ (Figure 3.90).

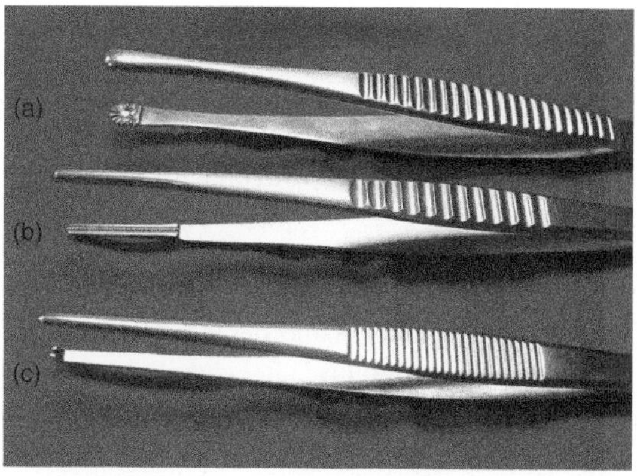

Figure 3.89 Thumb tissue forceps (a) Russian, (b) Debakey, and (c) 1 × 2.

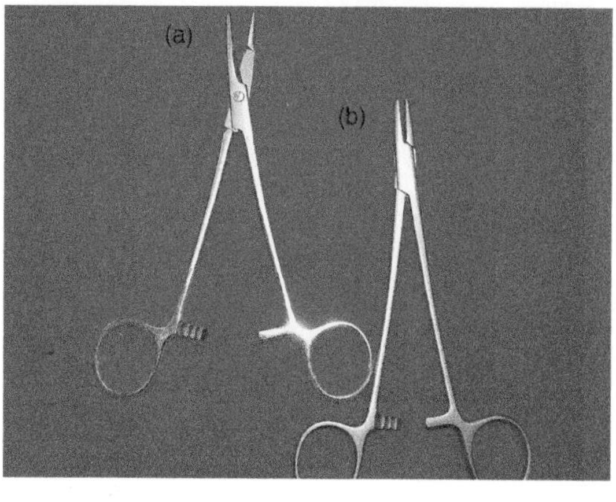

Figure 3.90 Needle holders: (a) Olsen-Hegar and (b) Mayo-Hegar (note gold rings indicating tungsten carbide inserts).

Mayo-Hegar A Mayo-Hegar needle holder is one of the most common styles of needle holder used by surgeons. The tips of this instrument connect directly to the box lock of the instrument. This instrument has ring handles at the end of each shank which allows the surgeon to use either the traditional ring finger/thumb grip or the palmed grip. This needle holder most often is used with larger, heavier needles due to the wider jaw of the instrument.

Olsen-Hegar The Olsen-Hegar needle holder looks identical to the Mayo–Hegar with only one major difference. With this instrument, scissor blades are found between the tips and the box lock. This feature allows the surgeon to cut the suture without having to use an additional instrument. A word of caution, however, to the less experienced surgeon: careful placement of the needle in the tips of the instrument must be observed. Poor placement can result in the inadvertent cutting of the suture before it should be cut.

Crile-Wood The Crile-Wood needle holder also looks very similar to the Mayo-Hegar. The defining characteristic of this instrument is the much narrower, more delicate jaw. This instrument may be chosen by the surgeon when working in smaller more confining surgical field or when using smaller needles.

Derf The Derf needle holder is a cross between the Mayo-Hegar and the Crile-Wood. The jaw shape is smaller than a Mayo-Hegar but is larger than a Crile-Wood. Derf needle holders are limited to shorter lengths 4–5″ and are often chosen for smaller mammals or exotic patients or extraocular procedures (Figure 3.91).

Mathieu The Mathieu needle holder is very different from all other needle holders described thus far. The tips and jaw are most similar to the Mayo-Hegar, but at the end of the shanks, there are curved corners that form a ratchet lock mechanism. The absence of rings makes this instrument easiest to use by surgeons who prefer the palmed grip (Figure 3.92).

Hand-Held Retractors

This type of retractor requires an assistant physically using this instrument to retract tissue for the surgeon. Unless there is another sterile person scrubbed in for the procedure, these instruments have limited applicability. The advantage of the use of handheld retractors is that the pressure exerted on the tissue can be monitored and regulated by the person holding the instrument (Figure 3.93).

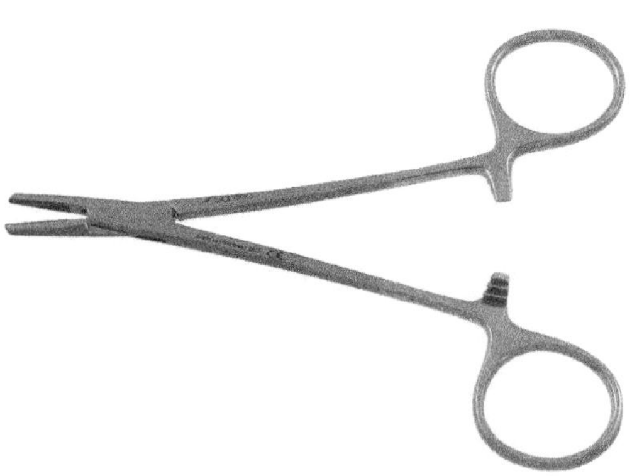

Figure 3.91 Derf needle holder.
Source: Courtesy of Sontec Instruments, Inc. (Cat. # 132-364).

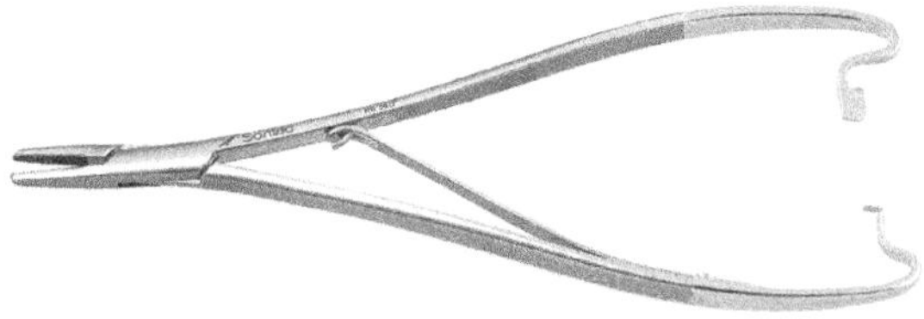

Figure 3.92 Mathieu needle holder.
Source: Courtesy of Sontec Instruments, Inc. (Cat. # - 1100-091).

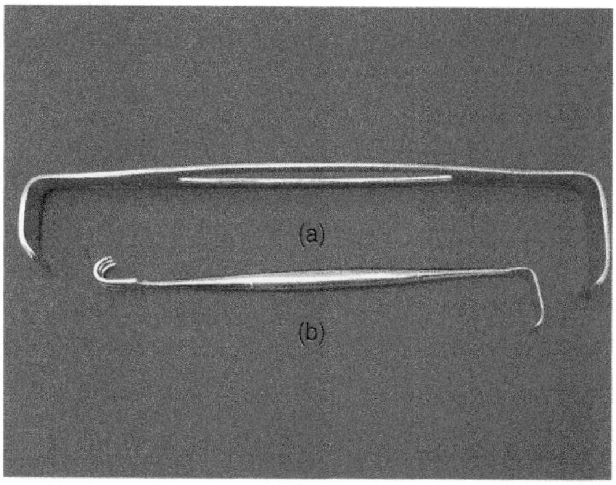

Figure 3.93 Hand-held retractors: (a) U.S. Army and (b) Senn double ended.

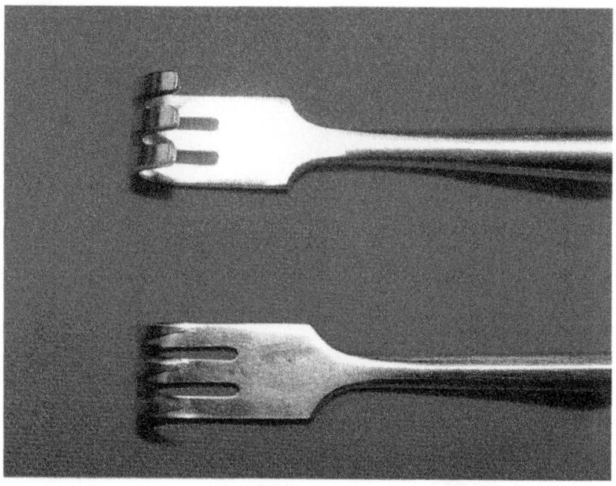

Figure 3.94 Senn double-ended retractor ends: sharp and blunt.

Senn The Senn double-ended handheld retractor has one end with a blade and the other end has a rake. The rake end has three separate prongs that can have either blunt or sharp tips (Figure 3.94). The tissue being retracted will determine whether a sharp or blunt style is used. The narrow blunt blade is only about 1″ in length, so use is limited to small muscle masses or superficial tissues. The two ends of the Senn retractor point in opposite directions from one another.

Army-Navy The Army-Navy retractor (sometimes called the US Army retractor) has blunt, wide blades on either end. Both blades point at each other. One blade is about 2″ in length while the other blade is about 1″ in length. The wider, sturdier blade allows for deeper/larger tissue retraction.

Miscellaneous Instruments

Snook Spay Hook

This instrument has a long (~8″) handle with a blunt hook at the end. Some surgeons use this instrument to exteriorize the uterine horns when performing an ovariohysterectomy on either a canine or feline patient.

Dowling Spay Retractor

The Dowling retractor was designed with the veterinary surgeon who must often work alone in mind. The instrument allows better visualization and stabilization by isolating the uterine horn.

Grooved Director

The grooved director is a useful instrument when making an abdominal incision. It is ~5″ in length with a deep groove on one side. After the surgeon makes the skin incision and then initial puncture on the linea alba, the grooved director is slipped under the created incision with the grooved side facing up. Keeping the instrument parallel to the linea, this instrument provides a "channel" for the surgeon to follow with the scalpel blade to avoid deviating from the linea as well as protecting the abdominal viscera from accidental incising (Figure 3.95).

Alligator Forceps

This instrument has ring handles, a long delicate shank, and a jaw that opens just at the very end of the shank. It is designed for narrow, deep cavities such as the ear canal or nasal passages. The tips have horizontal serrations for more secure grasping of tissue (Figure 3.96).

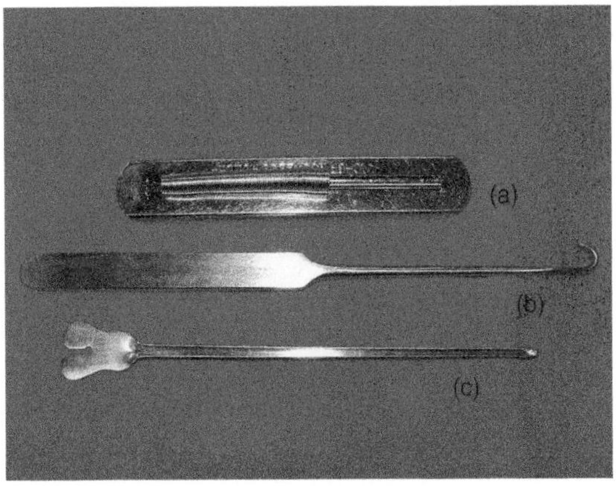

Figure 3.95 (a) Needle rack, (b) snook spay hook, and (c) groove director.

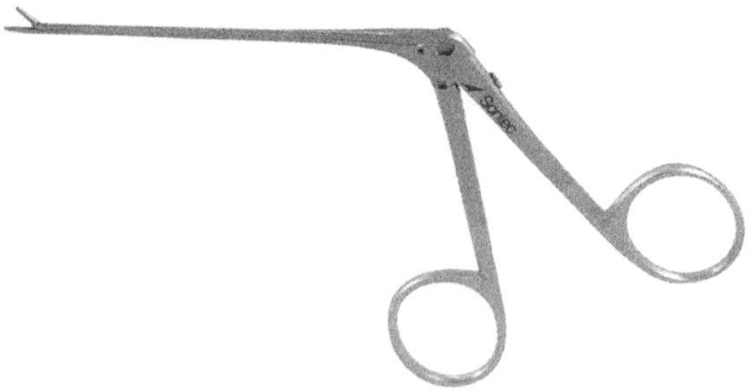

Figure 3.96 Alligator forceps.
Source: Courtesy of Sontec Instruments, Inc. (Cat. # 1100-328S).

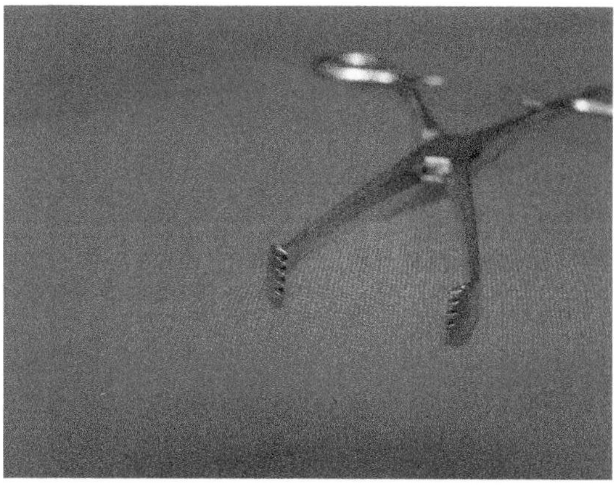

Figure 3.97 Allis tissue forceps.

Allis Tissue Forceps

The Allis tissue forceps is a very traumatic, ring-handled instrument. At the end of the shanks, the tips have interdigitating rows of 3×4 or 4×5 teeth. The large traumatic teeth are intended to grasp tissue that is very durable (i.e. linea alba, tendons, etc.) or tissue that is being removed from the patient, such as a tumor (Figure 3.97).

Needle Rack

The needle rack is a spring mounted on a flat platform. This instrument is intended to hold free suture needles within the pack so they do not get misplaced. Needles are merely pushed down between the coils of the spring to be held securely. The use of free needles in veterinary surgery is limited, however, some situations require them.

Abdominal Instrumentation

Retractors

Balfour The self-retaining retractor of choice for abdominal surgery is the Balfour retractor (Figure 3.98). This instrument has deep-sided cut-out blades that allow spreading of the abdominal wall to provide adequate visualization. This retractor also has a third blade option that can be placed on the cranial end of the incision to provide the surgeon better visualization. Balfour

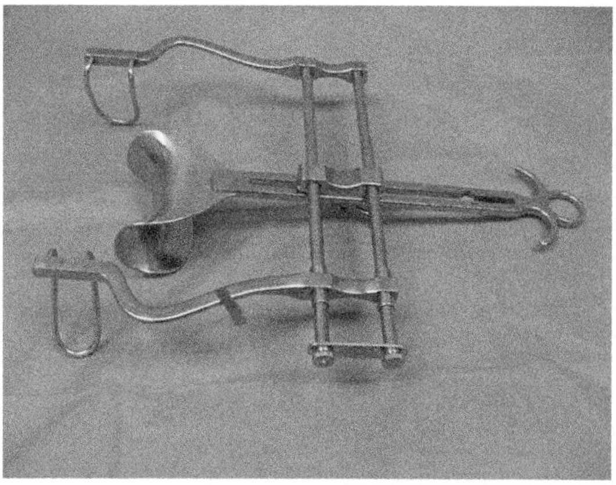

Figure 3.98 Balfour retractor.

retractors are also available in a small version for use with pediatric or smaller patients. The retraction is maintained using a tension mechanism as opposed to a box lock or hand crank (as seen with the Finochetto retractor).

Abdominal Intestinal Forceps

Babcock Intestinal Forceps The Babcock is a non-crushing forceps with a tip that has horizontal serrations. The appearance resembles an Allis tissue forceps, but the function is much different. Surgeons may use this to grab the stomach for manipulation during an abdominal procedure.

Doyen Intestinal Forceps The Doyen is a large, long forceps with longitudinal serrations in the jaw. The jaw length is approximately half the length of the entire instrument. It is a non-crushing instrument for use with the intestines, primarily during resection and anastomosis.

Thoracic Instruments

Retractors

Finochetto Probably the most frequently used self-retaining retractor for thoracic surgery is the Finochetto retractor (Figure 3.99). Available in two different sizes, it can be used with adult or pediatric patients. The smooth unserrated blades can efficiently retract ribs and delicate pleural tissue without trauma. Blades may have a window to decrease pressure. This retractor should be used with moistened laparotomy pads positioned between the blades and the tissue to avoid unnecessary pressure necrosis.

Malleable Malleable retractors are sometimes requested by surgeons to retract delicate lung tissue. A variety of widths from 1″ to 3″ allow the most efficient size to be chosen. As the name indicates, this type of retractor can be bent into the desired shape to achieve the desired effect. Solid blades allow for even pressure distribution. Assistants must take care to avoid excessive pressure when using this retractor. These retractors can also be used in abdominal surgery.

Thoracic Scissors

Thoracic scissors often are longer and have very short sharp-tipped angled blades. This construction allows for easy use in a deep thoracic cavity where minimal movement is desired.

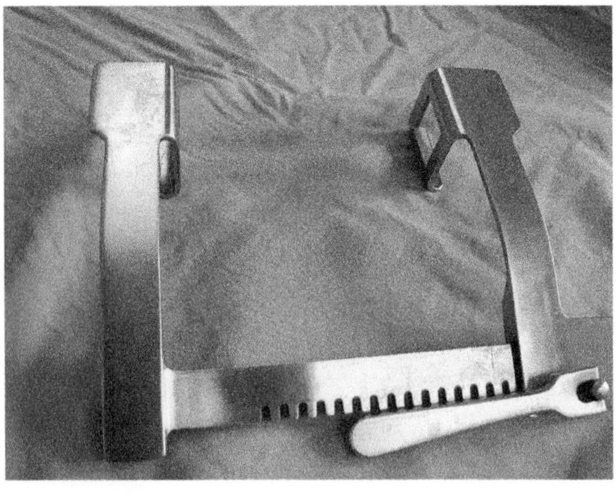

Figure 3.99 Finiochetto retractor.

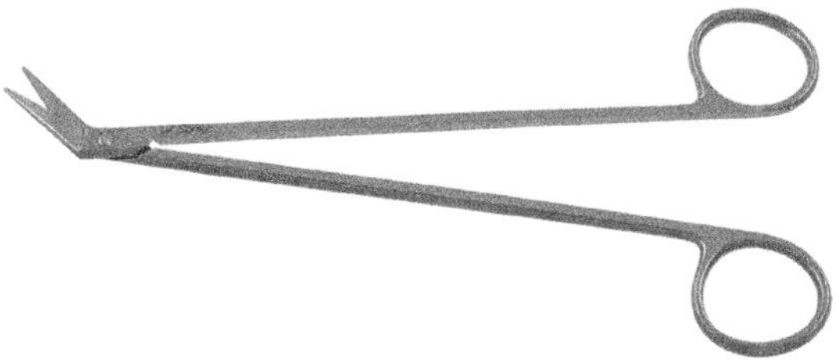

Figure 3.100 45° Potts Smith scissors. *Source:* Courtesy of Sontec Instruments, Inc. (Cat. # 440-210).

Potts Smith Scissors The blades are angled approximately 45° from the shank. This instrument may be used for delicate tissue or vascular dissection (Figure 3.100).

Thumb Tissue Forceps

Debakey The type of thumb tissue forceps most often used in thoracic surgeries is the Debakey thumb tissue forceps. Their delicate design allows atraumatic handling of tissue and vessels. They are available with regular or fine tips and a variety of lengths from 6″ to 12″. Longer instruments are especially beneficial for the surgeon working on a deep-chested dog.

Vascular Clamps

Mixter Vascular clamps have a unique design when designed specifically for use in cardiovascular procedures. One such clamp is the Mixter forceps. With serrations in a horizontal fashion, extending the length of the jaw, the tip of this forceps can form either a 90° or a 45° angle. This unique design facilitates vessel ligation with minimal disruption or manipulation of the vessel. When working with an especially friable or stressed vessel, this instrument can be invaluable (Figure 3.101).

Satinsky/Cooley

Other clamps often found in thoracic instrument packs are the Satinsky and/or the Cooley clamp. These specialized vascular clamps are used for clamping cardiac vessels. Due to their design, they are especially helpful in situations where traditional hemostatic forceps are not an option.

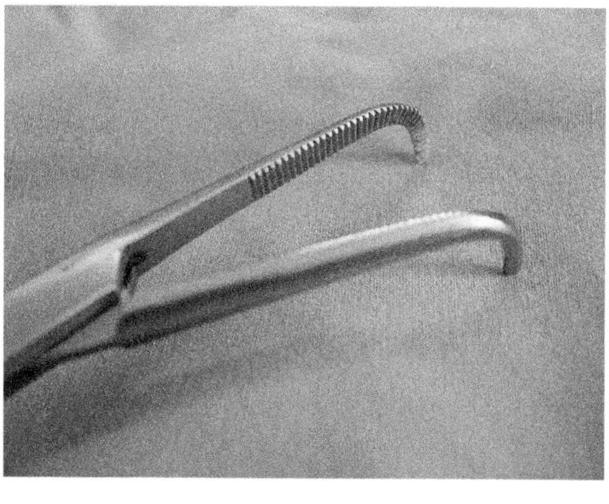

Figure 3.101 Right angle mixter forcep.

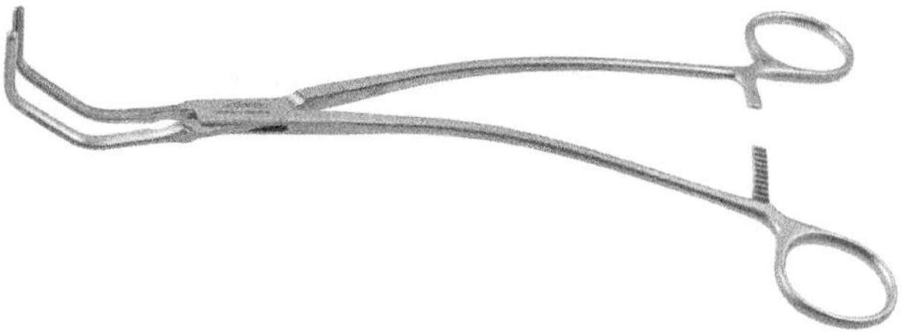

Figure 3.102 Debakey-Satinsky clamp. *Source:* Courtesy of Sontec Instruments, Inc. (Cat. # 2100-782).

The Satinsky clamps have a tip that can be straight, angled, curved, or tangential. A Cooley clamp has a semi-circular jaw. Satinsky clamps have a jaw with horizontal serrations the length of the tip, and a concave channel in the middle of the jaw (Figure 3.102). Vascular clamps are used to provide temporary occlusion of pulmonary and cardiovascular structures such as vessels or bronchi.

Orthopedic Instruments

Orthopedic surgeries require the most intricate and mechanical instrumentation. Advanced training on the use and care of this instrumentation is highly advised due to its complexity and value.

Retractors

Retractors used in orthopedic surgery can be either self-retaining or handheld in style. Often the surgeon is working alone, so the self-retaining styles are popular.

Gelpi Gelpi retractors are self-retaining and have two arms that end with sharp points. They are available in small or large sizes and deep or shallow angles. The smaller retractors are often used during joint surgeries or fracture repairs of small (~15 kg) patients. The larger shallow style is commonly used for fracture repairs, femoral procedures, humeral procedures, etc. The large deep angled retractors are generally reserved for large-breed hip surgeries or procedures where retraction of large deep muscles is required. Deep Gelpi retractors can also be used during neurologic/spinal surgeries, especially in cervical cases (Figure 3.103).

Weitlaner Another type of self-retaining retractor is the Weitlaner. The Weitlaner also has two arms, but at the end of the arms are multi-pronged blades. The pronged blades can be either a

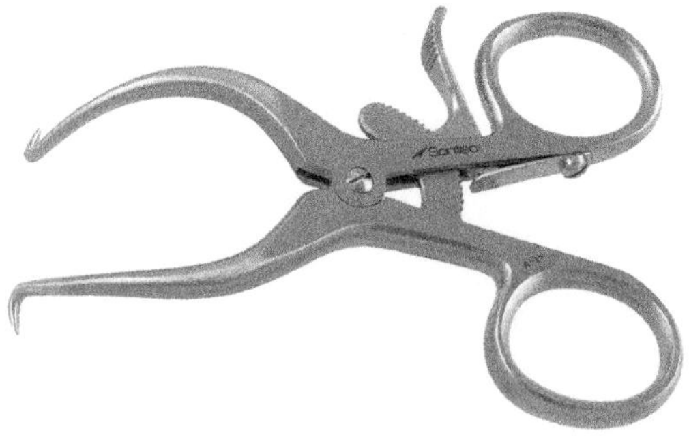

Figure 3.103 Gelpi self-retaining retractor. *Source:* Courtesy of Sontec Instruments, Inc. (Cat # 1100-629).

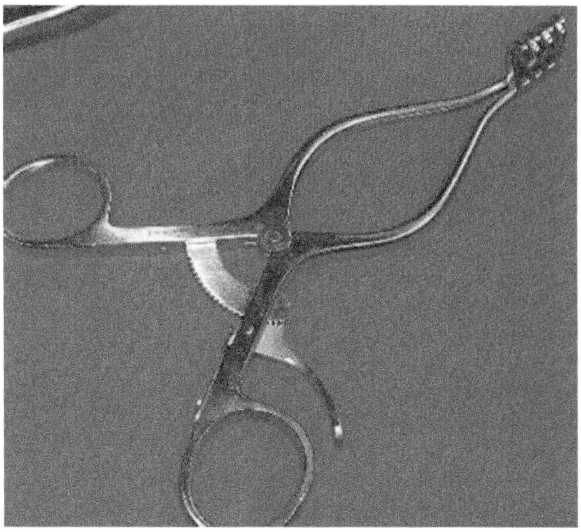

Figure 3.104 Weitlaner self-retaining retractor.

sharp or blunt tip style. This retractor can be used in almost all of the same situations as a Gelpi retractor, however, larger surgical incisions are better suited for the Weitlaner. Also, if nerves or large blood vessels are present in the dissected area, a blunt Weitlaner is a better choice as any sharp retractor may damage the nerve or vessel (Figure 3.104).

Meyerding Handheld retractors may be a better choice depending on the procedure. If the procedure involves large muscle masses in the pelvic area Meyerding retractors may be used (Figure 3.105). The Meyerding is a retractor with a wide blade that is positioned 90° to the handle. The end of the blade has teeth from side to side to better grip the muscle. Pressure must be monitored to avoid damage to the muscles and nerves. The Langenbeck retractor is the same style as the Meyerding with the exception of the teeth on the blade. The Langenbeck had a smooth blade tip and therefore may prove more challenging to retract large muscle masses without the tissue slipping.

Hohmann Hohmann retractors are specific orthopedic handheld retractors that are not used in any other situation. The Hohmann has a curved tip, with a broad plate just after the tip. The handle narrows a little after the plate to better fit into the hand of the person using it. The plates can be of various widths, from ½″ to 2″ (Figure 3.106).

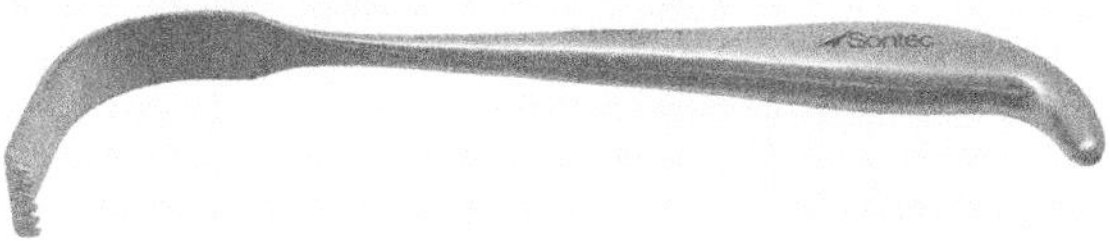

Figure 3.105 Meyerding retractor. *Source:* Courtesy of Sontec Instruments, Inc. (Cat. # 207-411).

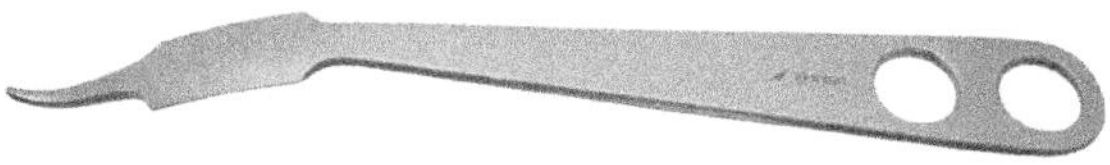

Figure 3.106 Hohman retractor. *Source:* Courtesy of Sontec Instruments, Inc. (Cat. # 1100-673).

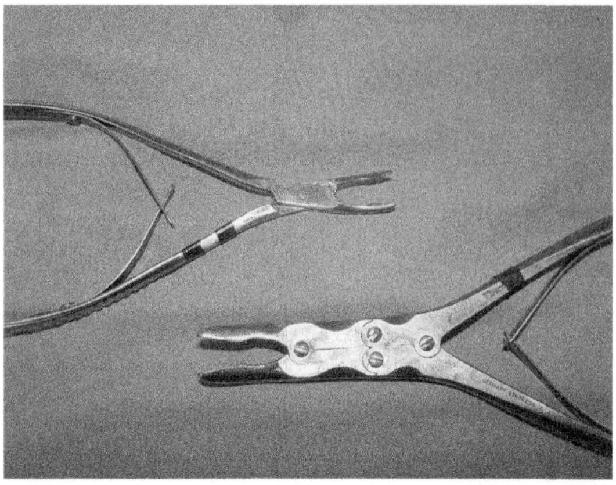

Figure 3.107 Single- and double-action ronguers.

Ronguers

There are multiple styles of ronguers that the surgeon may use during an orthopedic surgery depending on the procedure being done. The ronguer is an instrument that has squeeze handles with cupped tips that have cutting edges. A single action ronguer allows the tips to close as the handles are squeezed (Figure 3.107). Generally having a finer tip than other types of ronguers, the single action can be used for crushing bone pieces for autogenous bone graft implantation. It can also be used for removing small projections of hyperplastic bone. The double-action ronguer had a joint that bends out as the tips come together when the handles are squeezed. This ronguer has a larger cupped tip and is more appropriate for removing larger pieces of bone. In addition to the standard construction, there is also a duck-billed style that is a double-action ronguer with a body style that resembles the alligator forceps.

Periosteal Elevators

Periosteal elevators are designed to elevate the periosteum from the bone (Figure 3.108). They are often used during internal fixation of fractures and other orthopedic surgeries. The look of a periosteal elevator can have the tip being rounded or squared, narrow or wide. The edge of tip is sharp in order to easily remove the periosteum. The tip of the elevator can be straight or curved (Figure 3.109). Some of the more commonly used elevators are the Freer, AO, and Adson.

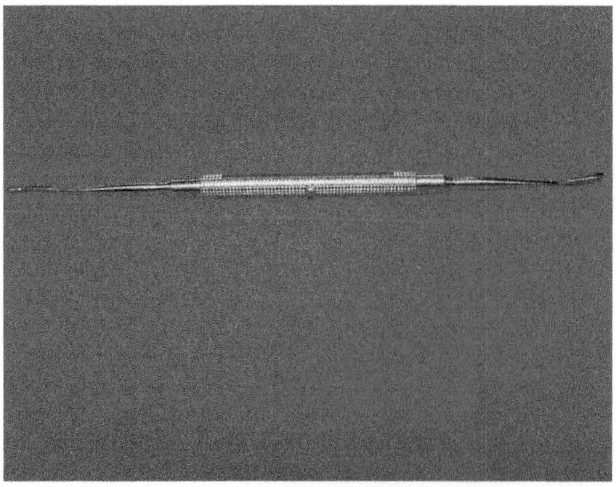

Figure 3.108 Freer periosteal elevator.

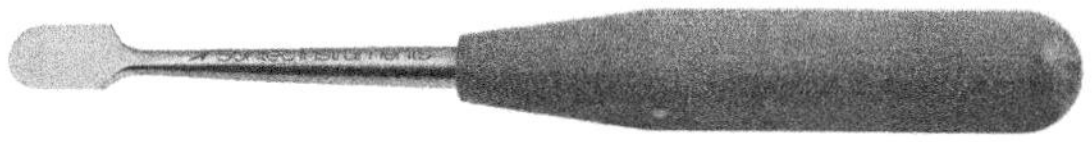

Figure 3.109 14 mm Round-edge straight AO elevator. *Source:* Courtesy of Sontec Instruments, Inc. (Cat. # 335-275).

Osteotomes

Osteotomes are long-handled instruments used for cutting bone. They can be ½″–2′ wide and have a beveled side on either side of the tip. Osteotomes can be used to shave off smaller pieces of bone or remove larger pieces (i.e. femoral head during a femoral head and neck osteotomy). They can also be used to remove bone for cortical bone autographs or for creating access for cancellous bone autograph collection. Osteotomes are non-electric and must be used with some type of mallet. Some osteotome handles are flat, whereas others are octagonal in shape to better fit into the hand of the user. The cutting end of the osteotome can be curved or straight (Figure 3.110).

Chisels

Chisels are very similar looking to osteotomes with the exception of having only one beveled side. Chisels are generally used in similar situations as osteotomes.

Mallet

A Mallet is an orthopedic hammer used to advance osteotomes and/or chisels. Most are two headed having either metal or replaceable plastic heads (Figure 3.111).

Bone Holding/Reduction Forceps

Bone holding/reduction forceps are instruments used to internally stabilize bone fragments until permanent stabilization of the fracture is achieved (Figure 3.112). These forceps can have ratchet locks or speed locks to secure the instrument to the bone (Figure 3.113). The tips may be pointed or blunt and have teeth or serrations (Figure 3.114). Often the forceps used is determined by the type of fracture, the location of the fracture, and the surgeon's preference. Many of the bone holder/reduction forceps are available in both small and large sizes. Some types of bone forceps commonly used are Kern, blunt reduction, sharp speed lock, and Verbrugge (Figure 3.115).

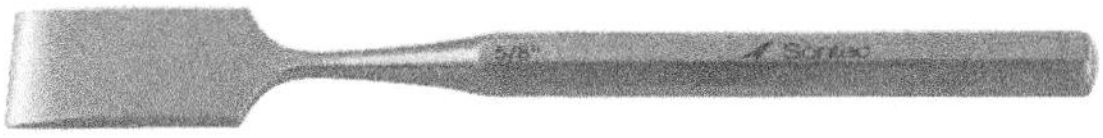

Figure 3.110 Hibbs osteotome. *Source:* Courtesy of Sontec Instruments, Inc. (Cat. # 330-553).

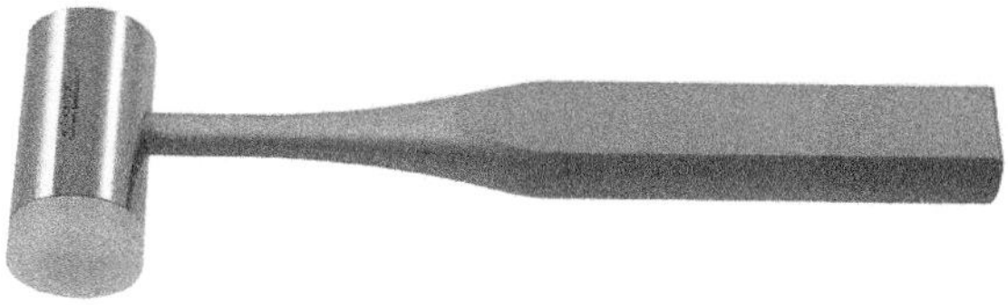

Figure 3.111 Sontec combo nylon mallet. *Source:* Courtesy of Sontec Instruments, Inc. (Cat. # 1100-462S).

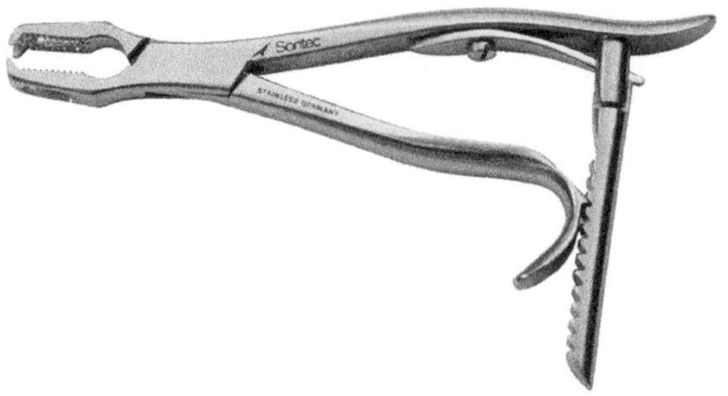

Figure 3.112 Kern bone clamp. *Source:* Courtesy of Sontec Instruments, Inc. (Cat. # 305-332).

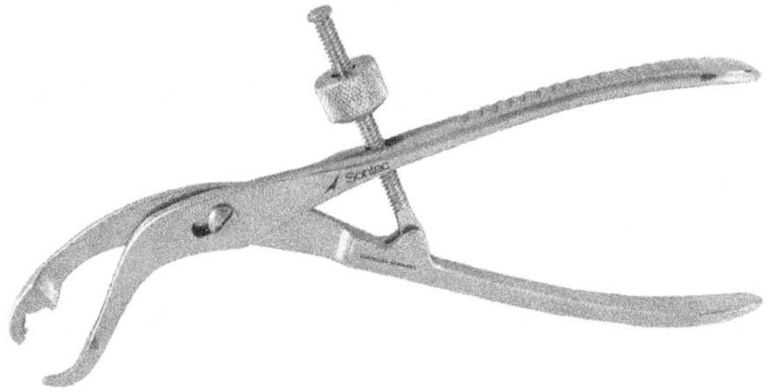

Figure 3.113 Verbrugge bone clamp. *Source:* Courtesy of Sontec Instruments, Inc. (Cat. # 1103-074).

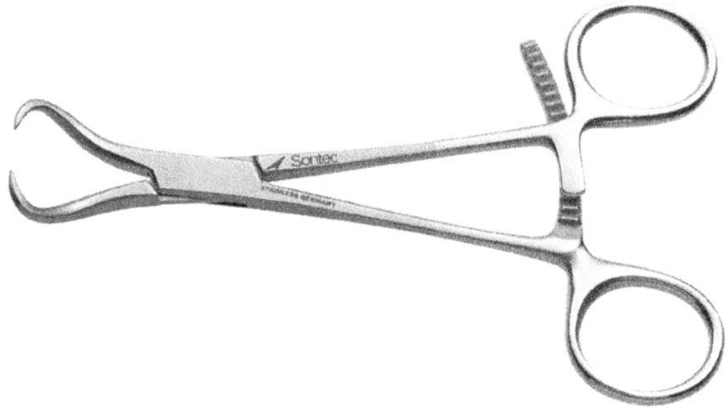

Figure 3.114 Bone reduction clamp. *Source:* Courtesy of Sontec Instruments, Inc. (Cat. # 1103-040).

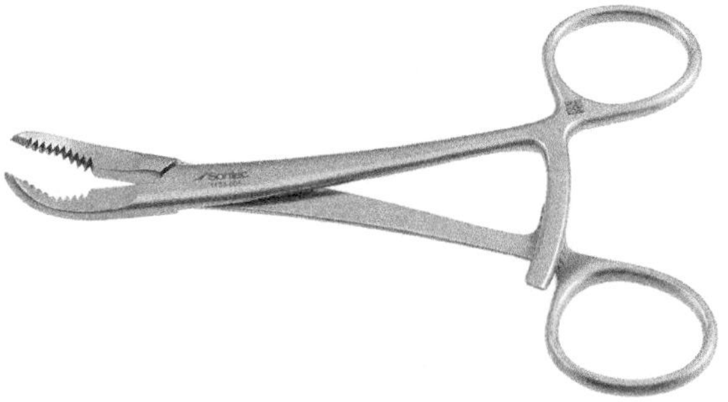

Figure 3.115 Stefan mini bone-holding forceps. *Source:* Courtesy of Sontec Instruments, Inc. (Cat. # 1103-005).

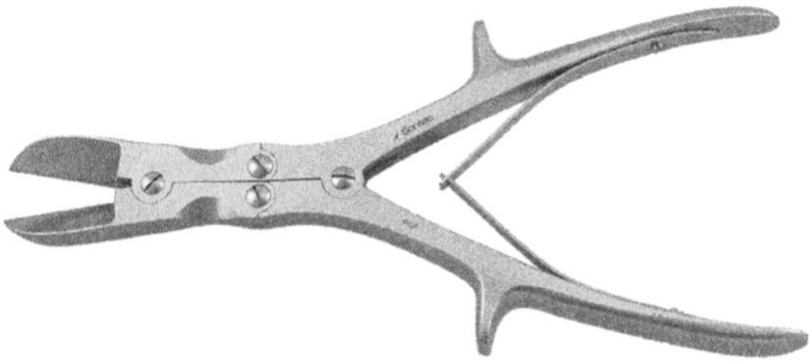

Figure 3.116 Straight Stille-Liston bone cutting forceps. *Source:* Courtesy of Sontec Instruments, Inc. (Cat. # 315-754).

Bone Cutters

Bone cutters are double-action, squeeze-handle-designed instruments with cutting edges on the inside of the blades on the tip. Bone cutters are used with the same hand motion as rongeurs but have flat tips as opposed to the cupped tips of a rongeur (Figure 3.116). Removal of small pieces of bone is the most common use.

Jacob's Chuck

A Jacob's hand chuck is a handheld "drill" that can be used for simple intramedullary (IM) pin placement or K-wire placement (Figure 3.117).

Power Equipment

Many styles of power equipment are available for use by the orthopedic surgeon. Some are electric, some are pneumatic, and others are battery operated. Electric devices obviously must be sterilized with ethylene oxide and therefore have limited feasibility in practice. Pneumatic equipment is run by connecting a hose to a nitrogen tank and can be steam sterilized (Figure 3.118). Battery-operated drills can be steam sterilized. The battery is inserted poststerilization and may either need to be covered by a sterile wrap or placed into the drill using a device to protect against contamination from the non-sterile person. Regardless of the brand of drill, almost all are equipped with multiple accessories. Drill bit adapters, either quick connect or chuck-style drill bit attachments, and mini wire drivers are common extras. Some also include a sagittal saw adapter (Figure 3.119). Some of the companies that have drills available are Synthes, 3M, Securos, and Arthrex. Power equipment is necessary for almost every orthopedic case, whether it is used to place bone screws, perform osteotomies, or secure intramedullary pins.

Figure 3.117 Jacob's chuck.

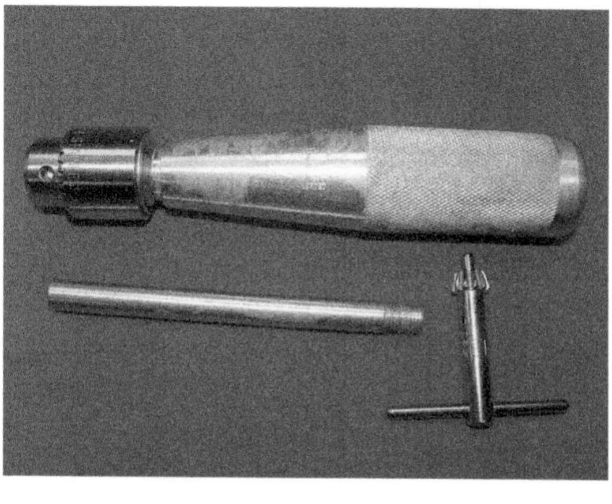

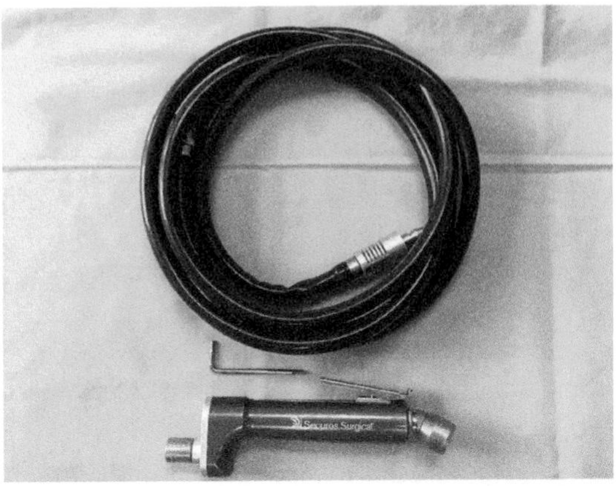

Figure 3.118 Securos Surgical® TPLO saw.

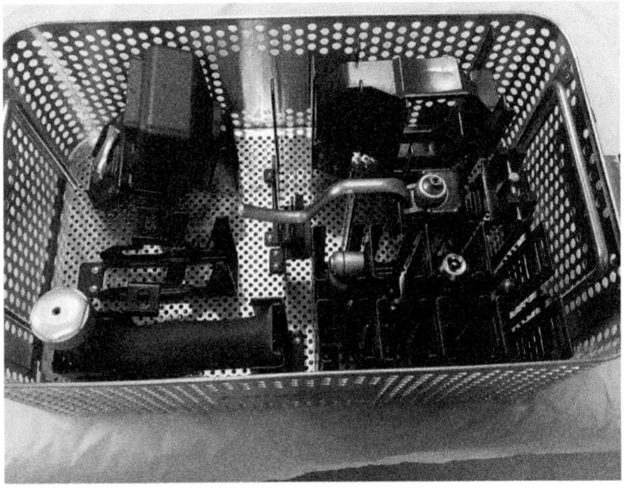

Figure 3.119 Arthrex® power system.

Internal Fixation Implants

There are many types of internal implants available for use by veterinary surgeons. Some implants are used for fracture stabilization and repair, some are for stabilizing bones postlengthening or corrective osteotomy for deformity repair. Intramedullary pins, orthopedic wire, bone plates, bone screws, and interlocking nails are the most commonly used implants.

Intramedullary Pins

Intramedullary (IM) pins are implants often used for repair of diaphyseal fractures in many bones except the radius. Surgeons may choose an IM pin due to the advantage of the ability of the implant to resist bending loads. Conversely, they have the disadvantage of no resistance to rotational loads and do not have an interlocking fixation with the bone. Pins are available in many sizes, from 1/16″ to ¼″ width. They are made of 316l stainless steel and are round in appearance. The ends can both be pointed (double armed) or have one end blunt (single armed). The most common style of points is either a trocar point with three cutting edges for easy movement through cancellous bone or the chisel point, which is a double-cutting edge, better for use with cortical bone. The ends of the pin

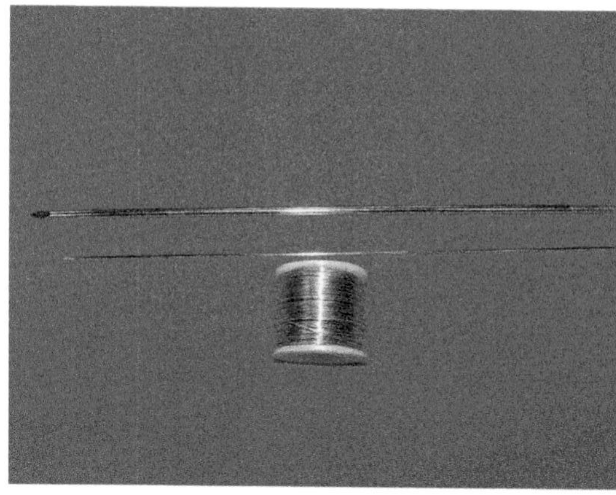

Figure 3.120 Intramedullary (IM) pin, K-wire, orthopedic wire.

may be smooth or threaded. The use of threaded pins was originally thought to increase the holding power of the pin in the cancellous bone, however, that theory is controversial. Kirschner wires are small (0.035–0.062″) pins that are smooth and generally have a trocar point. Too small to stabilize a fracture when used alone, they are often used to cross-wire fractures to supplement stabilization by another means (Figure 3.120).

Orthopedic Wire

Orthopedic wire used in the repair of fractures can be used alone or in addition to other internal implants. Wire is available on spools that can be autoclaved or in pre-cut lengths with a pre-formed loop on one end. Orthopedic wire is available in sizes from 18 to 32 ga and is made of a pliable form of 3161 stainless steel material. Cerclage wire is the term used for wire placed around the entire circumference of the bone, while hemi-cerclage is the term for wire passed through holes drilled in the bone. Spiral fractures or reconstructed oblique fractures are the most common procedures where wire is used. However, mandibular symphyseal fractures of the feline are often repaired with wire alone.

Wire Twisters

Wire twisters are instruments used to twist the orthopedic wire to secure its placement (Figure 3.121). Wire twisters can be as simple as an old needle holder or pliers, or they may be specifically designed wire twisters. Generally, when looped cerclage wires are employed, a

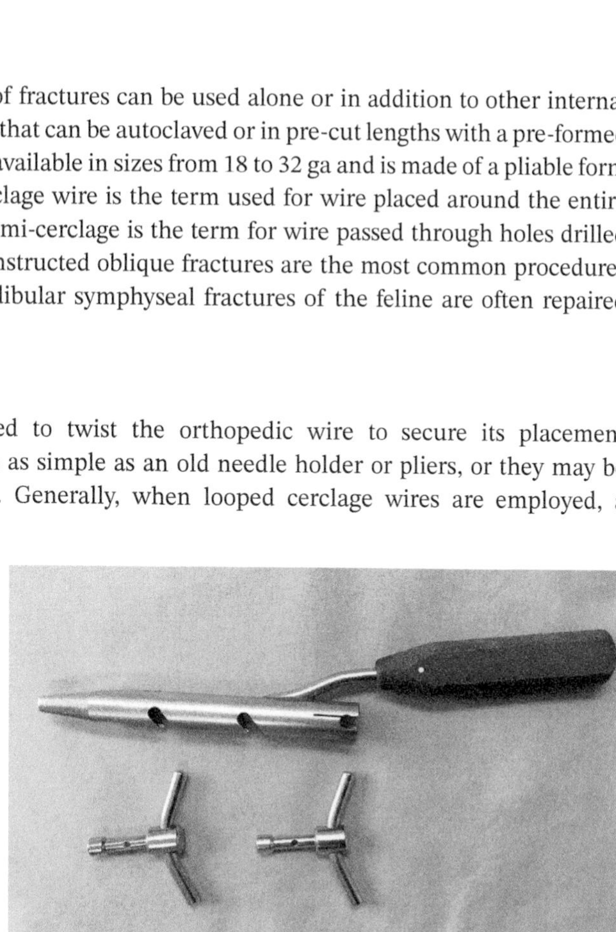

Figure 3.121 Wire twister.

specifically designed wire twister is used to attain appropriate tightness and placement. If using an old needle holder, it is imperative that the instrument be identified as a wire twister to avoid placement in a general surgery pack. The tips of the needle holder get quite damaged when used as a wire twister and could prove to be a very frustrating situation if it was used as a true needle holder.

Pin/Bolt Cutters

Pin cutters are handled instruments designed for cutting small intramedullary pins, K-wires, or sometimes orthopedic wire. Generally, these are squeeze-handle-designed instruments that require the sharpness on the tips of the instrument to be maintained. A fair amount of hand strength is required for operation of a pin cutter, so dull cutting edges will further impede proper use. Pin cutters can have the cutting edge on the end of the instrument (Figure 3.122) or a cutting edge on the side of the instrument (Figure 3.123). A bolt cutter, which is generally sterilized by EtO methods so it does not rust, will be needed for larger pins (Figure 3.124).

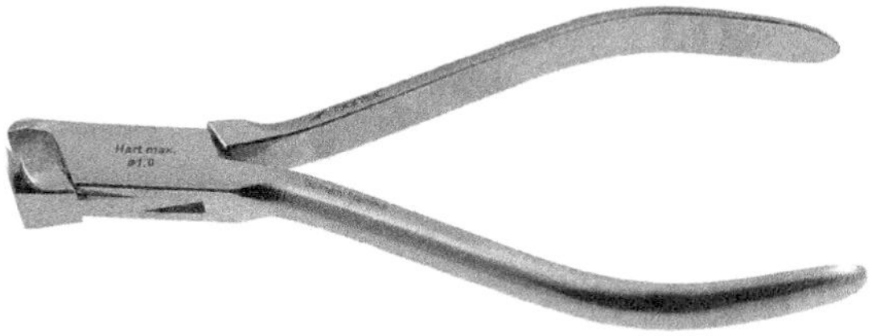

Figure 3.122 Wire end cutter.
Source: Courtesy of Sontec Instruments, Inc. (Cat. # 1103-110).

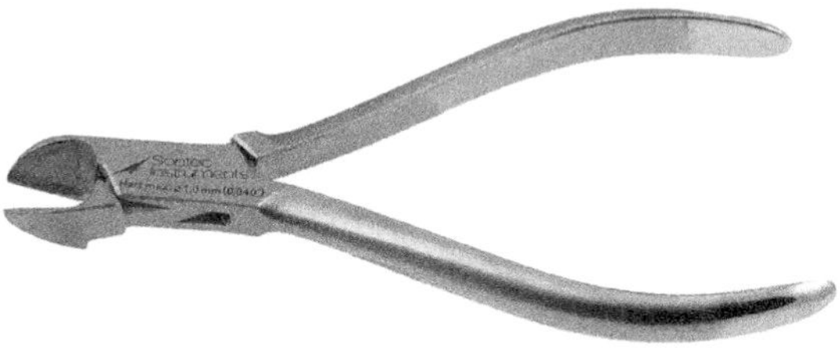

Figure 3.123 Wire side cutter.
Source: Courtesy of Sontec Instruments, Inc. (Cat. # 1103-115).

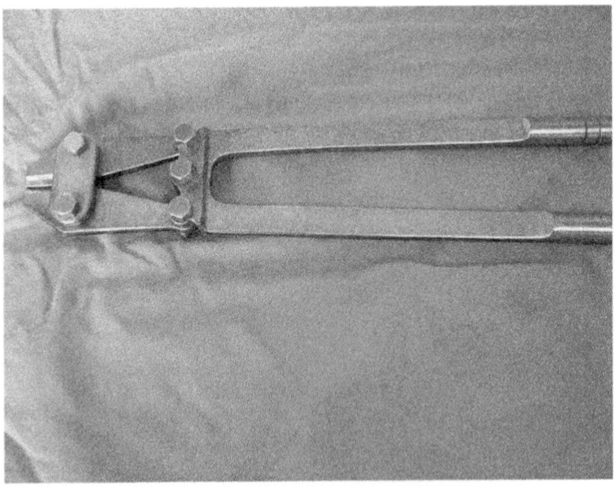

Figure 3.124 Bolt cutter.

Interlocking Nails

Interlocking nails are implants placed in the medullary canal of a fractured bone. This implant has a design that allows resistance to all forces that may be placed on a fracture. It is primarily indicated for use in femoral, humeral, and tibial mid-diaphyseal fracture stabilization. The implant is designed with screw holes at either end of the nail to allow screw placement for additional support. A variety of sizes, 4.0, 4.7, 6.0, 8.0, and 10.0 mm are available to permit use in many animals. There are also multiple lengths for each diameter size. Each size pin has a specific size screw that accompanies that pin. The 4.0 and 4.7 pin use 2.0 mm screws. The 6.0 mm pin uses a 2.7 or 3.5 mm screw. The 8.0 mm pin uses a 3.5 or 4.5 mm screw while the 10.0 mm pin uses only the 4.5 mm screw. In addition to the implant itself and the screws, there are multiple pieces of equipment needed for proper placement of the nail. The drill guide jig is used to align the drill bit with holes in the nail. The extension piece is used to attach the drill guide jig to the nail. Drill guides are used to protect surrounding tissue from the rotation of the drill bit. The drill bits are used to drill a hole in the bone for placement of the bone screw and the reamer is used to prepare the medullary canal for the placement of the nail.

Bone Plates

There is a wide variety of bone plates available for use in veterinary surgery. The plates are very specific to the needs of the fracture or surgical case. Although the ultimate decision for the size and type of plate to be used in a procedure is determined by the surgeon, it is critical that technicians understand the various types of plates and all the accompanying equipment. Sizing of bone plates includes two different characteristics of the plate. First of all, the width of the plate is expressed in millimeters (mm). Plates are available in the following sizes: 1.0, 1.4, 1.5, 1.6, 2.0, 2.4, 2.7, 3.5, 3.5 broad, 4.5, and 4.5 broad (Figure 3.125). The number on the plate refers to the size screw that will be used with the plate. In the case of the "broad" labeled plates, it merely means that the screw size is the plate size, however, it is a "wider" version of the original plate, hence the addition to the name of the term "broad." Also involved in the sizing of the plate is the length of the plates. The length of the plate is determined by the number of holes in the plate: a 7-hole plate has 7 screw holes, a 10-hole plate has 10 holes available, etc. Therefore, the complete name of a bone plate would be a 9-hole 3.5 plate, meaning there are 9 holes, each sized to accept a 3.5 mm screw, in the plate.

Plates may also have the type of screw hole configuration included in the name. Screw holes can be DCP which stands for dynamic compression plate; LC-DCP which means limited-contact dynamic compression plate; or LCP which means locking compression plate. Depending on the type of screw hole, a different function of the plate will occur. In the DCP hole, the principle is that an oblong hole with beveled edges to accept a conical head-shaped screw will allow compression

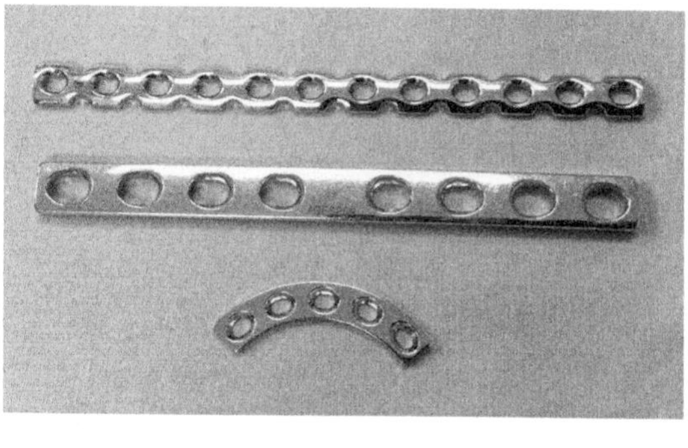

Figure 3.125 Examples of bone plates: 12-hole reconstruction, 8-hole DCP, and 5-hole acetabular.

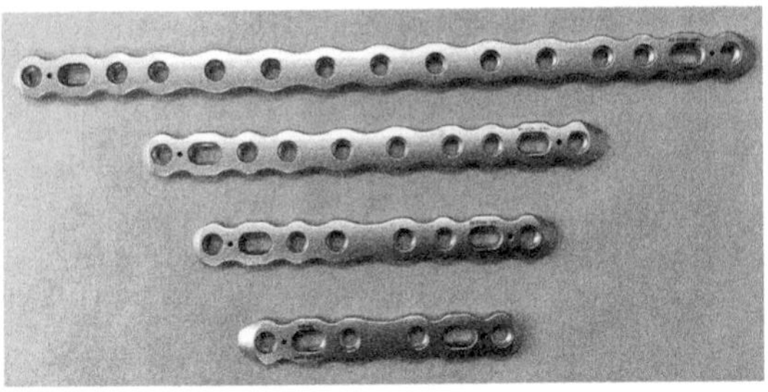

Figure 3.126 Locking plates.

on the fracture site. In the LC-DCP hole, the same principle of the DCP hole is true, but the plate construction has cut out of the plate on the underside, therefore allowing less contact with the bone. The LCP hole also has threaded holes in addition to the beveled hole edges. The threads allow for use of either a traditional bone screw or a locking head screw (Figure 3.126).

Other types of plates that are available are reconstructive plates, veterinary cuttable plates, acetabular plates, distal tibial fracture plates (also known as T plates), and tibial plateau leveling osteotomy (TPLO) plates. The reconstructive plates have areas of the plate cut out along the edge between the holes to allow for 3D bending and manipulation to fit the bone. Not only can they be bent up or down but they can also be bent sideways. The cuttable plates are available in lengths up to 50 holes and can be custom designed in length for each case. Veterinary cuttable plates (VCP) are available in two sizes – 1.5/2.0 and 2.0/2.7 mm. Cuttable plates are the only plates used in a stacking fashion when bridging a comminuted fracture to provide additional stability. Acetabular plates are specifically designed to match the varied configuration of the acetabular bone. Distal tibial fracture plates or "T" plates are also specific to use in canine distal tibial fracture repair, although originally they were designed for carpal arthrodesis. TPLO plates are designed for use during the TPLO procedure to repair the instability of the stifle following a rupture of the cruciate ligament. TPLO plates are specific to the side (left or right) that is having surgery as well as the design best suited for each individual patient – short, standard, and broad (Figure 3.127).

The function of the plate can be determined by appearance, as already discussed, or by application. Depending on how the plate is applied to the bone, it may be a compression plate, a neutralizing plate, or a buttress plate. Any plate can serve any function, depending on how it is applied by the surgeon.

Bone Screws

There are two types of bone screws. One is a cortical bone screw and the other is a cancellous bone screw. The name indicates the placement of the threads of the screw, either in cortical bone or cancellous bone. Cortical bone screws are fully threaded, meaning the threads of the screw are present the

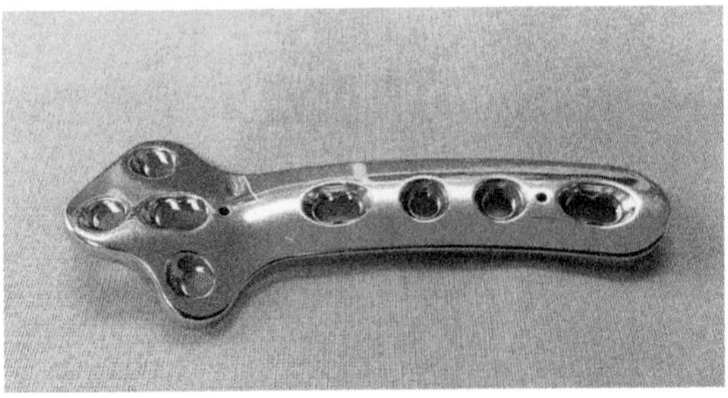

Figure 3.127 TPLO plate – right or left standard, etc.

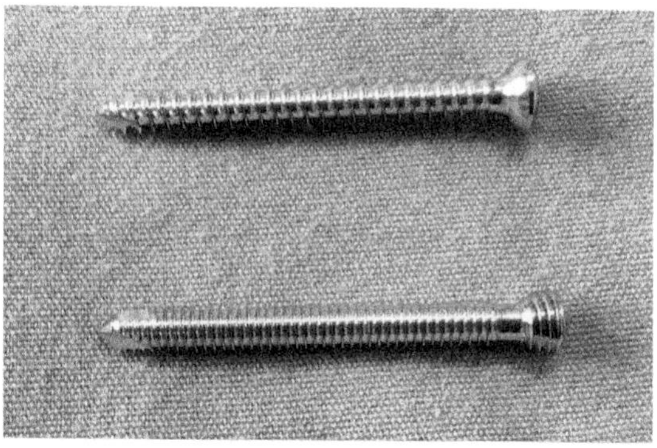

Figure 3.128 Bone screws: regular head – top, locking head – bottom.

entire length of the screw. The pitch, or the number of threads per inch, is greater than the cancellous screw, thereby allowing a greater number of threads to contact the cortical bone. Cancellous bone screws have a greater thread height than the cortical screw. The thread height is determined by the difference between core diameter and the outer diameter of the screw. A larger thread height means the threads are allowed to go deeper into the cancellous bone to hold the screw stable. Cancellous screws can be fully threaded or partially threaded, which means there are threads on only about one-third of the length of the screw at the most distal end. As with plates, screws are generally made of 316l stainless steel or titanium. Most cortical bone screws used now are self-tapping. They can also have a regular-style head or a locking head style (Figure 3.128). As described previously, regular head screws sit on top of the hole in the plate, whereas locking head screws screw into the threads in the plate hole to attach the screw to the plate. Self-tapping style screws have threads that tap the bone on its own for secure placement. Screws can be used by themselves, along with pins or orthopedic wire, or with a plate. Regardless of the function of the screw, the placement requires basically the same equipment. First of all, the surgeon will use a drill bit and drill guide to create the screw hole. The size of drill bit used is determined by the screw size being implanted. The inner core of the screw is the determining factor of drill bit size (i.e. a 3.5 mm screw has a 2.5 inner core diameter so a 2.5 mm drill bit is used). Along with the drill bit a drill guide is used to center the screw hole in the hole in the plate. The drill guides may have either a neutral or a load end. Depending on the intended function of the screw, the surgeon will choose the appropriate end to use. When creating the hole for a screw, the drill bit is passed through the closest bone cortex and then the other. There is a bit of a "give" in the resistance of the drill bit when the far bone cortex has been passed through. The drill bit is removed and the depth gauge is then used to determine the length of the screw needed. The hook end of the depth gauge is placed in the hole and then hooked on the far cortex. The sliding sleeve of the depth gauge is slid down until contact with the bone. The length in millimeters is then read from the scale on the instrument. The screw is inserted by using a screwdriver and is tightened to a "fingertip" tightness to avoid stripping the screw hole.

Lag screws are placed using the same equipment; however, multiple drill bit sizes will be needed by the surgeon to place the screw properly to act as a lag screw is intended (to compress a fracture line between two fragments). Another additional piece of equipment needed for lag screws is a countersink. The countersink will be used after the drill bit but before the depth gauge. The countersink creates a bevel at the screw hole opening to allow the screw to sit deep in the screw hole.

Although technicians are not routinely responsible for placing screws, it is quite frequent that they will be involved in the drilling of the holes or stabilization of the bone while the surgeon drills the hole. Technicians assisting in orthopedic surgery must be very comfortable with the equipment and the order in which the instruments will be used to place the screw to be of the most use to the surgeon.

Other implants and equipment that are needed for specific orthopedic procedures (i.e. TPLO, TTA, and joint arthroplasty) will be discussed in Chapter 5.

Arthroscopic Instrumentation

Arthroscopy in small animal surgery is a very common procedure. It often will be done in an attempt to forego the need for a more invasive procedure. Multiple advantages include faster patient recovery time, less patient discomfort, better visualization and assessment of the joint, and earlier diagnosis of joint disorders. The care of this delicate and expensive instrumentation is a critical skill that the veterinary surgical technician must possess (Figure 3.129).

The arthroscope itself can be varied depending on length, angle, and diameter. Arthroscopes are available in both short and long lengths. Most surgeons will choose the short length. The angles of arthroscopes available are 0°, 30°, and 70°. Sometimes a scope with an angled tip will be used for better visualization of the joint. Most frequently that will be the 30° scope. The diameters used most frequently in small animal veterinary arthroscopy are 1.9, 2.3, and 2.7 mm. The size used for the procedure will ultimately depend on the size of the patient and the size of the joint. In addition to the scope, usually a camera that attaches to the scope is also utilized (Figure 3.130). Cameras can have one chip or multiple chips, with the major difference being found in the resolution of the picture. One end of the camera attaches to the scope eyepiece on the sterile field and the other end attaches to a control box which transmits the image to a monitor for all in the room to see. Sometimes the camera will be sterile, but if not a sterile, clear plastic "Sleeve" can be placed over

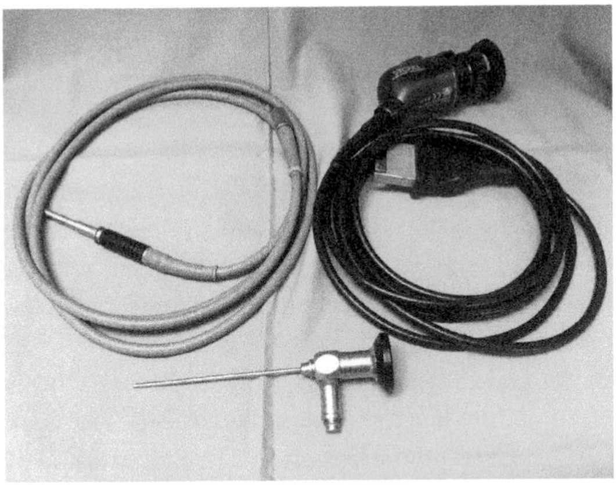

Figure 3.129 Arthroscope, light cable, and camera.

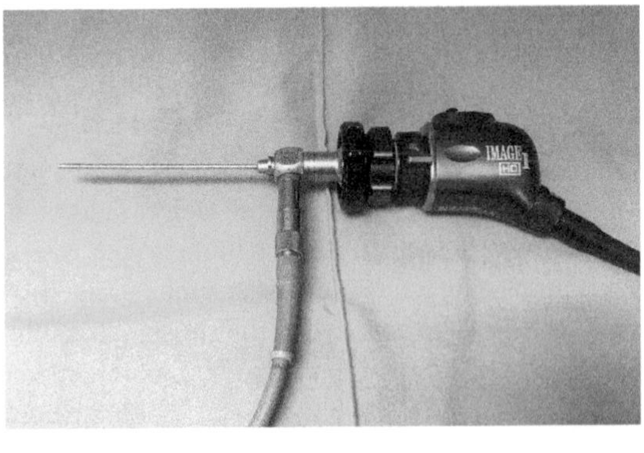

Figure 3.130 Arthroscope assembled.

the camera cord to allow use on the sterile field. The control box will allow modification of focus, white balance, etc. Another accessory for the arthroscope which is a necessity is the light source. A fiber optic cable attaches the light source to the scope and provides light via either a tungsten-halogen bulb or a Xenon bulb. A brighter light is provided by the Xenon bulb, but it is a more expensive bulb (Figure 3.131). Cannulas and obturators are also needed for placement and use of the arthroscope. Obturators are used to create a path into the joint to allow placement of the cannula. Various hand instruments such as probes, graspers, and curettes can also be inserted through the cannulas for use within the joint (Figure 3.132). Some procedures will require the use

Figure 3.131 Arthroscopy tower.

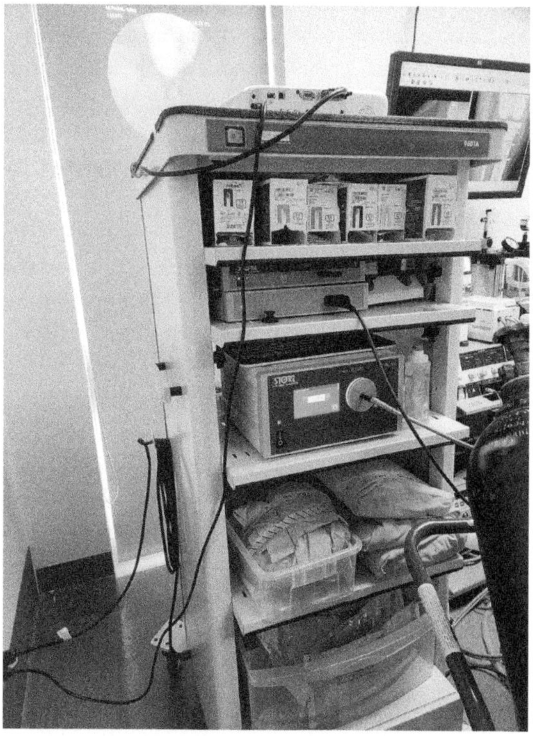

Figure 3.132 Arthroscopy instruments: obturators – top, cannulas – middle, and Egress plugs – bottom.

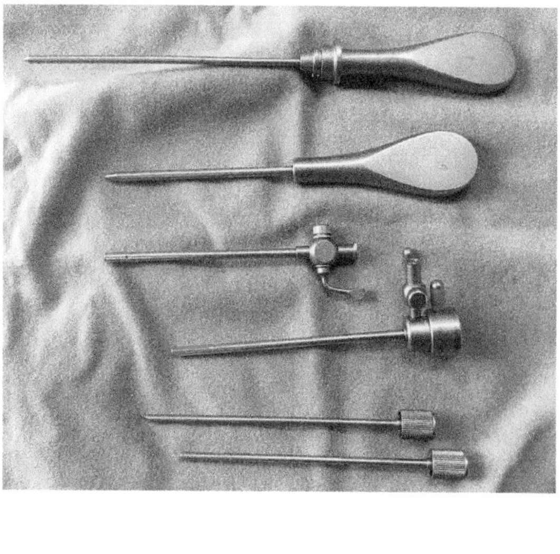

of a motorized shaver in the joint. Most shavers have the option of three modes of operation: oscillating, forward/reverse, and variable speed. A control box for the shaver allows selection of the desired mode. There are three types of tips available for use with a motorized shaver: a full radius blade, an aggressive cutter blade, or a bur. The blades are generally used for soft tissue removal with the shaver in the oscillating mode. The bur is used most frequently for bone removal with the shaver in the forward/reverse mode. Finally, a fluid source is required to allow free flow of fluid into the joint. The fluid infusion provides lubrication and flush and improves visualization. A gravity-assisted system may be used (with the assistance of a fluid compression bag) but does have its disadvantages. Foremost is the inability to provide high-pressure flushing when needed. Additionally, the lack of constant fluid pressures and attention by surgical staff makes this system less desirable. More often, a fluid pump is used to alleviate the aforementioned issues. A fluid pump maintains a constant pressure of delivery but does allow for variation in pressure when necessary. The initial cost of the unit, the specific tubing required, and the learning curve for mastering the set of the system are disadvantages worth considering.

Laparoscopic Instruments

Much like the arthroscopic instruments, the laparoscopic instruments are very expensive and require extreme care when being handled. Although the visualization tool is called a telescope, much of the other equipment and instrumentation is very similar to arthroscopic equipment. Either a 0° or a 30° rigid telescope is used, however, preference is for the 30° scope as it allows more evaluation of the cavity being scoped with less manipulation (Figure 3.133). A variety of lengths and sizes are available with patient size being the determining factor for use. In small dogs and cats, a 2.7 mm scope is often recommended. With larger dogs, a 5.0 mm telescope is best used. As with the arthroscopic equipment, laparoscopes require a light source that attaches to the scope via a fiber optic cable and then the cable is connected to a light source. Either a halogen or Xenon bulb is available commercially. A camera and monitor are a necessity in order for all members of the surgical team to view the procedure. Trocars and cannulae are also needed for placement of the scope and accompanying instruments. The trocar can be either sharp or blunt and is used to create path for placement of the cannula. Sometimes the surgeon may make a small incision to facilitate the placement of the trocar. The instruments and scope are then inserted into the cavity through the cannula to decrease irritation to soft tissue. Soft or flexible cannulas are recommended for thoracic endoscopy as they may decrease postoperative pain due to less rib nerve pressure associated with rigid cannulas. For abdominal laparoscopy, an insufflator is also required. CO_2 insufflation, via a Veress (insufflation) needle, is necessary to inflate the abdomen to allow visualization for the surgeon as well as provide distention of the abdominal

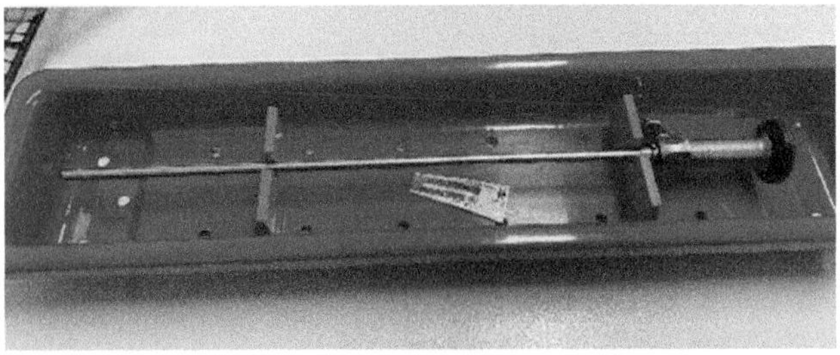

Figure 3.133 Laparoscope.

wall to minimize tissue trauma. Valved cannula will be used with the insufflator to control the infusion of the CO_2. An insufflator is not needed with thoracic endoscopy and the ribs provide adequate distention of the thoracic cavity without the need for any additional distention. Additional instruments such as biopsy forceps or punches, grasping forceps, or scissors are similar for both abdominal as well as thoracic endoscopy. Many of the instruments used are capable of being connected to an electrosurgery or radiosurgical unit. This type of instrumentation is advantageous as it minimizes the passage of different instruments in and out of the patient as well as providing hemostasis in the surgical field.

Neurologic Instrumentation

Equipment needed for neurologic procedures is quite varied. An air-powered drill is needed to make the approach, as well as the use of standard orthopedic instruments (Figure 3.134). Once the boney "roof" of the vertebrae has been removed or the craniotomy completed, the delicate instruments used in manipulating the spinal cord or brain are often the same instruments that may be used in an ophthalmic procedure.

Large double-action rongeurs, single-action rongeurs, and periosteal elevators may be used to remove large quantities of bone prior to the use of the pneumatic drill. Kerrison ronguers may be used to assist with bone removal as well.

The pneumatic drill is a cylindrical unit that is held like a pencil when being used. The trigger for the control of power is conveniently located on the side of the main piece. The drill bits available are either short or long in design and both require the use of a bur guard before being inserted into the drill. Tips can be broad in shape, often called a pineapple bur, or very fine and small (Figure 3.135). The broader tips are used for larger gross bone removal, whereas the finer tips are reserved for delicate bone removal when close to the spinal cord or brain. Instruments used for neurologic procedures are micro-instruments such as an iris spatula, Stevens tenotomy scissors, Iris scissors, Bishop-Harmon thumb tissue forceps, and Colibri thumb tissue forceps. Nerve retractors, ear curettes, and dural hooks may also be needed.

Retractors used in neurologic cases can be Gelpi self-retaining retractors or Weitlaner self-retaining retractors. Another type of self-retaining retractor limited to spinal surgery is a Frasier retractor. Similar in design to a Balfour retractor, the blades are similar to a Weitlaner with multiple blunt prongs fairly long and circular in shape (Figure 3.136).

Figure 3.134 Pnuematic drill for neurologic surgeries.

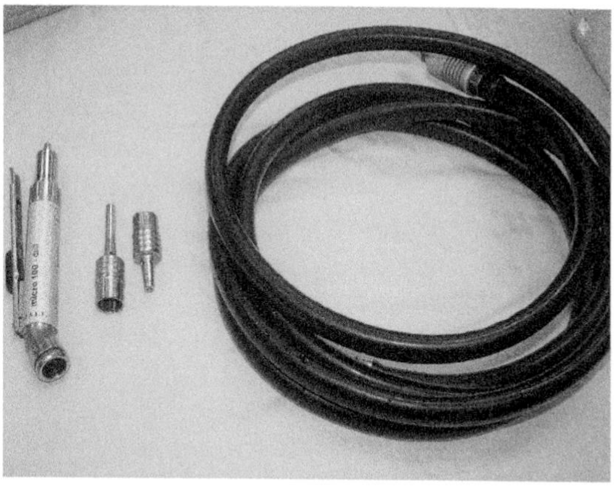

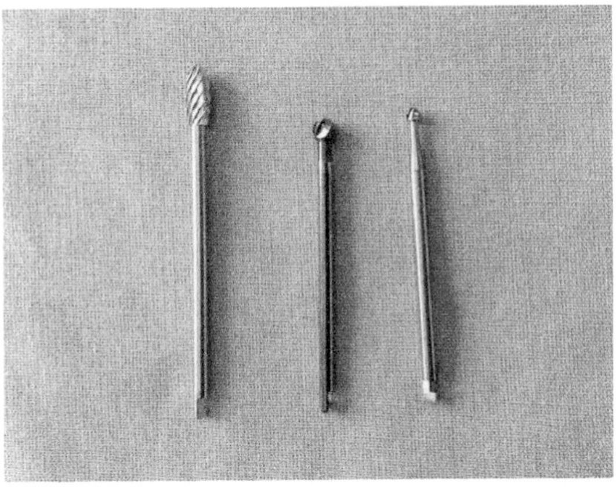

Figure 3.135 Hall drill burs.

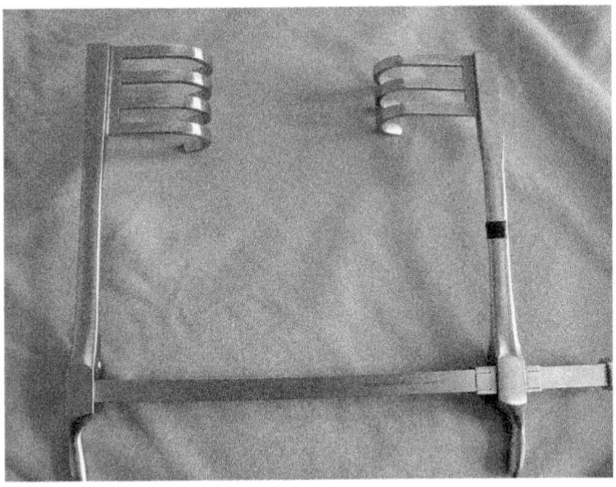

Figure 3.136 Frasier laminectomy retractor.

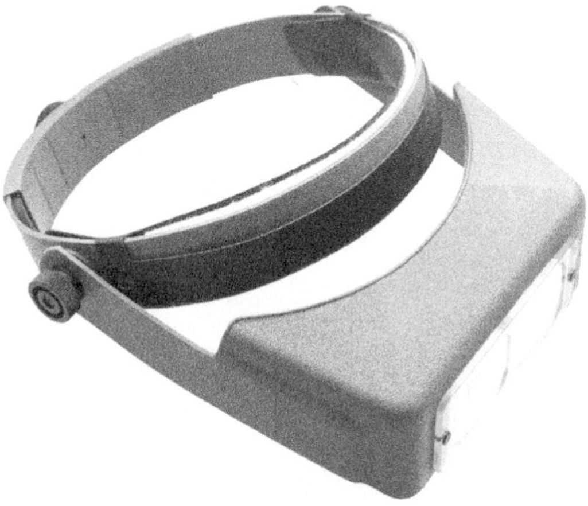

Figure 3.137 Optivisor binocular magnifier. *Source:* Courtesy of Sontec Instruments, Inc. (Cat. # 1103-400).

Ophthalmic magnifying head loops are also beneficial to the surgeon during neurologic surgery. Simple minimal magnification loops are easily available but lighted more powerful eye loops may be the surgeon's choice (Figure 3.137).

Ophthalmic Instrumentation

Ophthalmic instruments are as plentiful as all the other types of instruments. The very basic pieces will permit clinics to perform simple ophthalmic procedures. Speculums designed for use around the eye are very small and light. A Barraquer eye speculum (Figure 3.138) will retract the eyelids to allow exploration of the eye, foreign body removal, flushing, etc. A Castroviejo eye speculum (Figure 3.139) has the capability of adjusting the tension for retraction and is usually better suited for longer procedures. Lacrimal cannulas are employed for flushing when a lacrimal duct is blocked. Cannulas are available in a variety of gauges and can be straight or curved (Figure 3.140). A Jaeger lid plate (Figure 3.141) protects the eyeball when working on the eyelids of a patient. Instruments used during extraocular procedures may be smaller versions of general instruments or modified general instruments to better function with delicate eye tissue. Scissors such as Stevens tenotomy (Figure 3.142) and Iris scissors (Figure 3.143) are commonly used. Iris thumb tissue forceps (Figure 3.144) are often used with extraocular procedures. Intraocular instrumentation is much more delicate, as is necessitated

Figure 3.138 Barraquer wire speculum.
Source: Courtesy of Sontec Instruments, Inc. (Cat. # 10-1005).

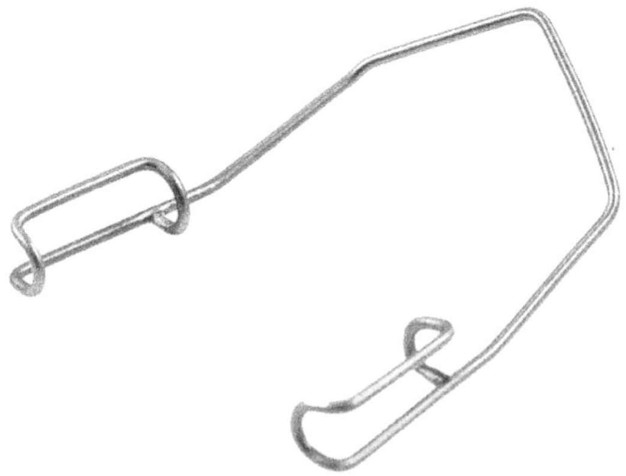

Figure 3.139 Castroviejo eye speculum.
Source: Courtesy of Sontec Instruments, Inc. (Cat. # 10-1703).

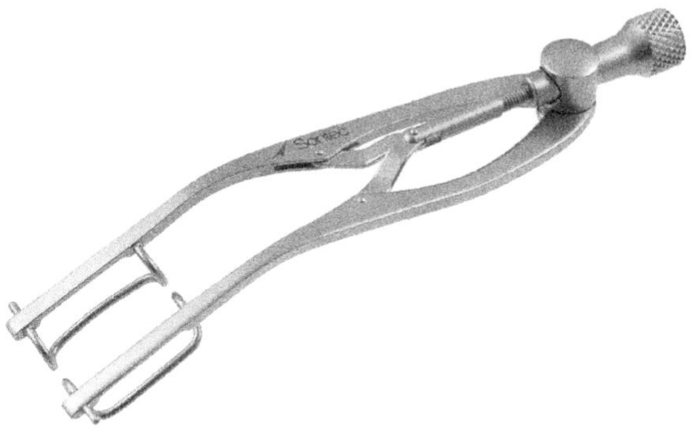

Figure 3.140 Lacrimal cannula.
Source: Courtesy of Sontec Instruments, Inc. (Cat. # 16-3290).

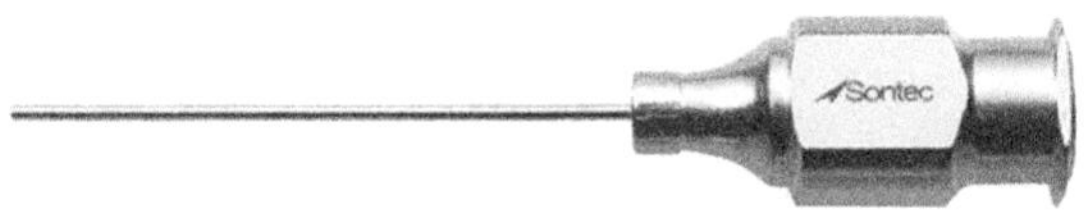

Figure 3.141 Jaeger lid plate.
Source: Courtesy of Sontec Instruments, Inc. (Cat. # 10-4520).

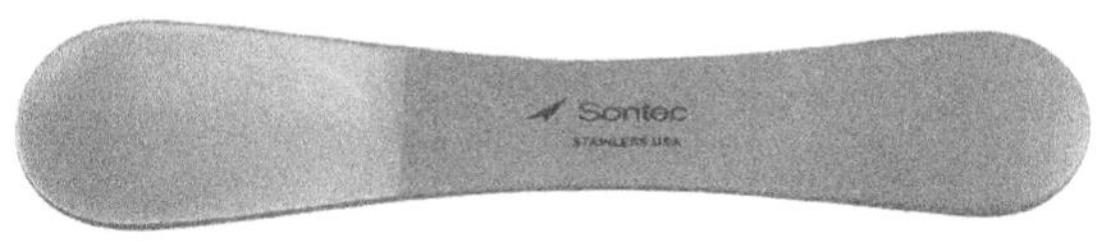

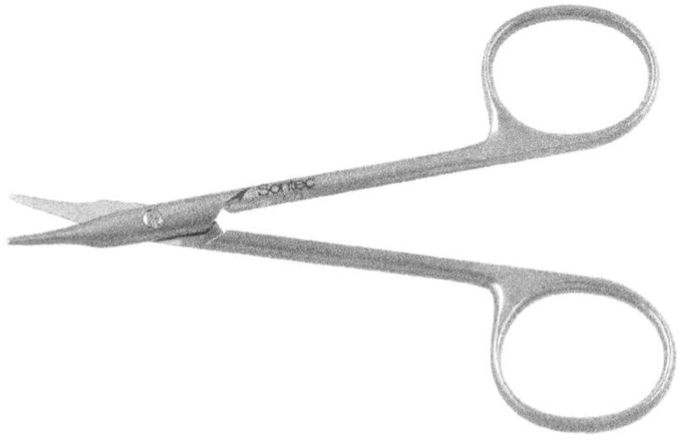

Figure 3.142 Stevens tenotomy scissors. *Source:* Courtesy of Sontec Instruments, Inc. (Cat. # 13-8810).

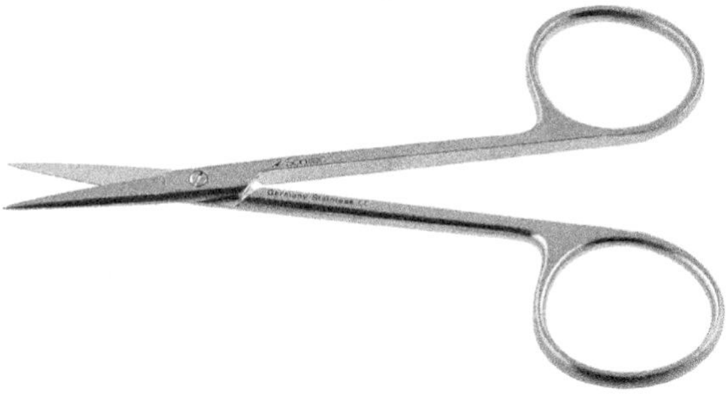

Figure 3.143 Iris scissors. *Source:* Courtesy of Sontec Instruments, Inc. (Cat. # 13-7700).

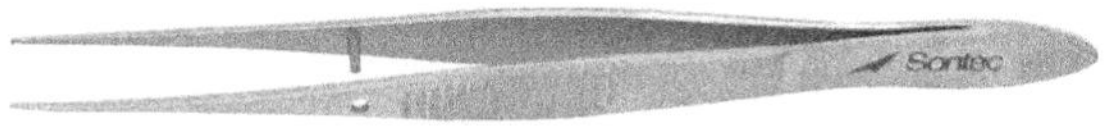

Figure 3.144 Iris 1 × 2 thumb tissue forceps. *Source:* Courtesy of Sontec Instruments, Inc. (Cat. # 14-4440).

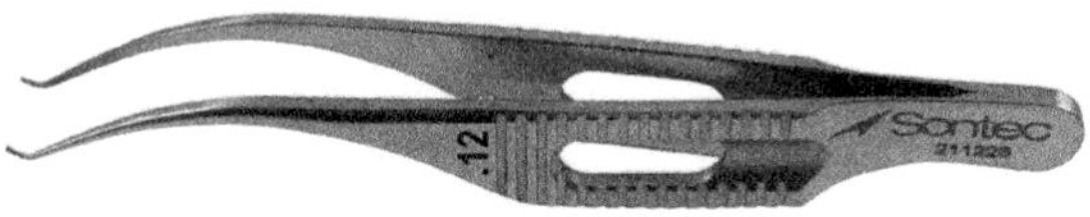

Figure 3.145 Colibri 1× 2 thumb tissue forceps. *Source:* Courtesy of Sontec Instruments, Inc. (Cat. # 14-1800).

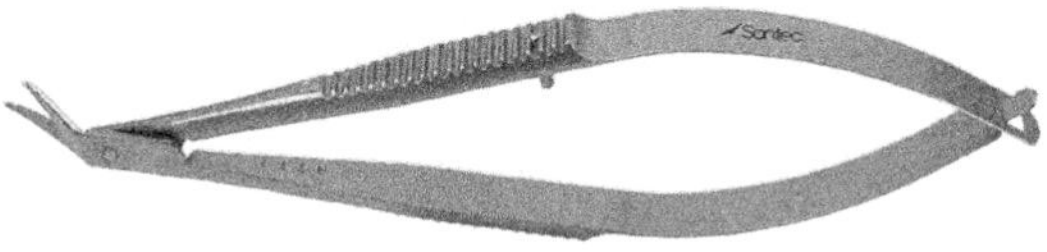

Figure 3.146 Castroviejo corneoscleral scissors. *Source:* Courtesy of Sontec Instruments, Inc. (Cat. # 13-1306).

by the fragile nature of the eye. Colibri thumb tissue forceps (Figure 3.145) and Castroviejo corneoscleral scissors (Figure 3.146) are examples of intra-ocular instruments.

Instrument Cleaning and Care

Proper maintenance of surgical instrumentation falls exclusively to the veterinary surgical technician. The value of the surgical instrument and implant inventory is a significant investment by the practice and requires the utmost care and attention. Knowledge of acceptable cleaning methods, inspection procedures, and required preventative maintenance will significantly affect the performance of the instrument as well as prolong longevity.

Manual Cleaning

Cleaning of surgical instruments should occur immediately after the procedure is finished. Allowing instruments to sit, unattended with blood, saline, and other fluids drying on them will cause great damage to the instruments. The presence of chloride ions from blood, pus, or other secretions will contribute to the corrosion of the instrument. If blood is allowed to sit on an instrument for longer than 20 minutes, the residue will mark and stain the instrument. If immediate cleaning is not possible, the instruments should be placed in a soaking bath of water and enzymatic cleaner. This soaking will permit the cleaner to begin removing the organic debris, thus making manual cleaning easier when time permits. Manual cleaning is performed with a soft bristle brush and a cleaning product approved for surgical instrument use. Cleaning agents such as dishwashing soap are alkaline based and will damage the instrument by pitting or corrosion. Other products commonly used in veterinary practices are chlorhexidine-based solutions or detergents, quaternary ammonium products, and surgeons' hand scrub products. These are examples of agents that will cause spotting and corrosion of the instruments, therefore they SHOULD NOT BE USED! Cleaning products should be neutral in pH (7–8 pH), enzymatic in nature, and designed with the specific use of cleaning surgical instruments (Figure 3.147). Products can be a powder formulation or liquid. When cleaning instruments manually, first rinse the instruments to remove the gross debris. If using a powder, dip the soft bristle brush in the powder and proceed to scrub all surfaces of the instrument including the jaws, serrations, box lock, and ratchet. After thoroughly cleaning, place the instrument in the basket of the ultrasonic cleaner that will be used. The basket should not be in the ultrasonic, but rather sitting in the sink where the instruments are being cleaned. Remaining instruments are cleaned in the same fashion until all are done. Instruments with multiple pieces must be disassembled prior to cleaning to ensure a thorough cleaning. Equipment with a lumen (i.e. suction tips, biopsy instruments, cannulas, etc.) should have a long brush (or pipe cleaner) run through the lumen to remove all gross debris.

Ultrasonic Cleaning

After hand washing, it is essential to follow cleaning the instruments with an ultrasonic cleaner. An ultrasonic cleaner is a device that is used to remove fine particles of debris that may be missed by

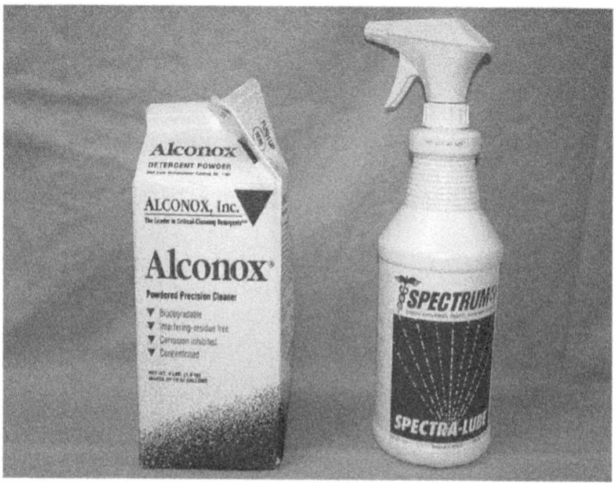

Figure 3.147 Instrument cleaning product and lubricant.

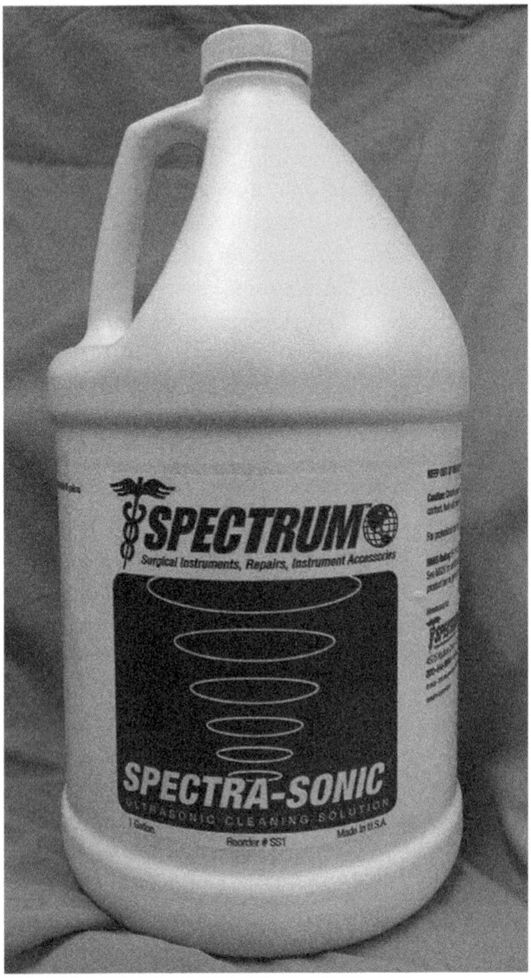

Figure 3.148 Ultrasonic cleaning solution.

other methods of cleaning. The use of cavitation – the physical vibration created by sound waves in a solution – is the premise of ultrasonic cleaning. Minute bubbles are created by the sound waves and as those bubbles come in contact with debris, they implode and remove the debris from its attachment. The debris is suspended in the solution, thereby rendering the instrument clean. The solution in the ultrasonic cleaning should be a neutral pH, ultrasonic-specific agent that has been properly diluted according to manufacturer's instructions (Figure 3.148). Upon dilution of the cleaning solution, the ultrasonic should be run for 10 minutes to "de-gas" the solution and remove pockets of solution. When placing instruments in the ultrasonic, there are a few things to remember:

- Take care to place heaviest instruments in the ultrasonic basket first, with lighter instruments on top.
- Instruments made of different metals (stainless, copper, chrome plated, etc.) should not be put in the same cleaning cycle.
- Instruments should be fully opened when placed in ultrasonic cleaner – box locks opened and ratchets opened.
- Do not overload the cleaner – instruments need plenty of room and should be completely submerged in the cleaning solution (Figure 3.149).

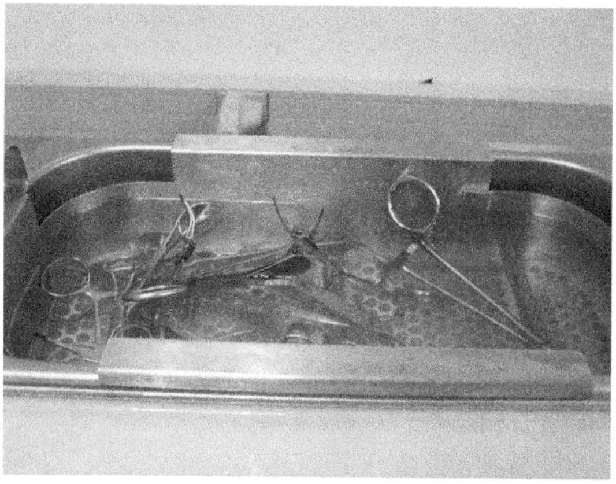

Figure 3.149 Ultrasonic cleaning unit overloaded.

Once loaded, the ultrasonic should be run for no longer than 10 minutes. Cycles longer than 10 minutes have not shown increased efficacy and may result in increased loosening of screws in some instruments. Also, the addition of heat to the ultrasonic tank has not shown additional benefits. Ultrasonic tanks should always be filled to within ½″ from the top and a basket must always be used when the ultrasonic cleaner is running. Solutions should be changed daily or upon appearance of cloudiness. Frequency of refreshing the solutions will depend on surgical caseload. Upon completion of the cycle, the instruments should be removed from the solution immediately and rinsed with distilled water. After being rinsed, the instruments need to be lubricated.

Instruments that cannot be cleaned by submersion in water must still be cleansed before sterilization. Power equipment and accessories cannot be submerged in any solution but must rather be wiped down with a cloth dampened with an instrument cleaning solution. Accompanying hoses must have the full length of the hose wiped down with the cloth as well. Large tabletop plate benders and other big pieces of equipment will also need to be processed with only manual cleaning. Any instrument containing optic fibers (endoscopes, arthroscopes, fiberoptic cables, etc.) must also be manually cleaned very carefully. Delicate handling of the instrument to avoid bumping or hitting the light end on a hard surface is imperative. Scope ends can be gently cleaned with a cotton ball and distilled water to remove any organic debris that may be present. Flexible scopes and light cables must be treated very gingerly and carefully. No bending of the item or abrupt trauma to the casing should occur.

Delicate ophthalmic or neurologic instruments can be manually cleaned and then processed in the ultrasonic cleaner, but should always be washed separately from other heavier instruments. The delicate nature of the instruments may necessitate reducing the ultrasonic time to 5 minutes.

Instrument Lubrication

Instrument lubrication, often referred to as "instrument milk," should be used after every cleaning. Instruments need to have all moving parts lubricated after every cleaning to keep them moving freely and to help eliminate rubbing and scraping against each other. Especially important are the box lock and ratchets. If the box lock is sticky while the surgeon is using it, after the instrument is cleaned, spray the box lock with lubricant and move the shafts of the instrument back and forth to aid in having the lubricant penetrate deeply into the joint. Only water-based lubricants, intended for surgical instruments, should be used (Figure 3.150). Mineral oil, WD-40, or other industrial lubricants are NOT to be used on surgical instruments. Current recommendation for lubricant

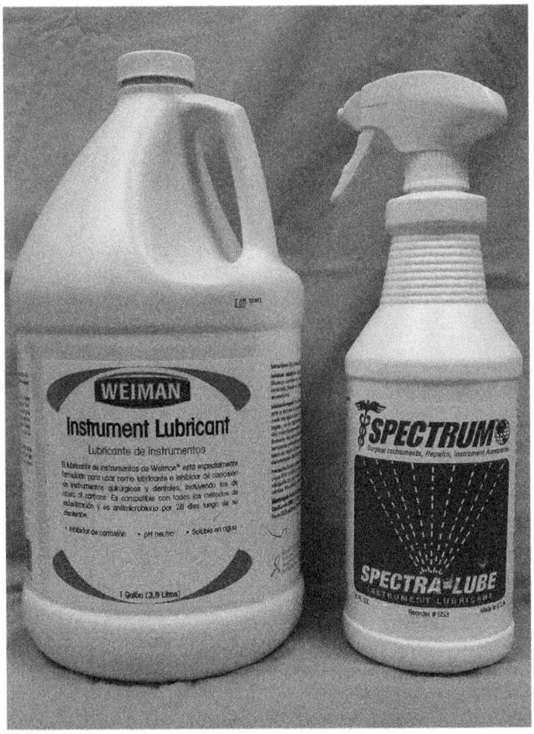

Figure 3.150 Instrument lubricant.

application is to spray it on rather than submersion in a bath. Lubricant baths may have been contaminated with bacteria from other instruments and may be left unchanged long after the recommended expiration of the solution. Spray-on lubricant is less expensive, easier to apply, and requires less storage/use space.

Instrument Maintenance

After cleaning and lubricating, but before packaging, each instrument must be inspected for appropriate function and condition. Certain types of instruments require more attention and maintenance than others. Scissors, for instance, are designed to be re-sharpened. After each use, the scissors should be opened and closed to ensure a smooth, gliding action between the blades. Any catching or rubbing indicates the need for repair. Scissor blade tips should be inspected for burrs or corrosion. Blades should be evaluated for chips, burrs, or cracks on the cutting edge. Screws in the hinge of the scissors should be inspected for retained debris and for cracks near the screw head. Ring handles should be inspected for cracks as well. Testing for sharpness may be accomplished by using commercially available test material for various lengths of scissors. Testing consists of making multiple cuts in the test material. On the last cut, the scissors are extracted. If there is no pinching or grabbing of the material, the scissors are sharp. If the scissors are not sharp, they will pull on the material. These scissors need to be sent to a qualified instrument repair company for sharpening. Stainless steel scissors will have the entire blade sharpened. Scissors that have a tungsten carbide insert cannot have the insert replaced or sharpened, but are sharper and stronger to begin with so will ultimately last longer than stainless blades.

Needle holders are another type of instrument that need special attention. The jaws need to be inspected for worn, cracking, or missing inserts and chipped or worn edges. If the jaws are smooth, close the ratchets all the way and look at a light through the jaw of the instrument. If light can be seen between the jaws, the instrument needs to be repaired. Jaws will wear out with normal suturing, so assessing the degree of wear is required after every use. The box lock should be inspected for cracking. Shanks should be straight, not bowed or angled. The ratchet action should be smooth and tight. Once closed, the teeth should not become disengaged until intentionally done.

Thumb tissue forceps should have the tips evaluated for proper teeth interdigitation if teeth are present. Edges of the tips should also be properly aligned. Hemostatic forceps must have the tips evaluated for wear, edge alignment, and ratchet security. Ratchets closed to the first position can be gently tapped on a hard surface. If the ratchet remains closed, the instrument is still in good functional status. If the ratchet pops open, the instrument needs to be sent in for repair.

Pack Preparation

Assembling packs for wrapping and subsequent sterilization is a detailed and important process that must be done meticulously to guarantee that the equipment the surgeon is expecting to be in the pack is actually there. When packing an instrument pack, it is often very helpful to have a checklist of items that belong in the pack. As the instruments are placed in the pack, they can be checked off on the sheet to show that the assembler did place the item in the pack. The checklist can be folded and placed inside the pack for use by the sterile person for an instrument count when the pack is opened. All instruments in a pack must have the ratchets open, the box locks open, and packed with enough room to allow circulation of the steam, gas, or plasma to touch all the surfaces of the instruments. This requires 3 mm of space between each instrument. Instrument racks that allow stacking of the instruments are the best option for achieving these requirements. Instrument rings can also be used, but because they only pass through one ring handle, the instruments are left hanging open with little support. Instrument stringers are designed to pass through both ring handles of the instrument, thereby keeping things neat and orderly. These devices lock closed so there is no chance of the instruments being dislodged during sterilization/handling (Figure 3.151). When placing instruments on the instrument-holding device, it is best to stack them from longest to shortest with the straight instruments first, followed by the curved instruments, with the curves up. If there are enough devices available, using two (one for straight instruments and one for curved instruments) is a nice option. Towel clamps should be placed on a separate device, with the non-penetrating towels on the bottom and the penetrating towel clamps on top since they will be used first.

Often metal trays or pans are used to contain the instruments in the pack. Metal trays/pans must have holes in the bottom of the pan to assist with adequate steam penetration during the sterilization cycle.

Folding linens for placement in a pack is very important skill. All cloth gowns and drapes need to be inspected before being used in a pack. The technician should check to see if there are any holes or worn spots on the gown or drape. Defective items are not allowed to be placed in surgical packs. Items should be inspected for lint, stray threads, or hair, and any debris should be removed before they are placed in a pack. If the items have a water-resistant property, there should be a grid

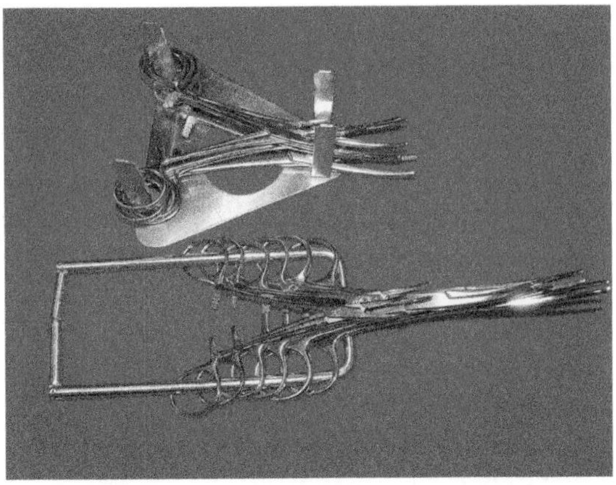

Figure 3.151 Holders for instruments in packs.

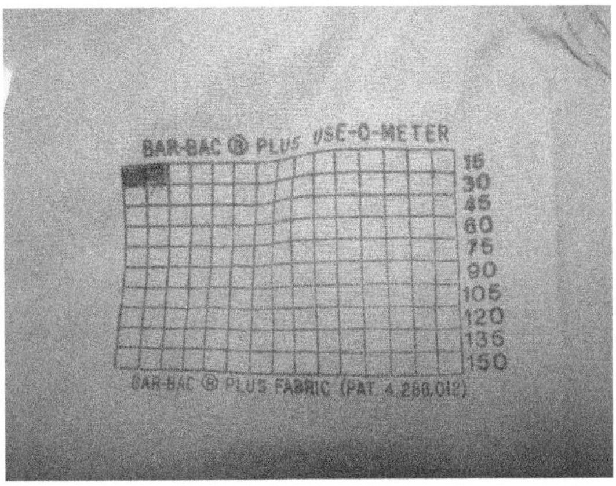

Figure 3.152 Washing grid on gown.

in one of the corners of the item (Figure 3.152). This grid is intended to track the number of uses of the items to ensure maximum water-resistant properties. Each time the item is used in a pack, one of the grid squares must be filled in with permanent marker. Once the grid is full, the item should be removed from use. Items must be folded in the same manner consistently so that those using the items in the pack will be familiar with what to expect. There are many ways to fold a gown, but the simpler the better. It is important to fold the gown so that the person putting the gown on will be able to recognize where their hands may or may not go to avoid contaminating the gown. Non-sterile back, or standard gowns, are used frequently in veterinary clinics. While providing a sterile field when facing the surgical table, the biggest disadvantage to this type of gown is that the back is not sterile. This significantly impacts the potential for movement of the sterile personnel in the room as well as limits the surgeon to only have surgical instrumentation on the instrument table. In the case of a fracture or other involved cases, back tables are often used for placement of sterile items. Without a sterile back gown, this scenario is impossible. Figures 3.153–3.159 shows the method for folding this type of gown. Wraparound gowns are a much better choice for all surgeries, especially for procedures that will involve using additional tables for equipment that will be located behind the surgical field.

Whether a hospital chooses to use cloth or paper surgical drapes, a process for folding must be established. It is important that the drapes are easy to unfold and aseptically placed on the patient.

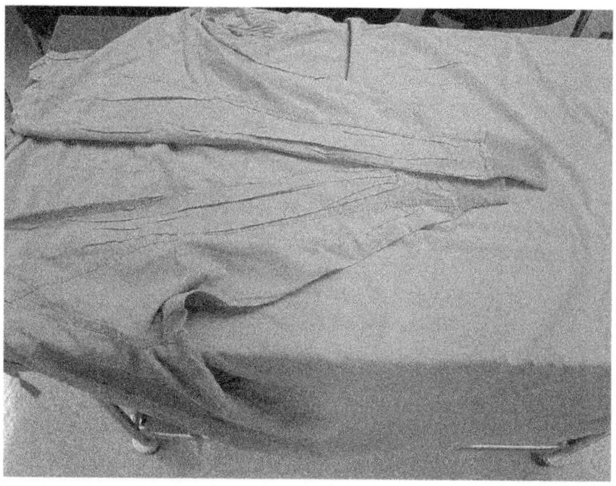

Figure 3.153 Lay the gown out on the table with the outside of the gown facing the ceiling and the neck of the gown to the left. Sleeves should be folded into the center of the gown.

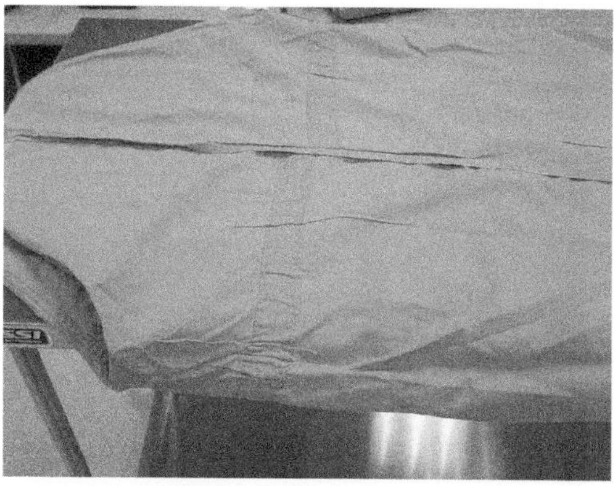

Figure 3.154 Grasping the seamed edge of the gown closest to the folder, fold the body of the gown up over the sleeves to the center of the gown. Reach over the gown and fold the opposite side in the same fashion.

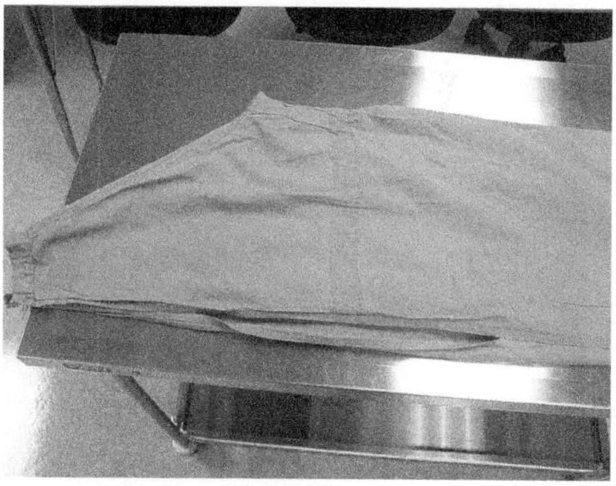

Figure 3.155 Pick up all layers of the neck with the left hand and all layers of the hem of the gown with the right hand and lift the gown into the air. The gown will fold in half. Lay the gown down on the table with the neck to the left and the raw edges of the gown facing the folder.

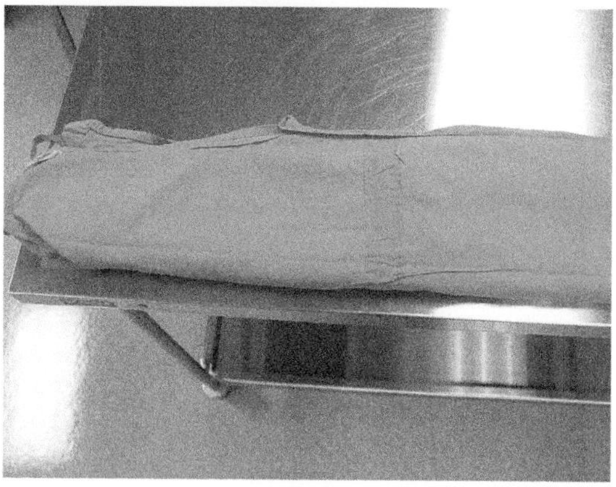

Figure 3.156 Picking up the edges closest to the folder, fold the gown in half lengthwise with the raw edges winding up away from the folder.

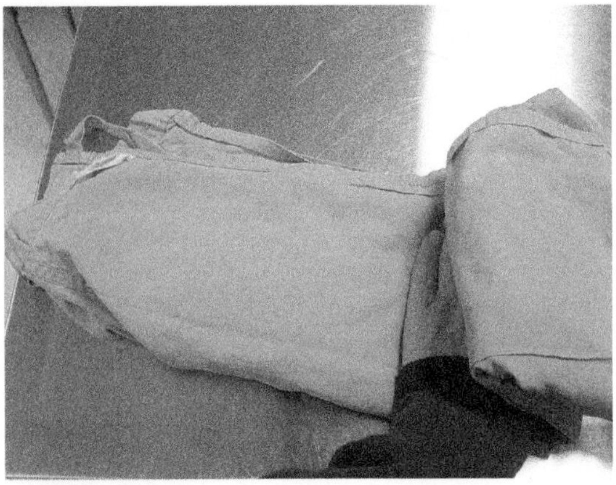

Figure 3.157 Place the left hand at the armhole of the sleeve, slide the right hand under the body of the gown, and fold the gown body up over the left hand.

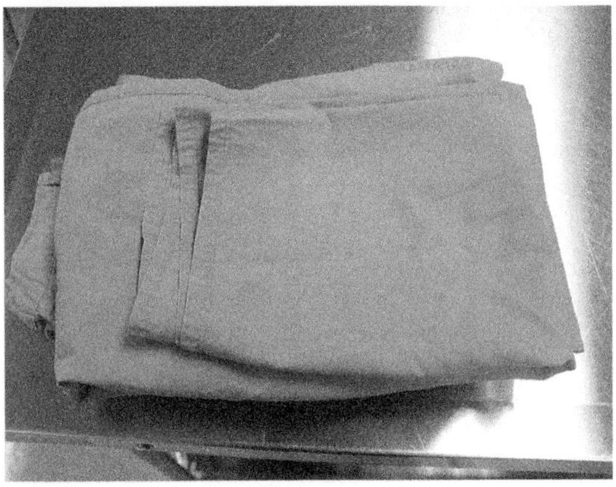

Figure 3.158 Continue the accordion folding until all of the body of the gown is folded.

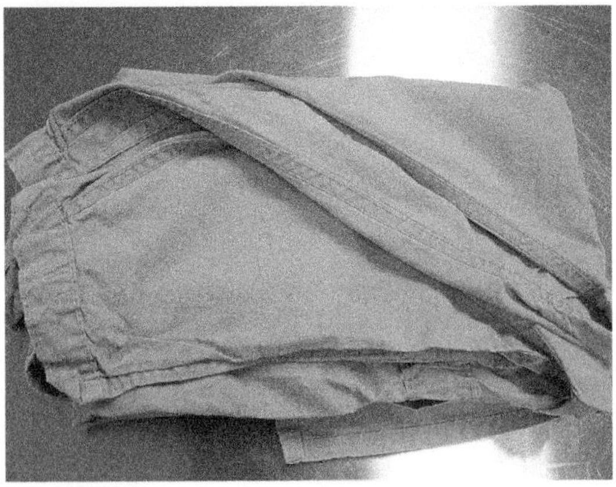

Figure 3.159 Turn the gown over so the seams of the armholes are found diagonally across the gown.

If paper drapes are used, it must not be a challenge for the surgeon to identify the area of the drape that will need to be cut to create the fenestration. Often surgeons will use "huck" towels or ground drapes. These drapes are used first on the patient as a primary layer and must be folded in a manner that facilitates easy opening and placement. Whether ground drapes, large paper drapes, or large cloth drapes are used, all folding should be identical. Figures 3.160–3.164 provides instruction on a folding option for all drape styles (Figures 3.160–3.164).

Figure 3.160 Folding the hand towel starts with laying the towel out on the table horizontally with the finished seam facing the ceiling. Grasp the long edge of the towel closest to the folder and bring it to the top of the towel, folding the towel in half.

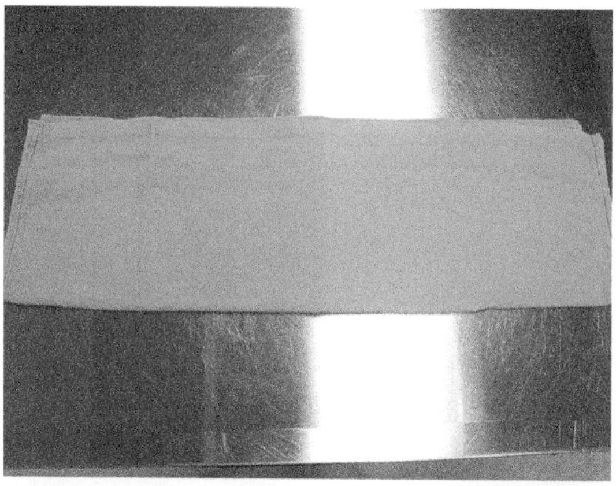

Figure 3.161 Grasp the top raw edge and fold it down so the towel is folded in half.

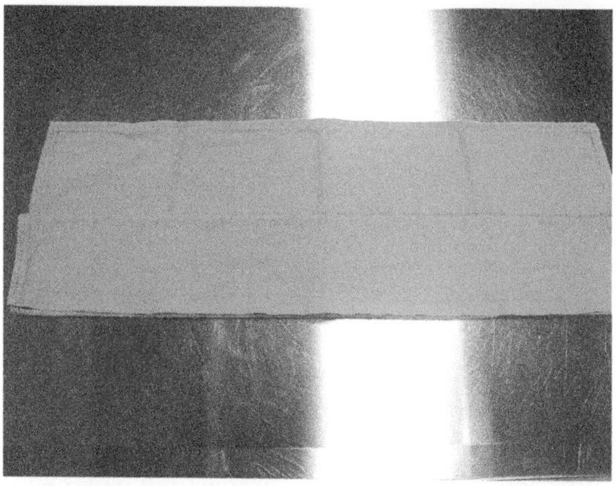

Figure 3.162 Pick up the towel on either short side to allow the bottom half of the towel to fold underneath.

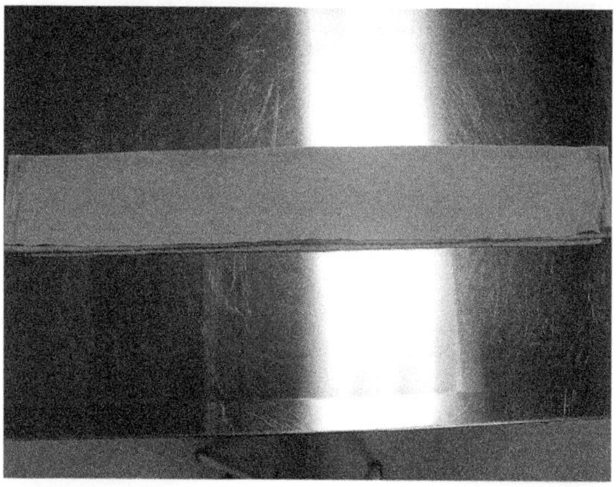

Figure 3.163 Fold the towel in half horizontally. Grasp the top two layers of the towel and fold it back on itself.

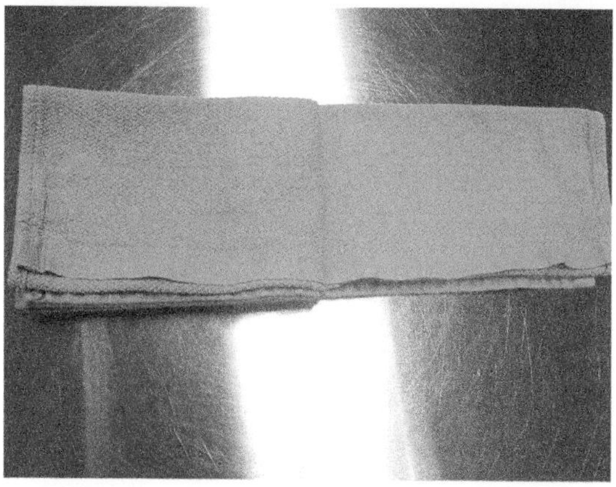

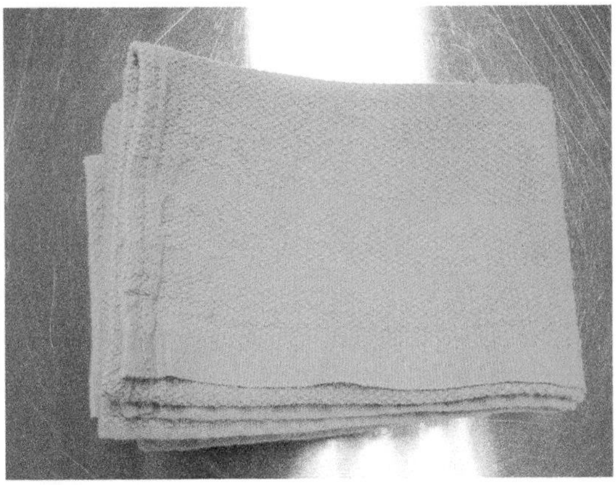

Figure 3.164 Pick up the towel so the bottom half folds underneath.

Pack Wrapping and Instrument Packaging

Unless being flash sterilized or chemically sterilized, all instruments and equipment required for surgery must be wrapped prior to sterilization. Instrument packs should be wrapped with either cloth or paper surgical wraps. Currently, there are no specific standards for cloth wrappers, but commercially available products are adequate. Cloth wrappers may be a greater initial cost to the hospital, but with life expectancies of around 50 washes, it will be more economical in the long run. Cloth wraps are more durable than paper wrappers and are not subject to the minute tears or trauma that can happen so easily with paper. Some manufacturers provide a use grid near a seam which allows for one square to be filled in each time the wrapper is washed. Once the grid is filled, the wrapper should be retired from use. Wrappers should be washed after every use to re-hydrate the material. Minimal soap and an additional rinse cycle are encouraged when washing surgical linens. Wrappers should be inspected after each washing to check for holes, areas of thinness, or other imperfections which would compromise the sterility of the item. Paper wrappers are also available to be used to wrap surgery packs. Paper wrappers should only be used once due to the high risk of trauma and subsequent sub-par performance. Paper may be less expensive initially, but only using them once will increase the overall cost. Peel packs are available for single instrument or small pack packaging and sterilization. Peel packs are plastic on one side and paper on the other. Peel packaging is available in pre-cut sizes as well as on the roll for more custom packaging (Figure 3.165). If using the pre-cut sizes, it is important to use a package large enough to comfortably hold the item without giving it too much room to move around. There should be about 1″ of space between the end of the instrument and the peel pack seal. Whenever placing an item in a peel pack, the ratchets should be opened, box lock opened, and the handle end of the instrument should be placed in the package first so the handles are by the end that is opened. If sharp tips are present on the instrument or piece of equipment, protective tips should be placed over the sharp end (Figure 3.166). Vinyl protective tips can be fenestrated or not. Items such as spinal needles, IM pins, and Gelpi self-retaining retractors are all examples of the types of instruments that should have a protective tip. Indicator strips are still required when using peel packages. After placing the item and indicator in the peel pack, the bottom edge is folded up and then the adhesive strip cover is removed. The adhesive edge is now folded up to seal the pack. It is not

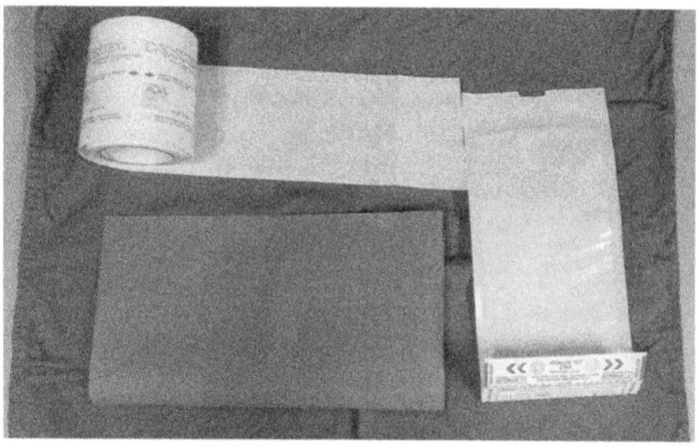

Figure 3.165 Peel packing options.

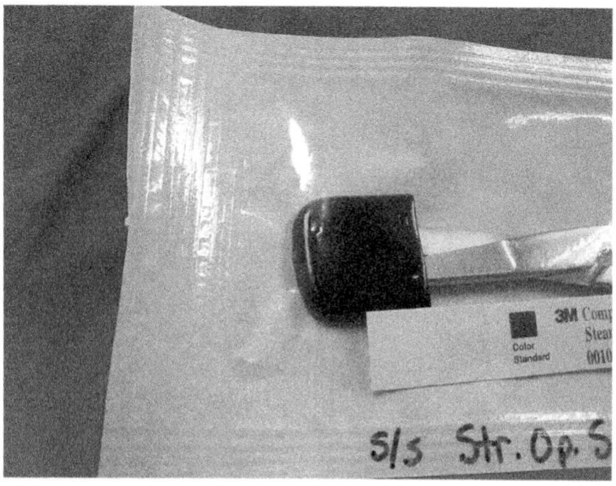

Figure 3.166 Protective end cap over sharp instrument; notice multiple seals on end due to thin sealing line.

acceptable to have folds or wrinkles in the seal (Video 3.6). When writing on the peel pack, information should only be written on the plastic side or on the seal that is over the plastic. Writing on the back paper side of the package permits migration of bacteria as the paper is a porous surface. If using the roll product, a heat sealer will also be needed. Peel packages should NEVER be sealed with paper clips, staples, tape, or other closure devices. A heat sealer will melt the plastic side into the paper side thereby creating a seal. If the heat sealer creates a very thin seal, multiple seals will be needed to ensure that the integrity of the package is maintained. If multiple items are to be packaged in the peel pack, double packing is indicated. Foremost, it makes it easier for the sterile person to grab a single package as opposed to multiple pieces. Second, it provides greater barriers to contamination and provides a stronger package for the items. The inside package should be placed film (plastic) side to film side to allow proper sterilization and visualization of the item inside. Double-peel pack items should have the inside item fit comfortably in the outer pack. Inside peel packs should not be folded. Extremely heavy items (i.e. osteotomes, mallets, curettes, etc.) should not be packaged in peel pack material as they will break through the paper. These types of items should be double wrapped in cloth wrappers. Items that are sterilized in a plasma sterilizer must have packaging specific to that system. Due to the nature of the sterilization process, no packaging products can be of organic nature.

Methods of Wrapping Packs

There are two main methods to employ when wrapping instrument packs or equipment for sterilization – the envelope style and the horizontal (or square) style. The envelope style is better suited for packs that will be held while being opened, or when placed on a surface to be opened, it is not important to cover the entire surface with a sterile field (i.e. gown packs). Wrapping packs using the horizontal style is generally reserved for packs that are very large, heavy, or long (plate sets, large instrument packs, etc.). When unwrapping horizontally wrapped packs, the packs are usually placed on a surface or table, and then as the packs are unwrapped, a sterile field that completely covers the table is created. Figures 3.167–3.172 show the procedure for wrapping packs using the diamond method (Figures 3.167–3.172 and Video 3.7). Figures 3.173–3.177 shows the procedure for wrapping packs using the horizontal method.

Any pack that is to be sterilized (using any method of sterilization) must have the correct information on the label. Using a black permanent marker is best when writing on the packs as pencil and ballpoint pen tend to fade drastically when steam sterilized, thereby making the label unreadable. Information on the pack label should include the date of sterilization, the size of the item wrapped (e.g. large), the name of the item wrapped, the autoclave and load numbers, and finally, the initials of the person making the pack. An explanation of the autoclave and load numbers will occur in the sterilization section (Figure 3.178).

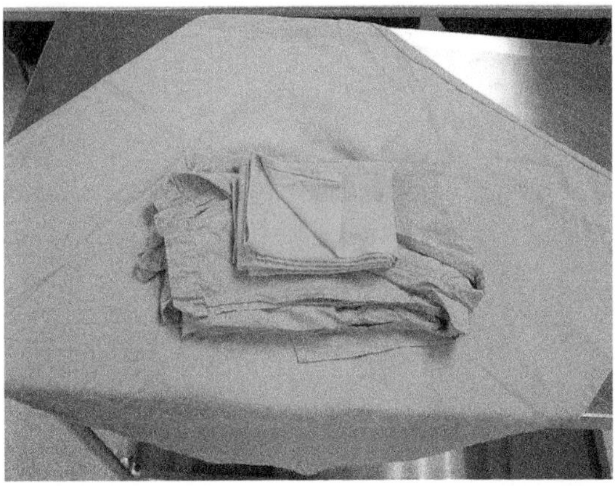

Figure 3.167 Lay the wrapper out on the table in a diamond formation to wrap a pack in the envelope style. Place the items for pack on the wrapper in this order: gown first, then sterilization indicator, and then hand towel.

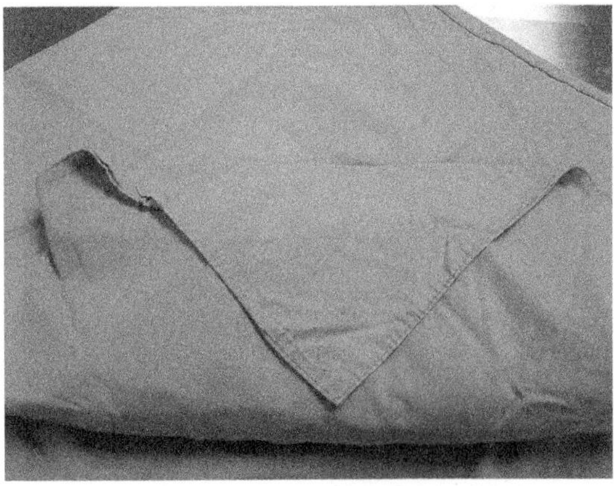

Figure 3.168 Grasp the point of the wrapper closest to the folder and fold it over the pack, then back on itself to form a "dog ear."

Figure 3.169 Grasp the point of the wrapper on either side and fold it over the items, and then back on itself to form another "dog ear."

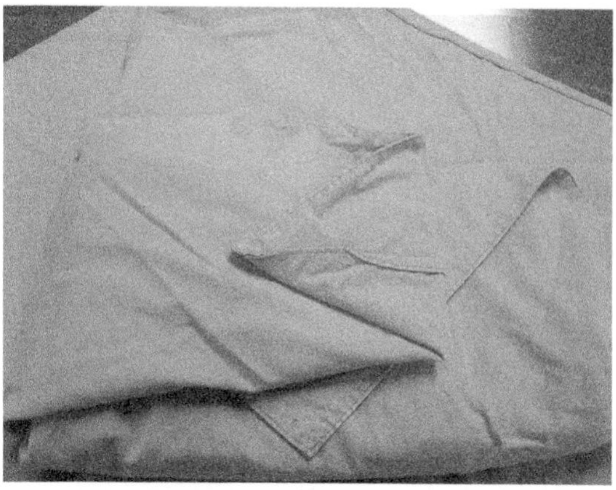

Figure 3.170 Grasp the point of the wrapper on the opposite side. Fold the wrapper over the pack and then again back onto itself to form a "dog ear."

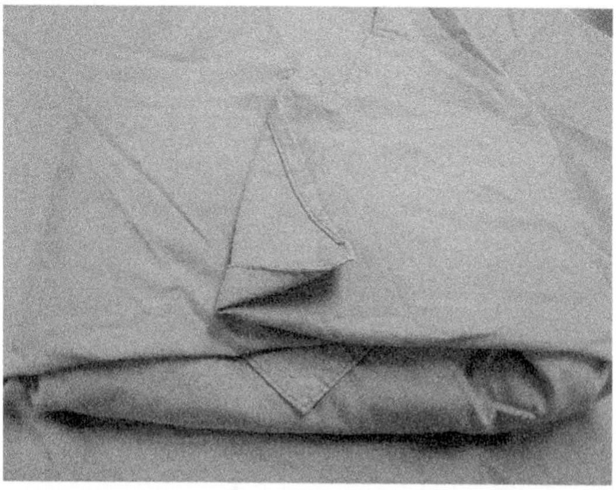

Figure 3.171 Grasp the final point of the wrapper, fold in the extra material, fold it over the pack, and tuck it into the pack.

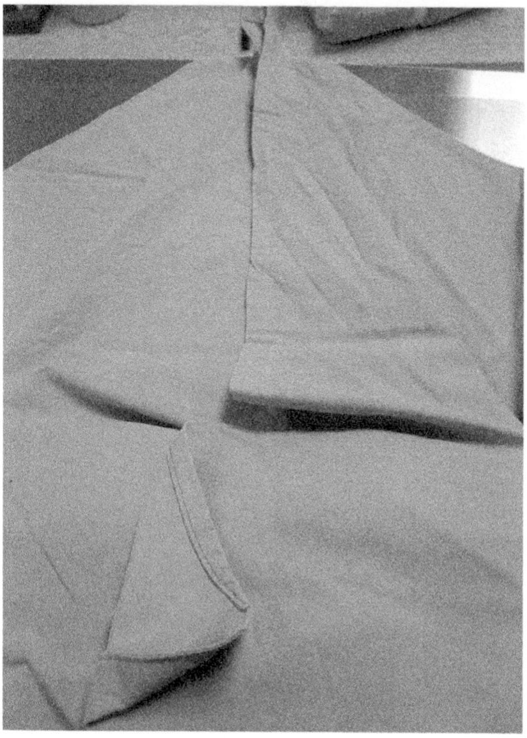

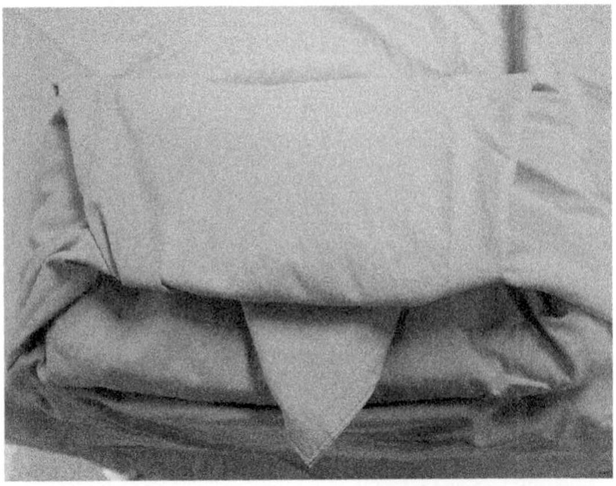

Figure 3.172 Repeat the wrapping with a second wrapper. Label the pack with the required information.

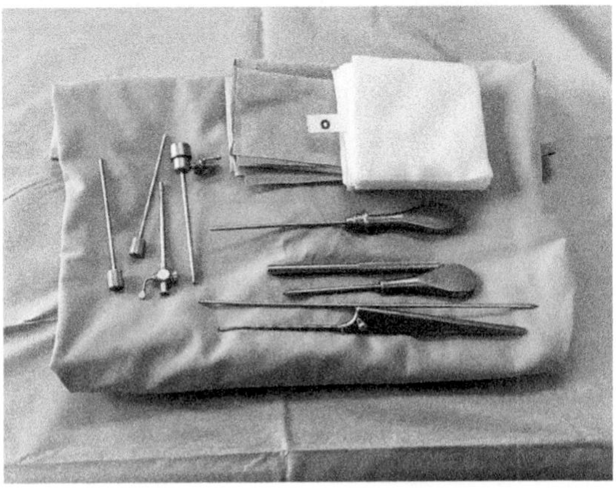

Figure 3.173 Items in center of wrap for horizontal wrapping method.

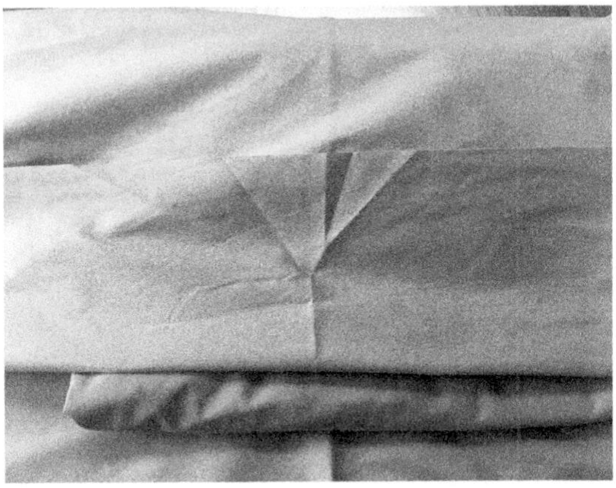

Figure 3.174 Farthest long edge of wrapper is folded over items and then back on itself to form a "dog ear."

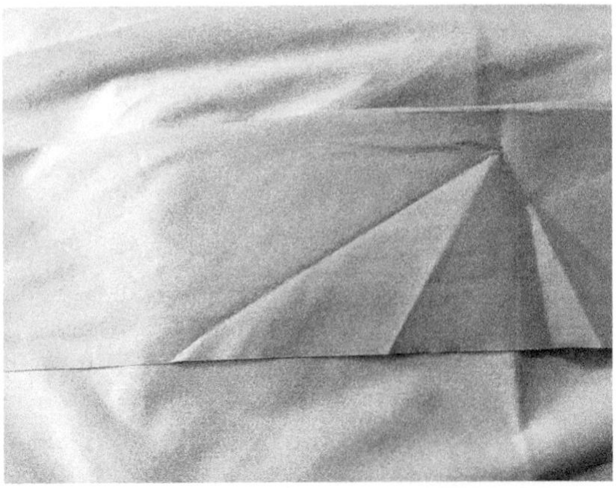

Figure 3.175 Closest long edge is folded over items and folded back on itself.

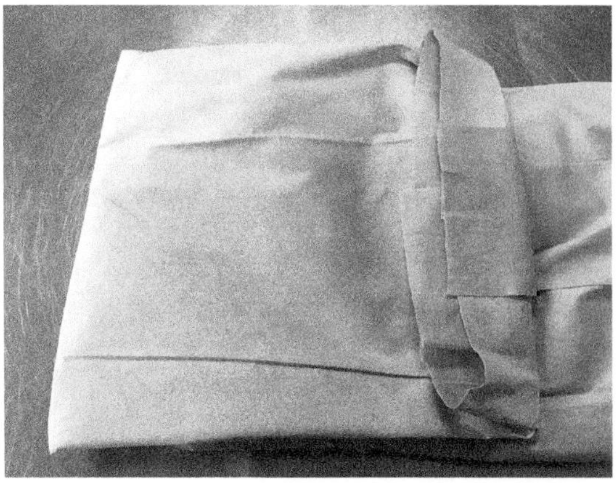

Figure 3.176 Side edge is folded over items and folded back on itself for a dog ear.

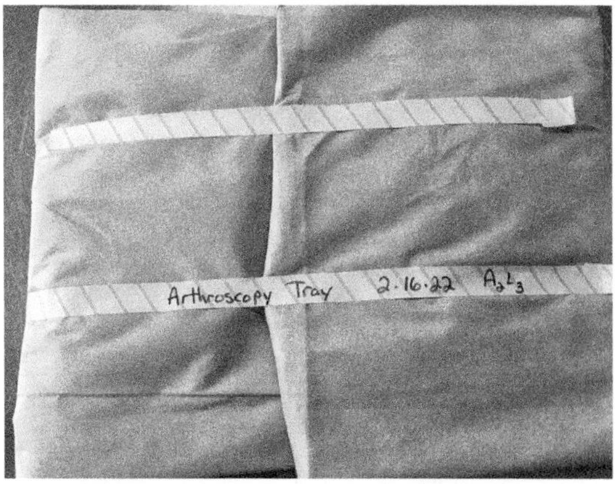

Figure 3.177 Opposite side edge is folded over and secured with tape.

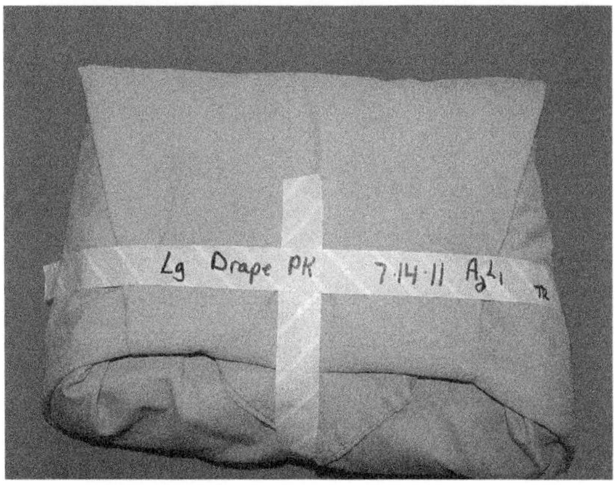

Figure 3.178 Properly labeled drape pack.

Sterilization

Sterilization is the process of using either physical or chemical means to kill all microorganisms on an item. There are a variety of options for sterilizing instruments and equipment for use in surgical cases. The method chosen will depend on availability, the operator's familiarity with the method of sterilization, the window of time available to sterilize the equipment, and the type of equipment that needs to be sterilized.

Chemical

The two most commonly used chemical, high-level disinfectants are *ortho*-phthalaldehyde solution and activated glutaraldehyde. Effective sterilization depends not only on the age of the solution but also on the dilution and the amount of organic material present. Solutions >2% and buffered to a pH solution of 7.5–8.5 have been shown to kill vegetative bacteria in less than 2 minutes. Fungi and viruses have been killed in <10 minutes and certain spores are killed in 3 hours. Strict monitoring of the solution is required to achieve the intended result. Solutions are approved for use for up to 14 days, but should be monitored before each use with a testing strip to ensure appropriate strength (Figure 3.179).

Either product is effective for high-level disinfection of devices and lensed equipment such as endoscopes, arthroscopes, and cameras when other options are not available. A container with a removable tray is used for manual processing of the equipment (Figure 3.180). High-level

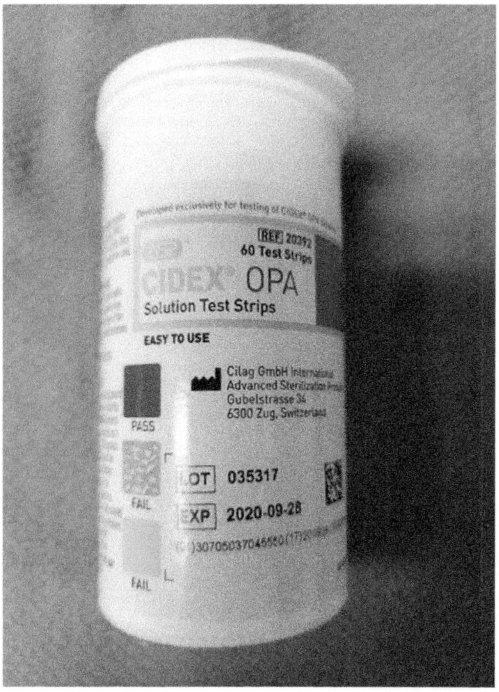

Figure 3.179 Testing strips for chemical high-level disinfectant.

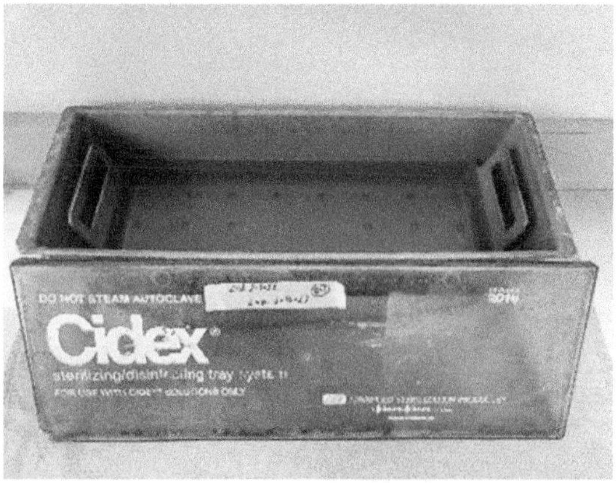

Figure 3.180 High-level disinfectant immersion tray.

Figure 3.181 Rinsing postimmersion.

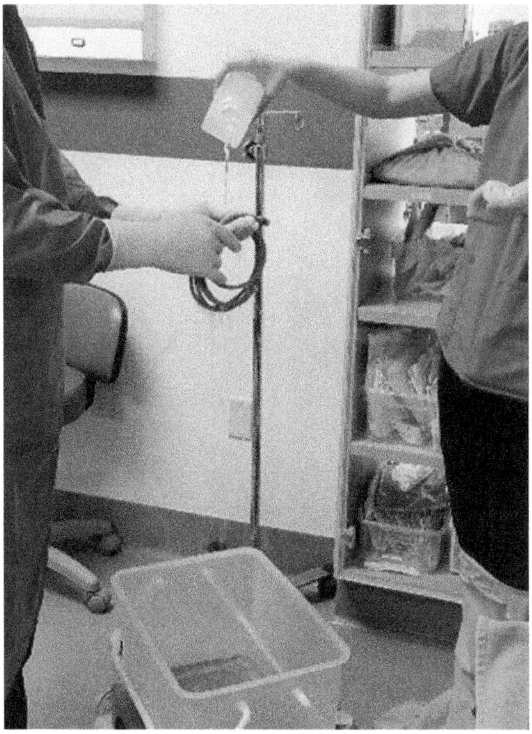

disinfection is achieved when equipment is immersed in the solution at 68 °F (20° C) for at least 12 minutes, provided a test strip confirms acceptable concentration for use. Upon completion of immersion, products must be rinsed with sterile water before contacting viable tissue (Figure 3.181). Surgeons collecting the items from the immersion tray should double glove to protect the gloves that will be worn for the surgery. These chemicals are a potential irritant to the eyes, nose, and skin so protective gloves (nitrile not latex), eye protection, and a respirator should be worn when working with this chemical. Disposal of the solution may be restricted by some municipal sewer systems, but neutralization with sodium bisulfate will render it safe for disposal.

Steam

Sterilizing instruments or equipment with a steam sterilizer, or autoclave, is the most common method of sterilization that is used in veterinary clinics and hospitals. Most surgical instruments and equipment are designed to withstand autoclaving. Items that are electric, fiberoptic, plastic, rubber, or other similar material are not to be steam sterilized. Steam sterilization requires three parameters to be met to consider items sterilized. Those three parameters are time, temperature, and pressure. If all three parameters are not met, it should be presumed that sterilization did not occur. There are two types of steam autoclaves – gravity displacement and vacuum assisted (Figure 3.182). With the gravity displacement autoclaves, as the steam enters the chamber, it pushes the air, or displaces it, out of the chamber, usually through the drain in the bottom of the chamber. The injection of superheated steam using pressure then allows for the penetration of the steam into the items in the chamber. Sterilization, or killing of the microorganisms, then occurs. At the end of the sterilization cycle, the steam and pressure are removed from the chamber, known as the venting portion of the cycle. The dry time portion of the cycle allows dry heat to dry the items in the autoclave but does not cool them. When the pressure reading reaches 0 psi, it is safe to

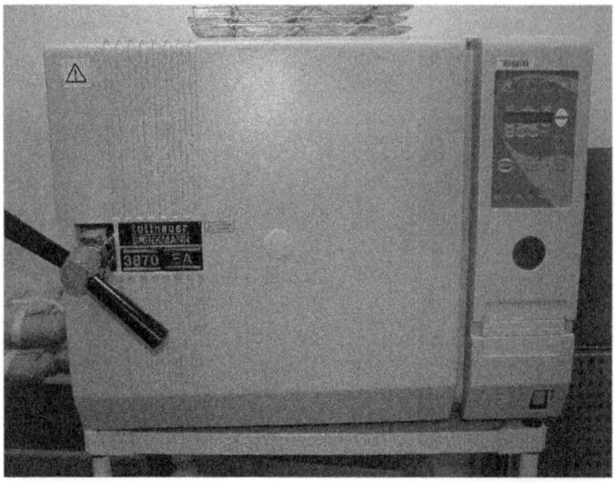

Figure 3.182 One style of autoclave.

open the autoclave. To avoid the possibility of burns, the operator should always stand behind the door of the machine as it is opened in the event the residual steam in the chamber escapes. The door should only be opened 1–2″ to allow gradual cooling. The door should be left ajar for approximately 15 minutes before the packs are handled. When cooled sufficiently to allow safe handling, the packs are removed and placed on cooling racks to allow for full drying and cooling. When completely cool and dry, the packs can be placed into storage.

The vacuum-assisted autoclave has the same parameters that must be met. The main difference in machine operation is that with a vacuum sterilizer, the steam is forced into the chamber which results in faster penetration of the packs. Similarly, at the end of the cycle, the vacuum evacuates the steam from the chamber resulting in faster removal of moisture creating packs that are less wet. Cooling of items in the autoclave should be the same process as described for gravity displacement machines. Items sterilized by steam sterilization may be wrapped in cloth, paper, or peel pack pouches.

Recommended sterilization cycle times depend on the type of machine being used, whether or not the items to be sterilized are wrapped or not, and the type of item being sterilized. Table 3.9 shows recommended cycle parameters. Pressure settings for sterilization cycles are inherent within the machine and will offer no option for altering the setting. It is important for the veterinary technician to be aware of what the expected pressures should be in the event the machine malfunctions. While these are recommended temperature, time, and pressure settings, it is important that autoclave manufacturer and equipment manufacturer instructions be read in the event different settings are required.

A unique sterilization option available only for steam sterilization is immediate-use sterilization. This used to be called "flash" sterilization, however, that term is not appropriate, so immediate-use sterilization is now the accepted terminology. Immediate-use sterilization is an option that should be reserved for only emergency situations where an instrument had been dropped during a procedure and needs to be re-sterilized. Ideally, inventory would be such that re-sterilization is not necessary, but realistically that may not be the case. Items to be sterilized for immediate use should undergo the same rigorous cleaning process prior to sterilization. Only gravity displacement autoclaves are used for this cycle. Recommended sterilization times are 3 minutes at 270 °F for metal or non-porous items, or items without a lumen. Instruments with a lumen or made of a more porous material (plastic and rubber) should have a sterilization cycle of 10 minutes. These items are not wrapped, so no dry time is needed. Once the sterilization cycle is complete, the circulating nurse can open the autoclave to allow the steam to escape.

Table 3.9 Sterilization guidelines.

Type of machine	Item being sterilized	Wrapped or unwrapped	Temperature	Time	Dry time	Pressure settings
Gravity displacement	Instruments	Wrapped	250 °F (121 °C)	30 min	15–30 min	15 psi
			270 °F (132 °C)	15 min	15–30 min	30 psi
	Textiles	Wrapped	250 °F (121 °C)	30 min	15 min	15 psi
			270 °F (132 °C)	25 min	15 min	30 psi
	Non-porous items only (i.e. routine metal instruments, and no lumens)	Unwrapped	270 °F (132 °C)	3 min	None	30 psi
	Nonporous and porous items (e.g. rubber or plastic items, items with lumens) sterilized together	Unwrapped	270 °F (132 °C)	10 min	none	30 psi
Pre-vacuum	Instruments	Wrapped	270 °F (132 °C)	4 min	20–30 min	30 psi
	Non-porous items only (i.e. routine metal instruments and no lumens)	Unwrapped	270 °F (132 °C)	4 min	None	30 psi
	Non-porous and porous items (e.g. rubber or plastic items and items with lumens) sterilized together	Unwrapped	270 °F (132 °C)	4 min	none	30 psi
	Textiles	Wrapped	270 °F (132 °C)	4 min	5–20 min	30 psi

While that occurs, the circulator should open sterile hand towels and don sterile gloves. Using the towels to grab the instrument and cover as best as possible, the item should be transported immediately to the operating room. The item will be hot, so care should be taken to avoid burns while handling. The item needs to be allowed to cool prior to use with the patient in order to avoid tissue trauma. Immediate-use sterilization is not permitted for any implantable item (plate, screw, drain, etc.).

Loading the Autoclave

Instrument packs to be sterilized in an autoclave can be placed flat on the tray if there are minimal items to be sterilized. This position inhibits air pocket formation and/or condensation, both of which can prevent complete sterilization. More efficient use of the autoclave chamber space is to load packs vertically, adhering to loading recommendations. Soft goods (cloth packs like gowns and drapes) wrapped for sterilization in an autoclave must be placed in the machine chamber vertically. This orientation allows better circulation of the steam and provides a greater possibility of adequate penetration of the steam. Wrapped packs should be placed with approximately 1″

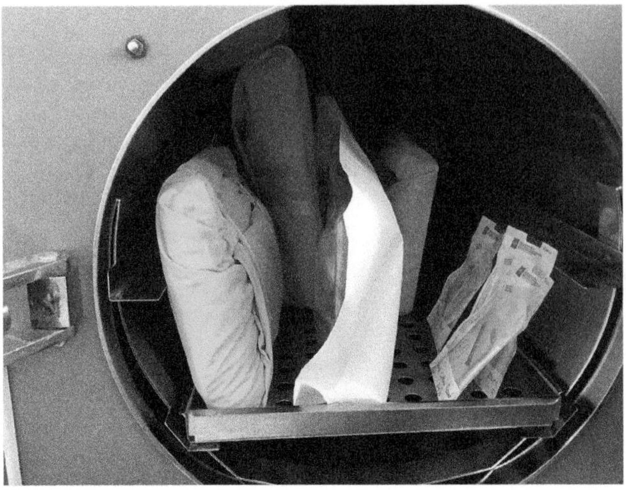

Figure 3.183 Properly loaded autoclave.

between items. Additionally, items should not touch the chamber walls or ceiling. Peel pouches should not be stacked on top of one another, but rather placed in a rack for security and appropriate loading. If a rack is unavailable, the pouches can be placed in vertical orientation with the paper of one pouch against the plastic of the next pouch. This provides the opportunity for appropriate penetration by the steam (Figure 3.183). Items loaded from plastic side to plastic side may not be sterilized as steam penetration may be inhibited. After the autoclave is loaded, the door must be closed tightly and the cycle may be selected. Each time the autoclave is run, the reservoir should be checked for an acceptable water level. Autoclave manufacturers will indicate on the machine what determines an appropriate level of water. If water needs to be added, only distilled water should be used. Water other than distilled can promote the buildup of minerals in the pipes and tubing of the autoclave that will eventually cause a mechanical failure of the machine. Recordkeeping of sterilization loads is imperative in the event of an inadequate cycle. A simple notebook by each sterilizer will allow the operator to list all the items placed in the load. If an inappropriate cycle is determined at a later time, each item run will be able to be easily retrieved from the shelf for re-processing. Each autoclave should be assigned a permanent number and each subsequent load is increased by a factor of 1. An appropriate load label on the pack label would read A_1L_1 – indicating autoclave 1 and load 1.

Autoclave Maintenance

Manufacturer's recommendations for autoclave maintenance should be strictly adhered to. In general, a monthly cleaning of the chamber is advised. There are products available that are added to the reservoir, and when a cycle is run, the chemical will move from the reservoir into the chamber and clean the surfaces while the cycle is running. Water left in the reservoir at the end of the week should be drained so that the chance of algae growing during non-use time is reduced. Lint residue buildup (a greater risk with paper wrappers/drapes than with cloth) can occur in the chamber, on the trays, and in the piping of the machine and can also cause equipment failure. Annual inspection by a qualified repair technician will assist in the diagnosis of potential problems with the machine before it breaks down – usually at the most inopportune time.

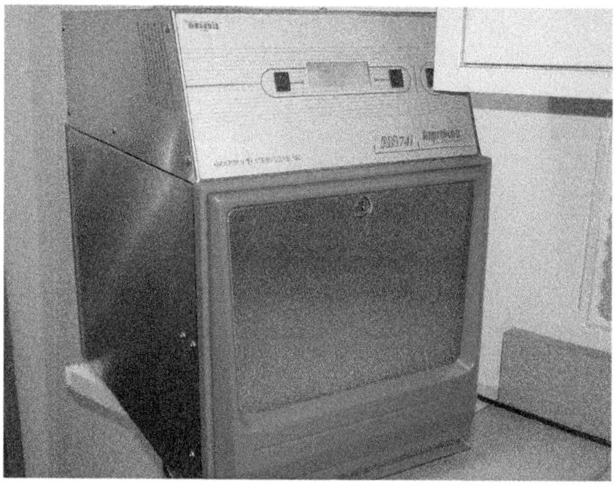

Figure 3.184 Ethylene oxide sterilizer.

Ethylene Oxide Sterilization (ETO, EtO, or EO)

Ethylene oxide is a toxic, flammable gas that uses low temperature and long periods of time to kill microorganisms on items by using alkylation to alter the DNA. Items that cannot survive steam sterilization should be sterilized with ethylene oxide (Figure 3.184). Fiberoptic cables, plastics, electric equipment, cameras, and rubber-based items are just a few examples of things that do well in an EtO cycle. Items prepared for sterilization by ethylene oxide MUST be completely dry prior to being loaded into the unit. Ethylene oxide cannot penetrate water molecules so all items must be void of any water droplets. The parameters that must be met for EtO are different from those for steam sterilization. Ethylene oxide requires the four parameters of time, temperature, humidity, and ethylene oxide gas concentration to be met in order for sterility to be achieved. Most items can be run for 12 hours, at a humidity of 20–40%, at a temperature of at least 68 °F, and using one of the available pre-measured EtO ampules. Larger ampules now available for larger loads require a run time of 24 hours. Tubing that is longer than 3 feet must be run for 24 hours using two ampules. Due to the dangerous nature of this chemical, it is imperative that personnel using the EtO sterilizers should be well trained in proper loading, operation, and troubleshooting. Companies that sell this type of sterilizer may offer training sessions for personnel. Items sterilized with EtO may be wrapped in cloth, paper, peel pack pouches, or polyethylene peel packs. One of the more commonly seen ethylene oxide sterilizers requires that items be loaded into a company-designed plastic bag. The ampule containing the ethylene oxide liquid is placed in the bag on top of the items and the bag is sealed. Once the bag is purged of air, the ampule is broken and the bag is slid into the unit. Then, the cycle (12 hours or 24 hours) is chosen, and the cycle begins. Proper aeration following the cycle must be acknowledged and adhered to. Adhering to the manufacturer's recommendations regarding operation of the unit is imperative for acceptable cycles and personnel safety.

Plasma Sterilization

Plasma sterilization is based on the theory of using ultraviolet photons and radicals to disrupt microorganisms. Hydrogen peroxide is the most common product used in vapor-phase plasma sterilization and is becoming popular due to the safety of its use. Unlike ethylene oxide, hydrogen peroxide is neither toxic nor dangerous for operators or the environment. Cost and machine size makes this method of sterilization more common in academic facilities. Smaller units are becoming available for use in private practice. Items prepared for sterilization by plasma must be completely dry. Special packaging must be used with products that are plasma sterilized as regular peel packs and linens are unacceptable. Items that are sterilized in a plasma sterilizer must have packaging specific to that system. Tyvek® packaging and polypropylene products are suitable for use with a plasma sterilizer. Due to the nature of the sterilization process, no packaging products can be of organic nature. The operation of a plasma sterilizer is very different from any of the other methods already discussed. Extensive training regarding cleaning, processing, packaging, loading, and sterilization is necessary for all individuals operating this system.

Monitoring the Sterilization Process

Monitoring the sterilization cycle is an important and often overlooked portion of the re-processing procedure. Not only is assessment of the machine function important but preventing the use of equipment that may not be truly sterile is critical to patient outcomes. Monitoring the efficacy of the sterilization process can be accomplished by combining any of the physical, chemical, or biological indicators that are available.

Physical Monitors

Physical monitors are those methods available that verify the sterilization parameters are met by the equipment. Things like recording charts, digital readouts, gauges, or printouts on the machine will perform this assessment.

Chemical Indicators

Chemical indicators are devices used to assess one or more parameters of the sterilization cycle. There are six classes of chemical indicators. Certain classes will be seen more commonly than others in veterinary use. Class 1 indicators are used externally. External indicators are used primarily to differentiate between processed and unprocessed equipment. This does not guarantee sterility, but rather merely that a pack was run through a sterilization cycle. Autoclave or EtO tape used to close packs is an example of a Class 1 indicator. Class 2 indicators are used to determine the sterilizer performance and are not used routinely with instrument packs. Bowie-Dick testing is an example of a Class 2 indicator and is used to detect air leaks, inadequate air removal, etc. from vacuum-assisted autoclaves. Class 3 indicators are internal indicators that are placed within a pack, generally at the most dense area of the pack. Indicators assess one of the parameters, such as whether or not the proper temperature was reached. These indicators are not common and may become obsolete. Class 4 indicators assess two or more parameters, such as paper strips routinely placed in the center of packs to be steam sterilized (Figures 3.185 and 3.186). Class 5 indicators are designed to assess all parameters needed for a sterile cycle. The rigor of testing is equal to a biological indicator. Class 6 indicators are designed for specific cycle parameters. The response from these indicators does not correlate with a biological indicator. These indicators assess isolated information for each pack. Again, because it assesses only limited information, it does not guarantee sterility of the pack. For example, if the autoclave is not functioning properly, the steam may penetrate the pack but the proper time parameter will not have been met. Indicators are dependent on proper use by the operator, proper placement within the sterilizer, proper functioning of the sterilizer, and proper loading of the sterilizer by the operator. Steam sterilization indicators assess the three parameters of pressure, temperature, and time, whereas EtO indicators are sensitive to the four parameters of time, temperature, humidity, and ethylene oxide gas concentration.

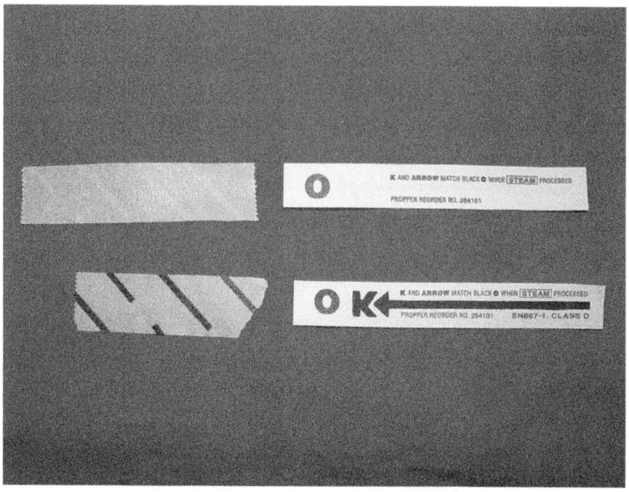

Figure 3.185 Before and after sterilization indicators for steam sterilization.

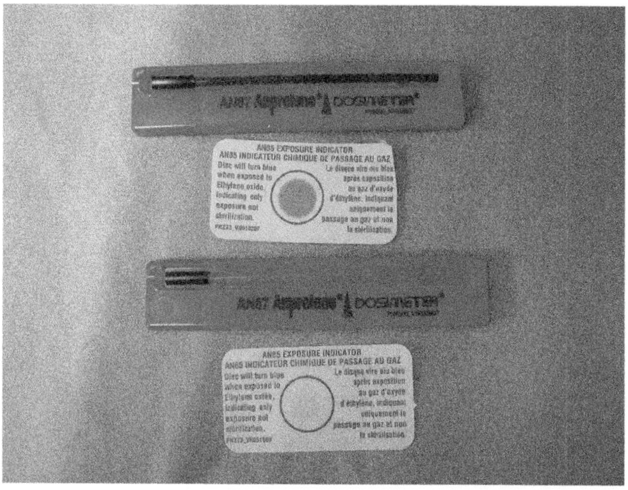

Figure 3.186 Before and after sterilization indicators for ethylene oxide sterilization.

Biological Indicators

Biological indicators are considered the closest available option to the ideal monitoring of sterilization cycles. Because one of the most resistant microorganisms (*Bacillus spores*) is used in the indicator vial, the indicators measure complete kill of a microorganism rather than merely assessing physical parameters of the sterilization cycle. The premise of a biological indicator is that with a concentrated large number of bacteria that are more resistant than most contaminants that may be found on equipment, the result of killing those pathogens will strongly suggest that other pathogens that may be present will also be eradicated. The indicators are placed in the most challenging area of the sterilizer and run through the cycle. At the end of the cycle, the small vial is cracked with the provided device and incubated at 135 °F. The results of the vial should be checked every 12 hours for 48 hours before assuming a final result. A color change indicates a positive growth result and the items within the load should not be considered sterile. Steam biological indicators use *Geobacillus stearothermophilus* and ethylene oxide biological indicators use *Bacillus atrophaeus* (Figure 3.187).

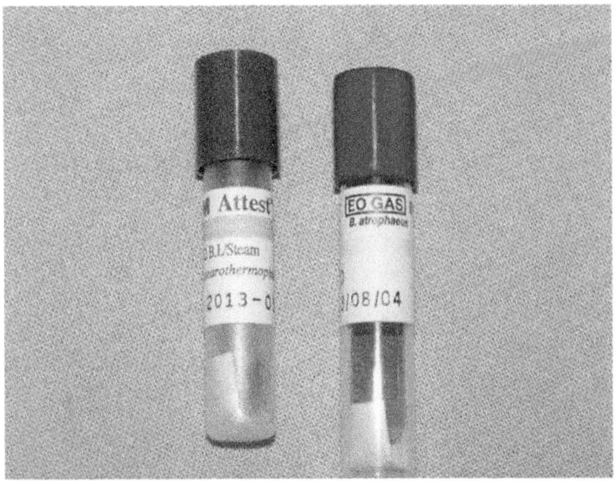

Figure 3.187 Unprocessed biological indicators.

Shelf Life

Date-related shelf life is falling out of favor. Event-related shelf life is becoming the accepted method of storing sterilized items. Time does not determine whether an item is contaminated, but rather handling and exposure to elements. More attention should be paid to storage conditions and frequency of handling rather than the calendar. Under ideal conditions, sterile items will remain sterile indefinitely. Storage should be in a closed cabinet to avoid dust contamination as well as exposure to air movement (Figure 3.188). Humidity should be less than 70% and a temperature of

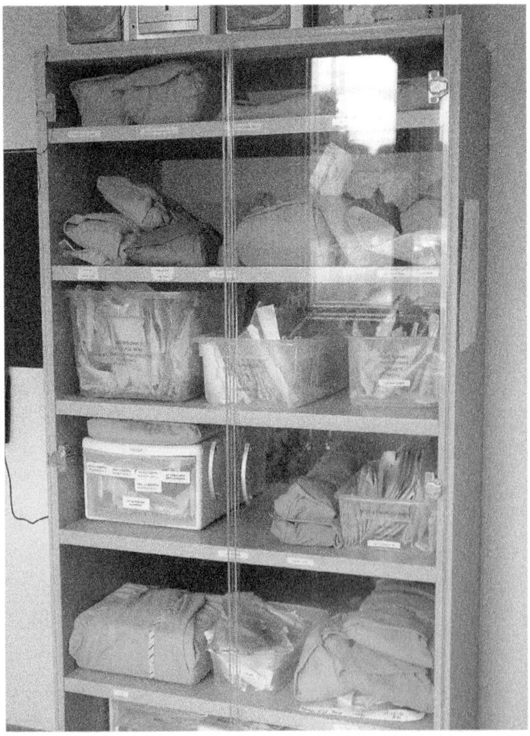

Figure 3.188 Closed cabinet for storage of sterilized items.

Figure 3.189 Avoid crushing peel packs and risking contamination.

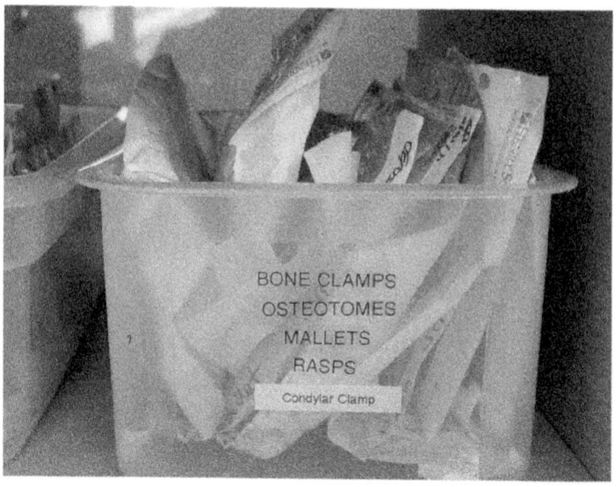

75 °F should be maintained. The storage area should be 8–10″ above the floor surface, 18″ below the ceiling, and 2″ from any outside wall. Items should be rotated so that the oldest item is the first one used. Excessive handling, rustling, and moving of the packs will add to compromise the integrity of the packaging. Especially with peel pack items, avoiding sliding, dropping, puncturing, or compressing the packing should be practiced (Figure 3.189). Items should be inspected before each use. Any question as to the integrity should warrant re-packaging and re-sterilization. Especially in the situation of large animal mobile veterinary services, extra care should be paid to sterilized packs. Storage in freezer Ziploc bags, plastic waterproof containers, or other such devices will greatly prolong the integrity of the packs.

Reference

1 Tear, M. (2012) *Small Animal Surgical Nursing – Skills and Concepts*, 2nd edn. Elsevier, St. Louis MO.

Webliography

1 Jaeger, M. (2017). Preoperative surgical site preparation. Clinicians Brief, Jan/Feb. 2017.

2 https://www.veterinarypracticenews.com/avoid-getting-in-trouble-with-heating-devices/#:~:text=Heated%20surgery%20tables%20and%20cages%20have,can%20put%20your%20patient%20at%20risk.&text=Heated%20surgery%20tables%20and,your%20patient%20at%20risk.&text=tables%20and%20cages%20have,can%20put%20your%20patient – Avoid getting in trouble with heating devices. Educate your staff on the use and risks of different heat sources to avoid harming your patients with inadvertent burn wounds [accessed on 15 February 2023].

3 Study finds fingernail length, not nail polish, increases bacterial counts. https://www.avma.org/javma-news/2018-05-01/study-finds-fingernail-length-not-nail-polish-increases-bacterial-counts [accessed on 16 February 2023].

4 Harrie Phillips PGCertClinEd, BAdVocEd (VocEd&Trng), RVN, DipVN (Surgical, ECC), DipTAE (Development & Design), DipBus, TAA, MACE – https://vetnurse.com.au/2018/03/07/surgical-skin-preparation/ [accessed on 25 February 2023].

5 ASP ™ Ortho-Phthalaldehyde Solution high level disinfectant for semi-critical medical devices IFU – https://www.asp.com/en-us/products/high-level-disinfection/cidex-opa-solution [accessed on 3 March 2023].
6 Autoclave temperature time and pressure chart – http://www.theratronics.ca/PDFs/Autoclave_Temperature_and_Time_Pressure_Chart.pdf [accessed on 3 March 2023].
7 Low temperature sterilizer – frequently asked questions. – https://tuttnauer.com/sites/default/files/2022-05/ebook_plasma%2003_10_21.pdf [accessed on 3 March 2023].

4

Intraoperative Surgical Assistant and Circulating Nurse

Teri Raffel Kleist and Cassandra Simmons*

College of Veterinary Medicine, Purdue University, West Lafayette, IN, USA

One of the areas of the clinic or hospital that frequently goes unsupported by veterinary technicians is the surgical suite; neither as an anesthetist nor as circulating nurse, but rather as a surgical assistant for the surgeon. Surgeons working alone are at the mercy of fate when it comes to speed and timely completion. Surgeons who work with a qualified and efficient assistant can attest to the benefit of the extra knowledgeable body. Working as a team, with the patient's best possible outcome as their goal, the surgeon and the assistant will set the tone and pace for the procedure.

A surgeon with a well-qualified proficient assistant can reduce the surgical procedure time significantly. Technicians who perform as assistants must be familiar with all instrumentation to be used and the process with which the surgeon will advance through the procedure. Assistants must master the skill of anticipation and have the instrument/equipment in the hand of the surgeon before he/she even knows it is needed. Sometimes, the surgeons' needs are made known nicely, and other times, not so nicely.

Regardless of how the need is made known, it is the technician's job to have what the surgeon is requesting available.

Even before the patient is anesthetized, the surgical assistant is involved with the case. Making sure that the appropriate equipment and instrumentation are available is critical. Nothing can impede the progress of a surgery more than having to wait for equipment or instruments to be sterilized, or worse yet, not having the necessary item available at all. The assistant needs to be sure that the required instrument is functioning and ready for use.

The circulating nurse/technician is an equally important member of the team. The circulating nurse is responsible for setting up the room with the necessary equipment, opening all equipment in an aseptic fashion, monitoring the procedure to ensure aseptic technique is not compromised, and documenting equipment used, implants implanted, and any complications that may occur.

---

* Madison College, retired.

Surgical Patient Care for Veterinary Technicians and Nurses, Second Edition.
Edited by Gerianne Holzman and Teri Raffel Kleist.

Companion website: www.wiley.com/go/holzman/patient

Patient Positioning

Once the patient is moved into the operating room, it is the responsibility of the OR tech to appropriately position the patient. For the procedure to be done efficiently, proper positioning of the patient is a critical step in the patient preparation process. If it is an abdominal, medial sternal approach thoracotomy, some orthopedic, or a neurologic procedure, surgeons require the patient to be positioned in a straight and anatomically correct fashion (Figure 4.1). One must consider the procedure being performed and the surgeon's positioning preference. For example, for stifle surgery, the patient is often positioned in dorsal recumbency with the instrument table over the chest of the patient (Figure 4.2). Conversely, for forelimb surgery and most thoracic or abdominal procedures, the instrument table is placed over the caudal end of the patient. If it is a procedure to remove a mass from an unusual location, the technician must be certain that the positioning of the

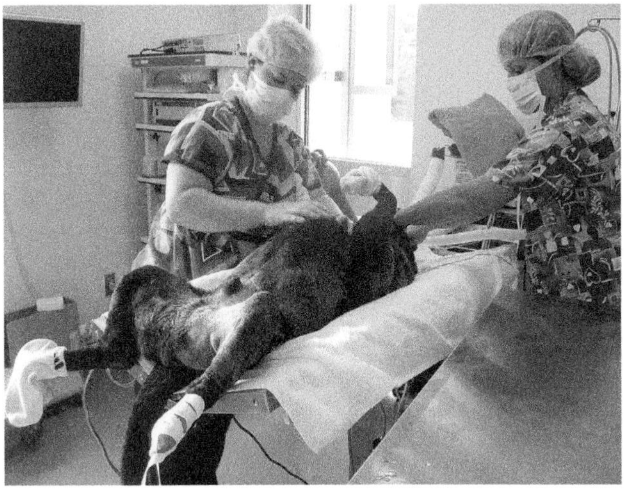

Figure 4.1 Positioning the patient on the surgery table.

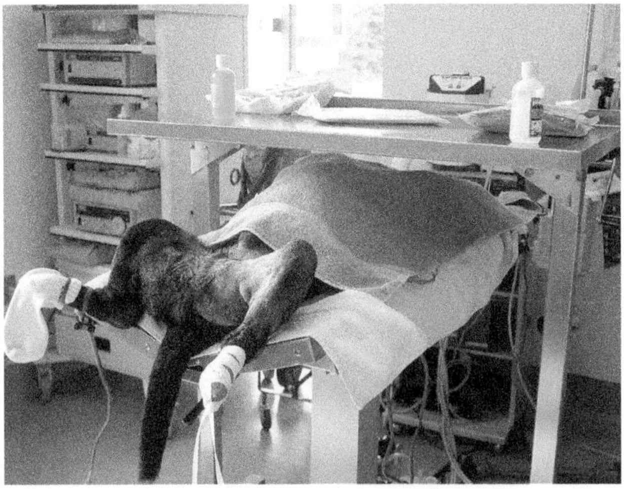

Figure 4.2 The instrument table over the chest of a patient having stifle surgery.

patient does not impede the surgeon's ability to perform the procedure. Often it is advised to have the surgeon verify the positioning of the patient on the surgery table before they scrub and before the final patient prep is performed. Patients in dorsal recumbency that are leaning to one side or another risk receiving an incision through the muscle layers of the abdominal wall instead of through the linea alba. Once a patient has been positioned to the surgeon's liking, the patient must not shift or move from that position until the end of the case.

The use of positioning aids will greatly assist in maintaining the animal in the desired position. Some surgery tables have a split top that allows either one or both sides of the tabletop to be adjusted (Figure 4.3). Positioning for the patient can be accomplished from a flat surface to a "V" position. For patients that need to be in dorsal recumbency, the use of the surgery table "V" may be all that is needed. For deep-chested dogs, long sandbags, as opposed to square sandbags, will be an effective method for supplementing the tabletop to maintain the patient in the proper position. Foam wedges may also be used but may slip and if contaminated by blood or other fluids, may be difficult to clean and disinfect. Additional positioning aids include vacuum beanbags or similar devices and leg ties. Both can be easily disinfected between patients by laundering or wiping down with a disinfecting solution. Vacuum positioning aids are extremely helpful in maintaining patients in unusual positions. These devices are especially helpful for ophthalmic procedures or thoracic cases that necessitate the patient be positioned in an oblique state, rather than a level lateral position. Because they can be conformed around the patient in any fashion, and then have the air vacuumed out to maintain the position, these devices are very unique. Leg ties are extremely common, and in most cases, it is the only positioning assistance that is needed. Soft ropes or commercially available leg ties are recommended. Roll gauze, IV tubing, or elastic bands are not recommended as they may apply too much pressure to the soft tissue and impede distal limb circulation. An adjustable loop on the leg tie should be placed just proximal to the carpus/tarsus and then have a half hitch placed just distal to those joints (Figure 4.4). Double placement as described aids in better distribution of pressure to reduce circulation issues. Most surgery tables have either brackets or side bar rollers on the side table rails that are used to secure the leg ties. Brackets require a figure 8 method of securing the leg tie with a half hitch on the last loop to secure placement (Figure 4.5). Rollers are easier to use and simply require the leg tie to be passed between the two rubber rollers to hold the rope securely (Figure 4.6). Care should be taken to avoid excessively extending the limbs. Limbs should be maintained in as anatomically correct a position as possible, depending on the position the patient is in. There are also specific procedure positioning aids available. Examples include an arthroscopy brace and a total hip arthroplasty (THA) brace. These items

Figure 4.3 A surgery table with the split top in a "V."

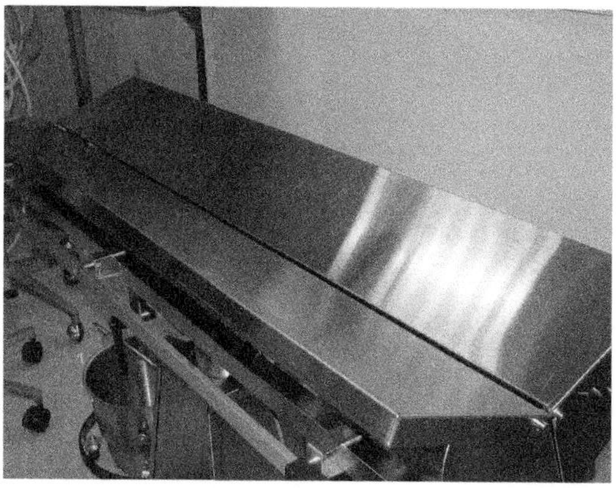

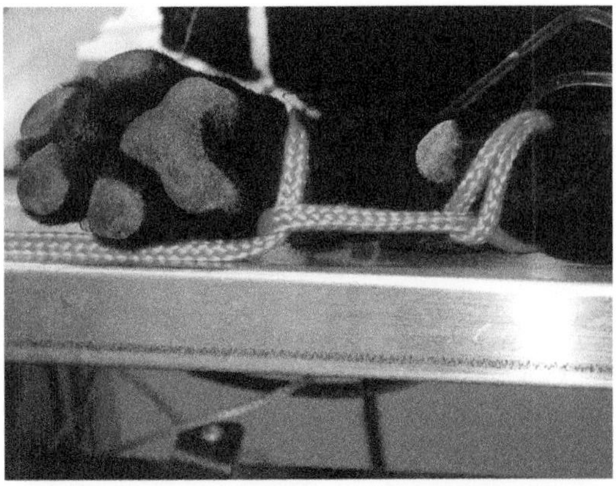

Figure 4.4 Leg with a half hitch.

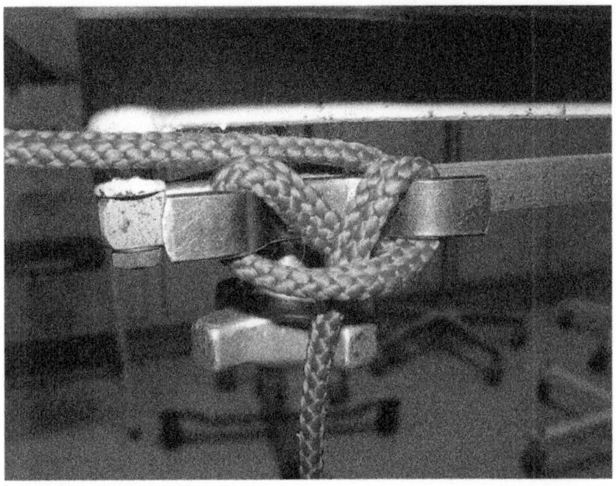

Figure 4.5 Leg tie as a figure 8 on a surgery table bracket.

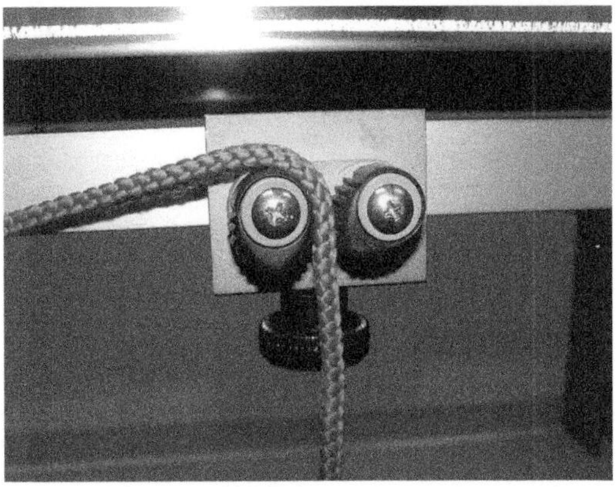

Figure 4.6 Leg tie through a roller-style bracket on a surgery table.

are used to position the patient in a specific manner relative to the procedure. Sometimes the brace must be covered by a sterile drape before the limb can be placed on it and other times the positioning aid is completely under the patient's drapes.

Patients undergoing spinal surgery are generally placed in ventral recumbency. The use of sandbags and/or vacuum aids is required in order to achieve and maintain proper positioning of the patient. Patients in this position must be monitored for adequate respiratory capability. The vacuum positioning aids are quite stiff and hard following evacuation of the air and are therefore not very forgiving at allowing expansion of the chest wall if conformed too tightly to the patient. It is important to remember that whichever positioning aid is employed, it should not be wrapped around or laid over the chest of the patient, but rather gathered or formed along the sides of the chest. It is impossible to describe all the potential positions for surgical patients, as it is so dependent on the surgeon's preference. It is even difficult to make the statement that all patients for a certain procedure (i.e. stifle surgery) are always placed in the same position (i.e. dorsal recumbency). Factors such as procedure being done, size of the patient, and surgeon familiarity all determine the positioning of the patient on a case-by-case basis. The most important thing to remember is that excellent communication must exist between the technician doing the positioning and the surgeon performing the procedure in order to avoid unnecessary delays.

Sterile Patient Prep

Following positioning of the patient, the sterile prep may begin. It is highly recommended that the patients have the clipping and initial skin prep (scrub) performed in an area outside of the surgery room. Once completed the patient is moved to the surgical suite, positioned, and a final sterile prep is done. A sterile surgical patient prep is done in a very similar fashion as the initial prep, with the major difference being the use of sterile products. Prep sets can be made a couple of ways, depending on clinic choice. A small instrument pan ($3'' \times 8''$) or a kidney (emesis) basin can be used as the pan. Two stacks of 10 4×4 gauze sponges are placed in the pan. An indicator strip should be placed in the middle of the sponges. A latex glove (size 7 or $7\frac{1}{2}$) can then be laid on top of the sponges (Figure 4.7). Some facilities prefer not to include the glove, which is an acceptable modification. The pan is double wrapped using the envelope style of wrapping, or peel packed, and is sterilized in the autoclave. An alternative to sterilizing prep sets is to purchase pre-sterilized non-woven gauze in packs of 10.

In addition to the sterile prep set, squeeze bottles of the prep solutions also need to be available. The solutions and prep set should be set up in the surgery room when the rest of the packs and equipment are placed in the room. Once the patient is positioned, the prep set can be opened. The pack is aseptically opened to reveal the sterile contents. Before proceeding, the caps of the solution bottles should be opened. If a glove was not included in the sterile prep set, a pack of appropriate sized gloves should now be aseptically opened, and using the open gloving technique, a sterile glove is placed on the dominant hand. If a glove was included, it is now aseptically put on. Having

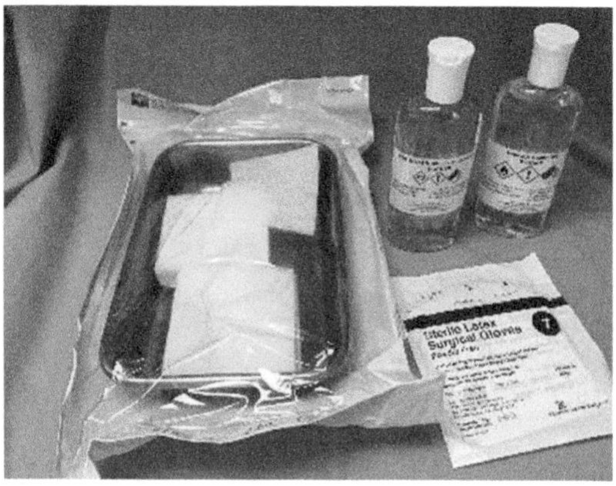

Figure 4.7 Sterile prep set and solutions.

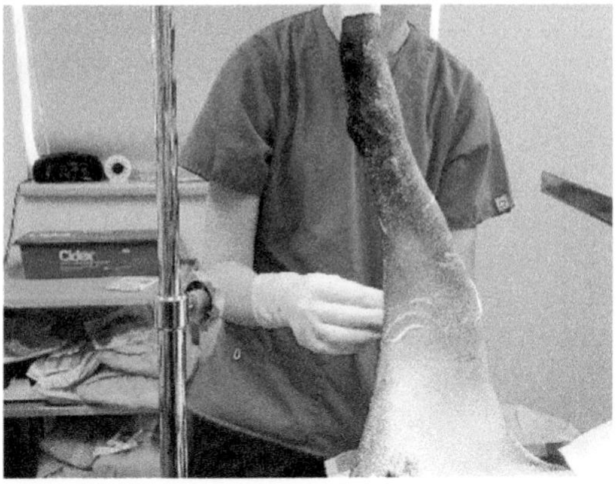

Figure 4.8 Sterile prep for orthopedic surgery.

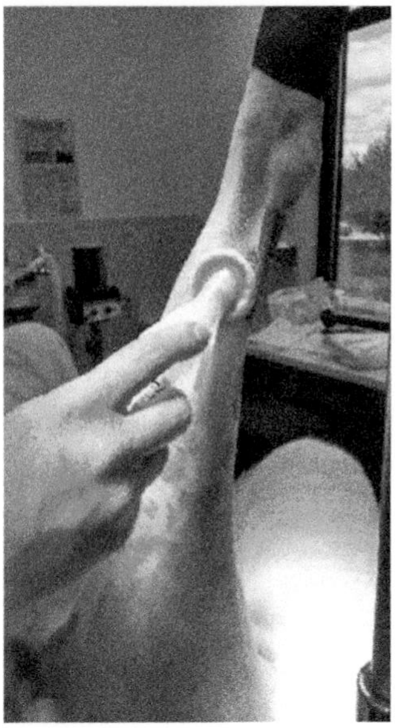

Figure 4.9 Chloraprep application for final sterile prep. *Source:* Courtesy of Heidi Reuss-Lamky.

one sterile hand and one non-sterile hand allows the technician the versatility to perform the sterile prep without assistance. The non-sterile hand is also available to stabilize the suspended limb during the prep for orthopedic cases.

With the sterile gloved hand, 1–2 sponges are picked up. The non-sterile hand picks up the surgical scrub bottle and aseptically applies some scrub solution to the sterile sponges. Care must be taken to ensure the cap of the bottle does not touch the sponges. The prep now continues using the same pattern that the initial scrub used (Figure 4.8). New prep sponges should be retrieved as needed. The rinsing agent is aseptically applied to the sponges in the same manner as the scrub solution. Be sure to save a few dry sponges to be used for the application of the final paint solution.

An alternative to this type of final prep is a One-Step Prep of chlorhexidine and alcohol (Chloraprep®) or povidone-iodine and alcohol (Duraprep®) (Figure 4.9). These products are available in 1.0, 1.5, 3.0, 10.5 and 26.0 ml wands. Chlorhexidine One-Step Preps are sold in clear, orange, or teal solution. A One-Step Prep is painted on as a final sterile prep. One should don a sterile surgical glove, using the open gloving technique, then break the inner tube of the One-Step Prep wand by compressing the wand tabs and shaking the wand to mix the chlorhexidine or povidone-iodine with the alcohol. Once the pad is saturated with the solution, the intended surgical site can be painted in the chosen pattern. Good technique will overlap each pass of the wand by 50%. The wand must be discarded once hair is touched. The prep solution must dry before the patient is draped.

Once the final paint is applied, the draping may begin. Every effort should be made to allow the final solution to dry prior to draping the patient to encourage optimal efficacy of the product.

Patient Draping

Once the patient has received the second "sterile" prep, draping can begin. Assistants must be thoroughly knowledgeable about the procedure and the approach the surgeon will use in order to effectively drape the patient. Depending on the procedure to be done, draping may need to include extra wide margins away from the incision. For example, draping to allow access to the exit of a chest tube for a thoracic procedure or allowing access to a bone graft site for harvesting a graft for a fracture repair.

Especially during the draping sequence, but throughout the entire procedure, the technician must be acutely aware of strict asepsis in the surgical suite and sterile field. According to Dr. Brian Beale, "the surgical assistant should be cognizant of the need for strict asepsis and act as the asepsis police in the operating room" [1]. Any question as to a break in aseptic technique must be treated as a valid break and corrective measures must be taken. Whether that means changing a pair of gloves, a gown, or an entire pack of instruments, it must be done. Although often times not very well liked by all members of the surgical team, the veterinary technician is acting as the patient's advocate and looking out for their well-being. Breaks in asepsis are not to be argued or debated but accepted and corrected.

Non-orthopedic Draping (Soft Tissue, Neuro, etc.)

Draping for non-orthopedic procedures is a fairly simple process. After the sterile drape pack has been opened aseptically by the circulating tech, and is available to the sterile team members, draping may begin using the four-corner draping method. Usually ground/field drapes (also known as quarter drapes) are placed first. It is important that before draping, all skin prep solutions (alcohol and paint solutions) have adequate time to dry/evaporate. Not only it is important for optimal efficacy of the prep products but it also decreases complications from the use of electrosurgery and/or lasers. Presuming the ground drapes are folded as described earlier, find the short side of the drape that has the open folds (Figure 4.10). Place the index finger of each hand in the outermost opening (Figure 4.11). Using the thumb and middle finger of each hand, hold the drape and lift it up (Figure 4.12). The long side of the drape with the folds should be facing the ceiling. Holding the drape in front, move the hands away from each other to open the drape (Figure 4.13). Lift the thumb of each hand to allow the drape to unfold. Once the towel has unfolded the thumbs should be returned to the previous position of holding the drape between the thumb and index finger (Figure 4.14). Drapes should never be flipped, shaken, or fanned as that action may release dust and/or lint into the air and potentially onto the sterile field. Holding the towel with the index finger and the thumb of each hand, rotate the hands so all the fingers and palms are facing the operator (Figure 4.15). Rotate the hands again so the palms are down and the edges of the drape cover the gloved hands (Figure 4.16). This action protects the sterile hands from becoming contaminated as

Figure 4.10 Short-side, open folds of ground drape towels.

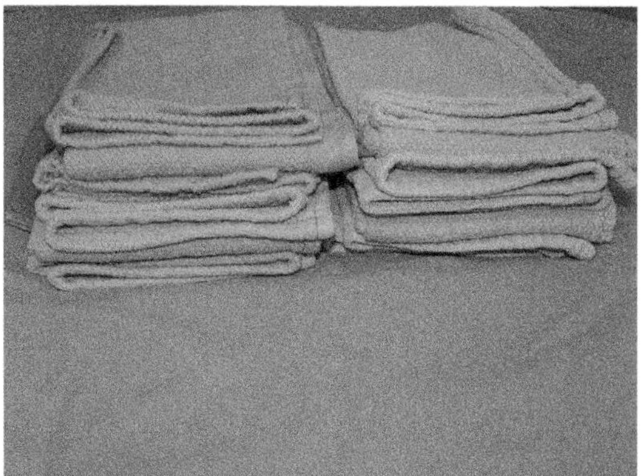

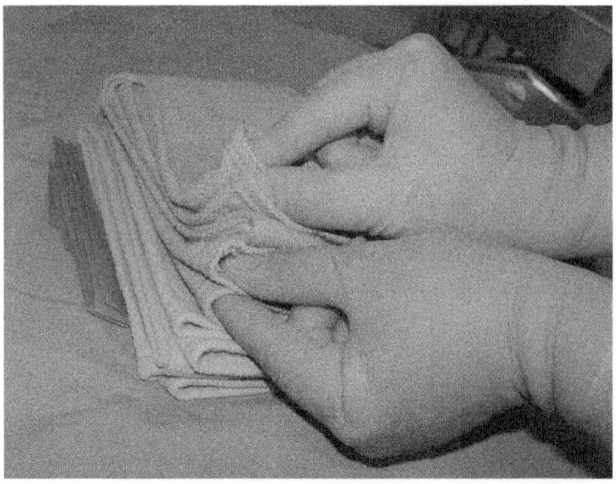

Figure 4.11 Fingers in the appropriate folds of the towel.

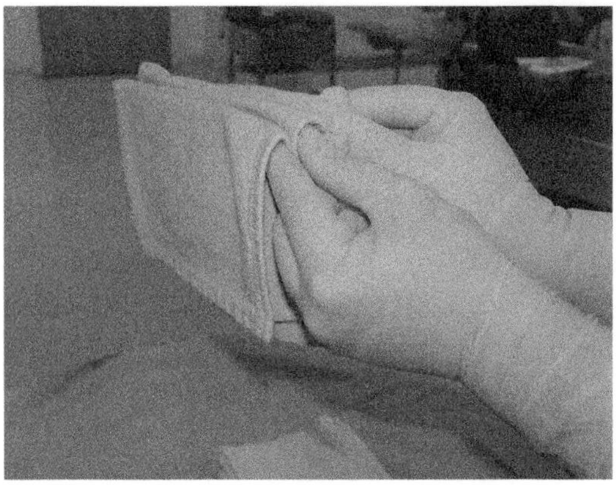

Figure 4.12 Picking up the towel.

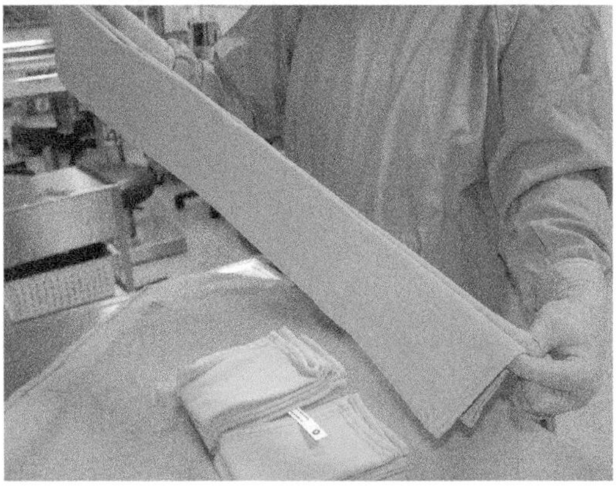

Figure 4.13 Opening the towel.

the drape is laid on the patient. This method of unfolding results in a crisp fold being closest to the incision, which helps the drape to lay as flat as possible. The side of the patient closest to the person draping should be draped first. As the drape is being placed, it is critical that no part of the sterile gown or sterile hands come in contact with a non-sterile surface. The folded edge of the drape should be placed ½″–1″ laterally to the proposed incision site. Communication with the surgeon prior to draping is strongly recommended in the event special draping needs may be requested by

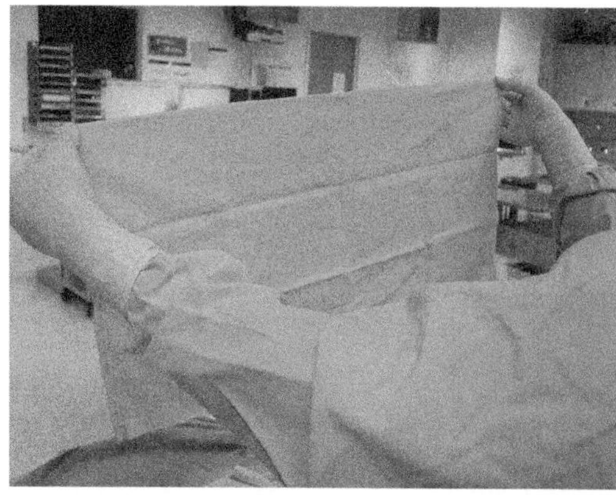

Figure 4.14 Lift each thumb and allow towel to open.

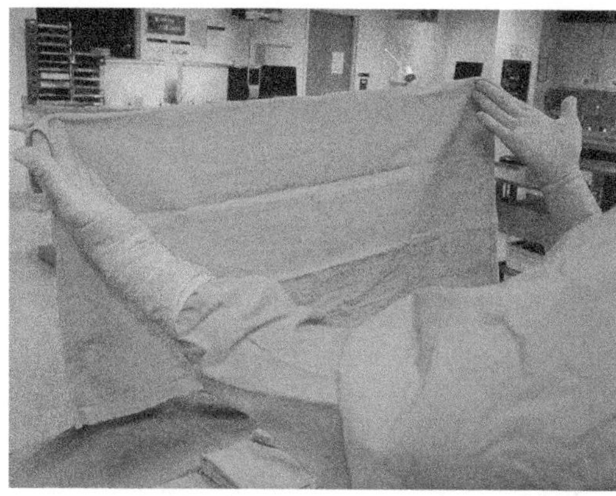

Figure 4.15 Rotate each hand so palms are facing the operator.

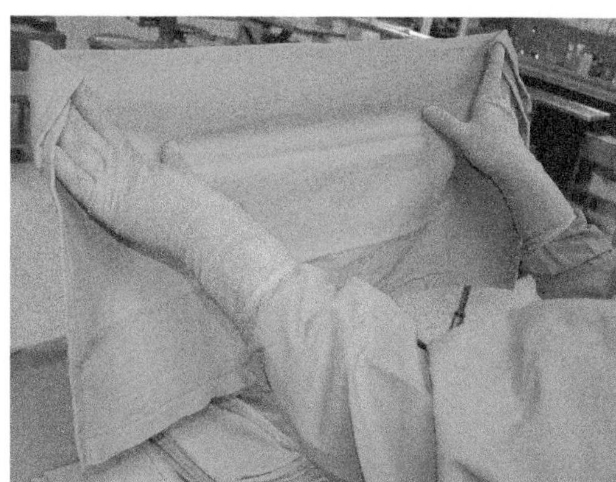

Figure 4.16 Pronate the hands so the fingers are protected by the towel.

the surgeon. Once a drape is placed on the patient, it cannot be moved or adjusted, therefore proper initial placement in imperative. The second drape is placed opposite from the first. The person draping must NEVER reach over the non-sterile area to place a drape. Walking around the table to place the drape is the only acceptable practice. The second drape should be placed in the same distance from the proposed incision site as the first drape. The third drape is placed on the cranial aspect of the proposed incision. As before, a ½″–1″ margin from the incision's cranial end should be followed.

When placing the third drape, care must be taken to keep the front of the gown facing the surgery table. The person draping should turn just the arms and shoulders to place the drape. Especially, with long-haired patients, arms may need to be elevated to avoid sleeve contamination from the fur. After the third drape is placed, penetrating towel clamps should be placed at the intersecting corners of the towels to secure them to the patient. Penetrating towel clamps are used to pierce the skin and securely hold the drapes in place. Depending on the area of the body being draped, caution must be taken to avoid penetrating a structure with the towel clamp (i.e. Jugular vein, nerve, etc.). The caudal drape is the last to be placed using the same physical stance as the cranial drape. The person draping the patient is not allowed to stand at the end of the surgery table to place the drape. In most cases, this would require reaching over the non-sterile table and that is a break-in aseptic technique. Penetrating towel clamps can now be placed in the two remaining intersecting corners of the drapes. After all four ground drapes are placed and secured, the same draping process is repeated with larger drapes. The top drapes need to be large enough to completely cover the patient and tabletop to reduce the risk of contamination. Some surgeons will choose to use a large fenestrated drape instead of the four top drapes. Still, other surgeons may choose a large non-fenestrated field drape that allows the surgeon to cut a custom fenestration the size of the four-corner draped field. The newly cut fenestration is then secured with towel clamps being placed over and around the box lock of the first set of towel clamps. If a single large drape is used, care must be taken to avoid any breaks in aseptic technique as the drape is laid on the patient. Care must be taken to avoid raising the drape too high and hitting the surgery lights, or conversely lowering the drape to watch placement, but then the bottom edge of the drape touches below the hem of the gown. Any of the options are acceptable, however, four-corner draping allows more flexibility, whereas the fenestrated drape is one finite size and will have to do no matter the size of the patient. Fenestrations that are too large risk overexposure of the patient's skin, increasing infection risk. Fenestrations too small may hinder the surgeon's ability to visualize as needed due to a smaller incision. Top drapes can be secured with either penetrating or non-penetrating towel clamps. Some surgeons may choose to use the povidone-iodine-impregnated sticky drape. In most situations, the sticky drape is applied after all the drapes are in place. Making sure the prepped area is completely dry before application of the sticky drape will provide the greatest opportunity for good adhesion of the drape.

Orthopedic Draping

When patients are having an orthopedic procedure and the limb has been suspended for the prep, the draping procedure is quite involved. After the drape pack has been aseptically opened for the sterile team, the first ground drape can be placed. In order to keep the limb feely moveable for the surgeon, the ground drapes are placed ~1″ onto the shaven area from the clipped margins at the proximal end of the limb. Ground drapes should be placed in the order which will allow the last drape place to be the one by the IV pole that is suspending the limb. The risk of contamination is higher when placing that drape, so it should be done last (Figure 4.17). After all ground drapes are placed and secured, the suspended limb will need to be cut down. The foot can then be grabbed by a sterile team member with a sterile drape. Another option is to grab the foot with sterile VetRap® and cover all the tape (Figure 4.18). Once it is verbally confirmed that the sterile team member has control of the foot, the tape should be cut by the circulating nurse close to the foot to avoid any non-sterile item from touching the prepped leg. It is imperative that the circulating tech not cut the tape until it is known that the sterile member has control of the foot. Lack of observation of this detail can result in the limb being dropped, the sterile drapes and potentially the sterile team members being contaminated, thus requiring re-draping and re-gowning/gloving of the sterile team members. The circulating technician can then move the IV

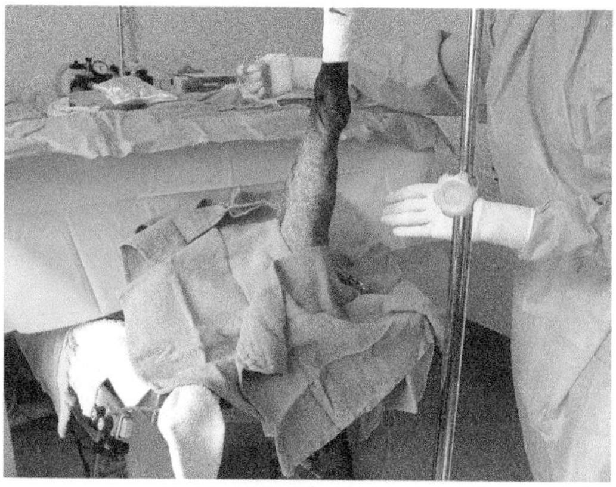

Figure 4.17 Securing ground drapes for an orthopedic case.

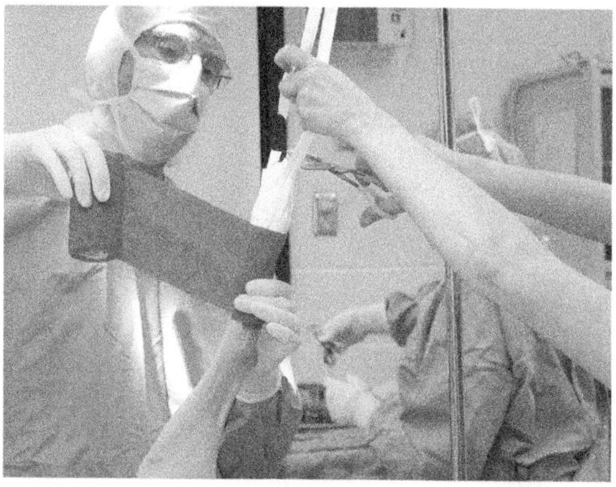

Figure 4.18 Surgeon grabbing the foot with sterile Vetrap® while the circulating nurse cuts down the suspended limb.

pole away while the sterile team member covers the foot with the sterile drape or other sterile foot covering (Video 4.1). Once the foot is completely covered, the drapes can be placed. If another layer of four-corner draping is used, the process is the same as what was used with the ground drapes (huck towels). If a fenestrated drape is used, the limb is fed through the fenestration and the drape unfolded to cover the patient, creating a sterile surgical field (Figure 4.19). A povidone-iodine-impregnated sticky drape can also be used for orthopedic cases. The application is the same as it is for a soft tissue case (Figure 4.20).

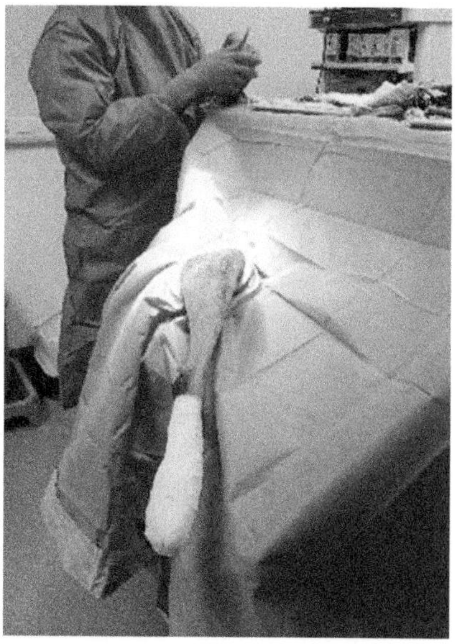

Figure 4.19 Completed draping for an orthopedic case.

Other Responsibilities

Other responsibilities of the surgical technician include setting up the "back" or instrument table, passing surgical instruments, and lavaging the tissue to ensure tissue viability, providing hemostasis with either manual

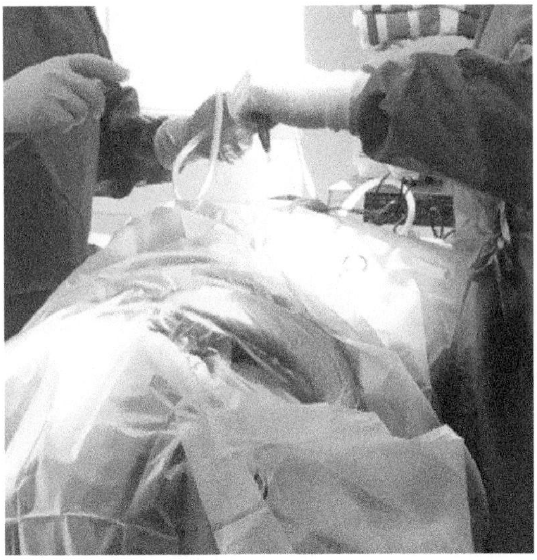

Figure 4.20 Iodine-impregnated adhesive drape used in orthopedic surgery.

pressure with a gauze sponge or use of electrosurgery, providing tissue retraction or limb manipulation as needed, and alerting the surgeon to any problem that may not have been noticed by the surgeon.

Setting Up the Instrument Table

The surgical assistant is in charge of the instrument table. The instruments should be laid out so the assistant can easily see the tips to quickly identify the instrument requested. For some surgical cases, the assistant will be standing opposite the surgeon on the other side of the surgery table. In other cases, they may be standing behind the instrument table at the caudal end of the surgery table. Some technicians like to assemble the instruments on the table so the "sharp" instruments (scalpel blades and scissors) are on one side and then progress across the table top to the "dull" instruments (hemostats). This order is logical and helps other sterile members find an instrument if need be.

Passing Surgical Instruments

Correctly and firmly passing an instrument to the surgeon or other sterile member is a critical skill. Communication or lack thereof, between the assistant and the surgeon, can greatly enhance or negatively affect the flow of the case. Instruments handed with less than a firm "slap," may result in the instrument being dropped.

Scalpel Handle and Blade

Handing a scalpel handle loaded with a scalpel blade must be done safely because the risk of injury to the surgeon is great. Using an overhand grip, the assistant should hold the handle with the blade facing them. The non-cutting edge of the blade should be facing the palm. The handle and blade should be firmly placed in the waiting hand of the surgeon (Figure 4.21).

Ring-Handled Instruments

Ring-handled instruments should be held at the box lock in a vertical position, tips to the ceiling, and ring handles to the floor (Figure 4.22). The instruments should be locked to the first ratchet so it is easier for the surgeon to grasp the ring handles. The instrument should be placed firmly in the

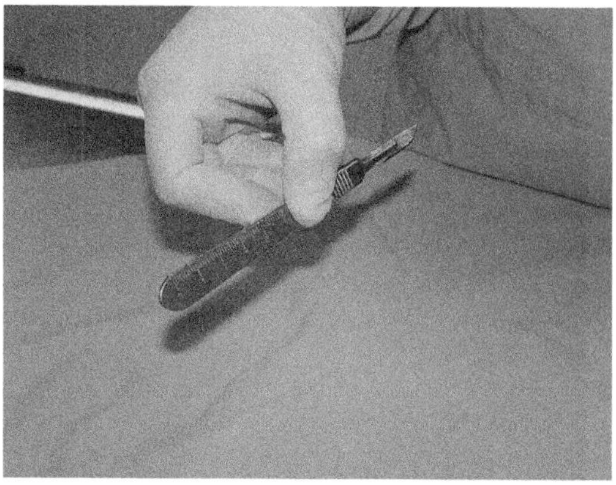

Figure 4.21 Proper method of passing a loaded scalpel blade and handle.

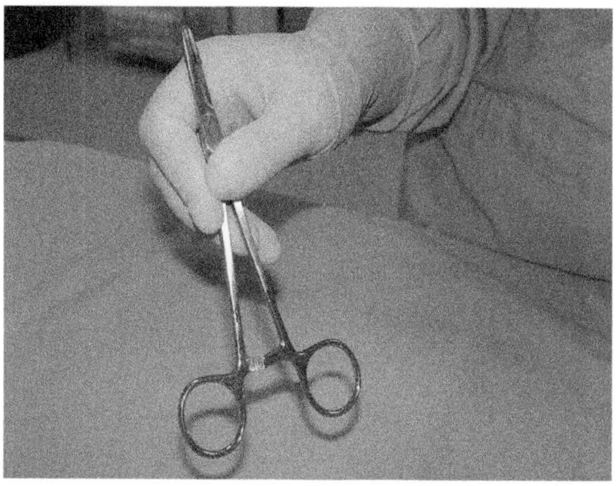

Figure 4.22 Proper method of passing a ring-handled instrument.

palm of the waiting hand with the ring handles hitting the palm. Loading the needle holder with a suture needle should also be the assistant's responsibility. The needle holder should be placed about three-fourth of the way on the needle curve, closer to the suture attachment. The needle holder should never be clamped on the needle at the needle/suture junction. The needle should have the curve up so the surgeon is ready to place the first stitch.

Thumb Tissue Forceps

Thumb tissue forceps should also be held in a vertical fashion when being passed to the surgeon (Figure 4.23). The assistant should hold the thumb tissue forceps at the fused end with the tips facing the floor. Using this method will provide the surgeon with an instrument they can use right away instead of having to flip it around.

Lavaging

Maintaining the integrity of the tissue is a critical role of the surgical technician. Sterile bowls should be filled, aseptically, with sterile saline and kept on the instrument table. The surgical assistant should hold the bowl off the sterile field to allow the circulating nurse to fill the bowl. The circulating nurse must be careful to not touch the bowl with the bottle of lavage fluid. Additionally, the bowl should not be overfilled to avoid spillage once on the table (Figure 4.24). The bowl should be readily accessible, yet out of the way so as to avoid repeated bumping and spilling. Bulb syringes,

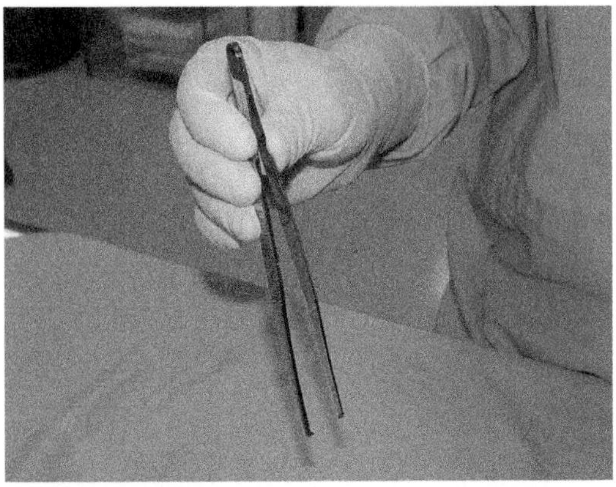

Figure 4.23 Proper method of passing a thumb tissue forceps.

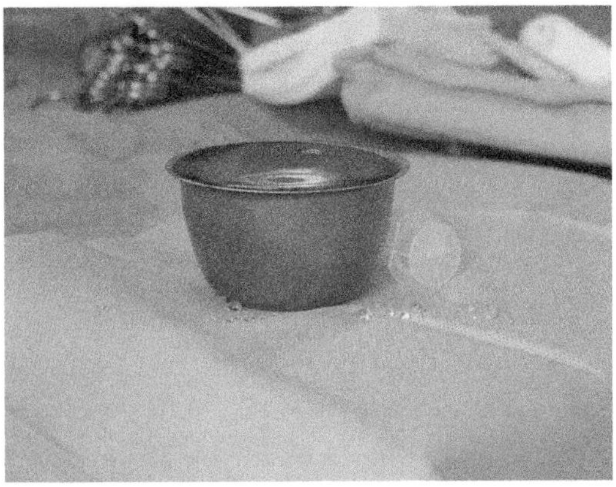

Figure 4.24 Fluid bowl too full.

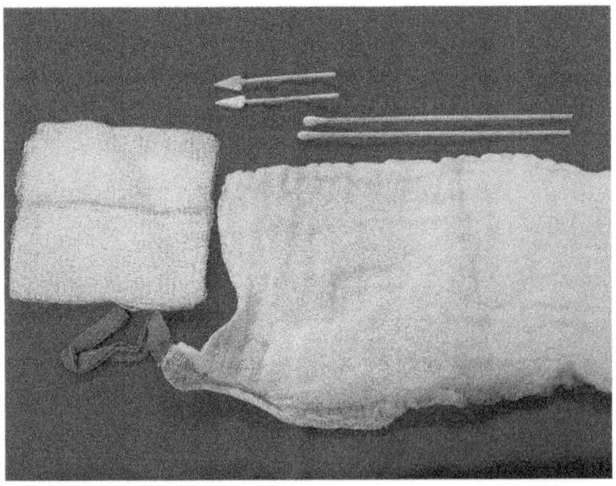

Figure 4.25 Options for hemostasis: radiopaque gauze sponge, radiopaque laparotomy pad, surgical spear, and cotton-tipped applicator.

regular syringes, or gauze sponges are most commonly used to apply sterile fluid to the exposed tissues. Tissue must be kept moistened at all times. Exposure to room air and heat from the surgical lights can lead to rapid dehydration and decreased viability. Tissues that may be exposed for long periods of time (exteriorized intestine, urinary bladder, etc.) should be covered with a saline-soaked radiopaque sponge or lap pad for increased moisture retention (Figure 4.25). Re-hydrating the sponge, without removing it, can be done with a bulb syringe or regular syringe saturating the sponge as necessary.

Hemostasis

Hemostasis can be achieved by using either energy or non-energy methods. Energy methods use either electrosurgery or electrocautery. Electrocautery is the use of a small amount of energy applied to a specific area with a handheld (usually battery-operated) device. This method is best for minimal bleeding in very superficial tissues. Electrosurgery is an energy method that requires equipment capable of generating a large amount of energy (500,000 cycles/seconds) to pass through tissue (Figure 4.26). This method is available in monopolar or bipolar options. If using a monopolar handpiece, a grounding plate MUST be used to complete the cycle of energy and remove the energy from the patient. The ground plate must have a conductive agent applied and most facilities use electrode gel (Figure 4.27). If using a bipolar handpiece because of its design (it looks like a tweezer), the current passes between the two tips, and the energy is removed from the patient in that circuit (Figure 4.28). Monopolar electrosurgery can be utilized by either touching the tissue/vessel directly with the electrosurgery handpiece or by touching an instrument clamping a vessel or tissue (Figure 4.29). Monopolar handpieces can be activated either with buttons on the handpiece or by using a foot pedal. Bipolar handpieces are activated when the handpiece is closed on the tissue. Technicians may be the person applying the electrosurgical pencil to the tissue or clamping the vessel with the hemostat. If electrosurgery is to be used, the cord from the handpiece must be secured on the sterile field to avoid having the handpiece slide off the field. Once the handpiece is on the sterile field, measure to allow enough

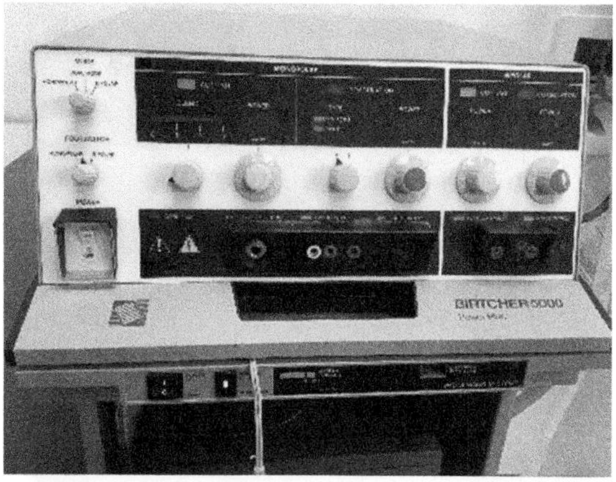

Figure 4.26 Electrosurgery unit.

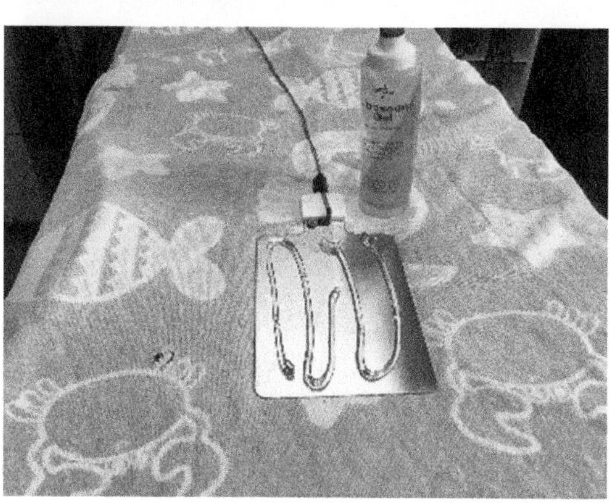

Figure 4.27 Ground plate with gel.

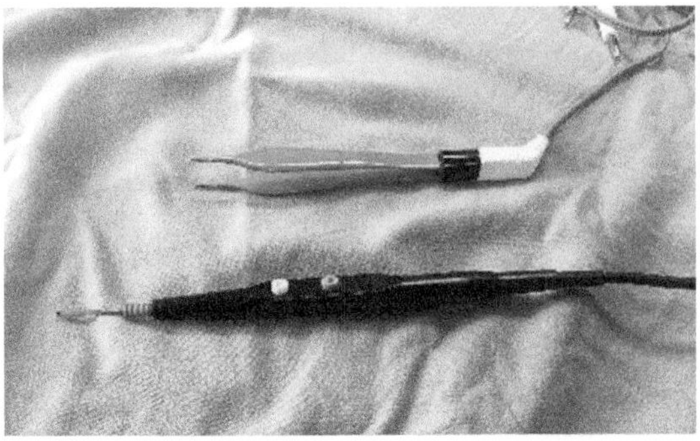

Figure 4.28 Bipolar (top) and monopolar (bottom) handpieces.

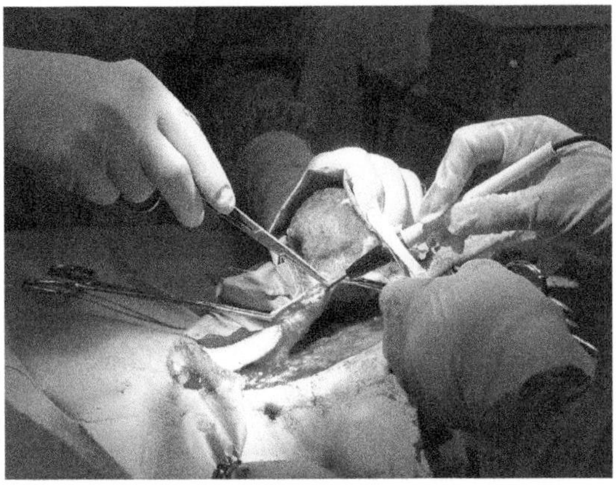

Figure 4.29 Electrosurgery handpiece touching instrument to cauterize tissue/vessel.

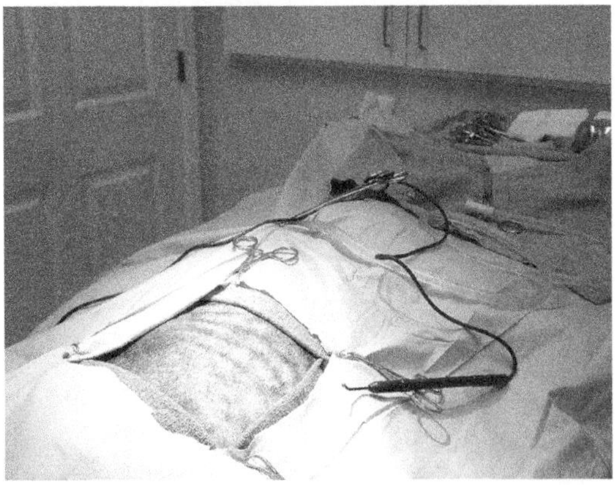

Figure 4.30 Electrosurgery pencil and suction tubing set up on the sterile field.

cord to reach all areas of the field. At the determined length, loop the cord in half and slip it through one ring handle of a towel clamp securing a drape. Then, take the loop and place it around the other ring handle of the same instrument (Figure 4.30). This will secure the cord without inhibiting electric flow to the handpiece. Then, the rest of the cord can be tossed off the sterile field so the circulating nurse can plug it in. Another popular energy-based hemostasis product is the Ligasure™ device. This surgical tool looks like an alligator forceps with ring handles, a long shaft, and an opposing jaw at the end of the shaft. This device uses pressure and energy to seal vessels up to 7 mm in diameter in 2–4 seconds.

Non-energy hemostasis can also be achieved by a variety of methods. The use of a cellulose product, gelatin sponge, or beeswax are all products available for use when electrosurgery is not feasible. Generally, these types of non-energy hemostatic agents are reserved for biopsies and other procedures where a defect that needs to be filled may be created in an organ. Small vessels or capillaries that are bleeding can often be controlled with pressure from a gauze sponge rather than using electrosurgery. When trying to control hemorrhage in an area, it is critical that either blotting or constant pressure be utilized. Wiping is contraindicated as it may disrupt a clot that is already forming on a microscopic level. A 16 ply 4″ × 4″ radiopaque sponge that is completely soaked will hold approximately 13 ml of blood. A 12″ × 12″ laparotomy sponge, soaking wet will hold ~65 ml. Radiopaque sponges should always be used with deep cavity surgeries as the radiopaque thread or strip in the sponge will allow for easy identification on a radiograph should a sponge be unaccounted for at the end of the procedure.

Suction

Hemostasis, as well as field vision, can also be controlled by the use of suction. A suction unit is a device that provides a vacuum, used via sterile tubing, to evacuate fluid from the surgical field. This unit can operate by an interfacility evacuation system or by electricity (Figure 4.31). There are canisters that sit in the unit to collect the fluid that is removed from the field. Sterile suction tubing must be opened for the surgical team. A suction tip will also be needed. The procedure being performed will dictate the type of suction tip that should be used. A Poole suction tip (Figure 4.32) is a two-piece tip that provided a basket with many holes that fit over the main suction tip. The basket assists with the prevention of trauma to tissue (i.e. omentum, lung, etc.) that may be trapped as the

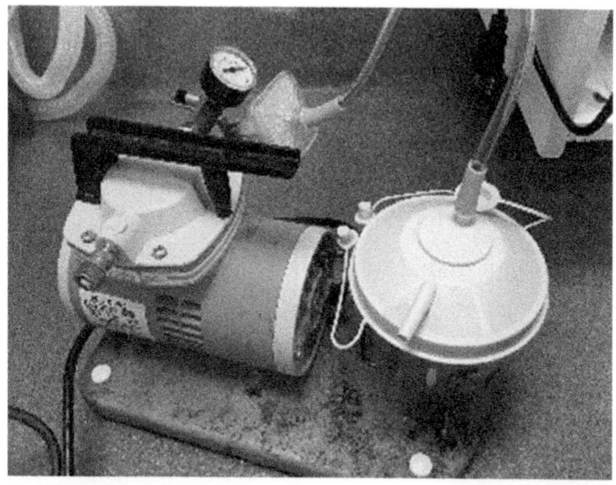

Figure 4.31 Suction unit.

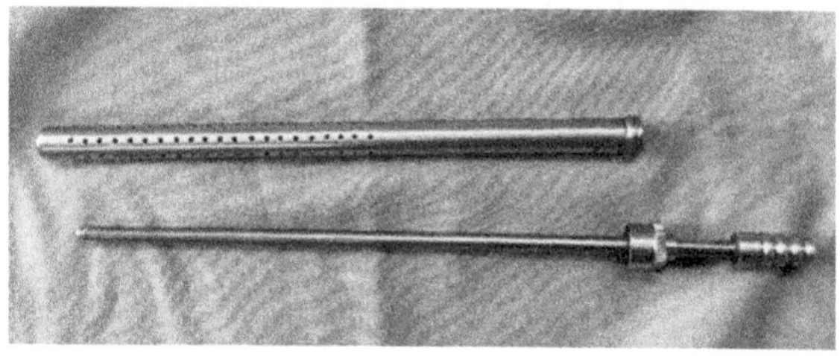

Figure 4.32 Poole suction tip.

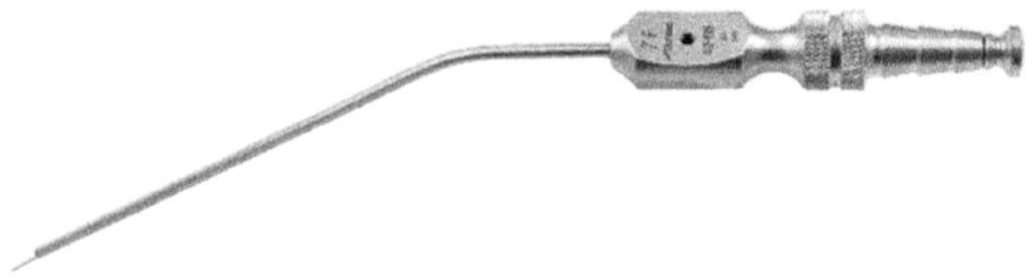

Figure 4.33 Frazier suction tip. *Source:* Courtesy of Sontec Instruments, Inc. (Cat No. 412–68).

fluid is evacuated. This tip is best used to quickly evacuate large volumes of fluid (lavage fluid, blood, and peritoneal fluid). Frazier suction tips are often used for orthopedic and neurologic surgeries (Figure 4.33). This tip is available in a variety of sizes ranging from 5 to 12 fr to best suit the need of the situation. Suction tubing is available for purchase as a sterile disposable product. Suction tubing, due to its length, is difficult to clean and should be disposed of after use. Suction tubing should be secured to the surgical field in a similar fashion as the electrosurgery handpiece. After determining the necessary length to remain on the sterile field, pass the tubing through one ring handle of a different towel clamp securing a drape, then pass it through the opposite ring handle of the same instrument. Make sure that the tubing is not kinked anywhere to compromise suction intensity. The rest of the tubing can be tossed off the table for the circulating nurse to connect to the suction unit.

Retraction

Excellent assistants will know exactly how much pressure can be placed on tissue with an instrument before damage occurs and will be able to recognize abnormalities in tissue appearance and will alert the surgeon. Ill-colored tissue, a decrease in blood pressure (evidenced by decreased oozing), and malposition of tissue or an organ are all examples of things that the surgeon may unintentionally miss. The surgeon is focusing on the problem of the patient that is to be corrected (as they should) and may not see "the whole picture" as the assistant does. In no way is it intended that the assistant insinuates the surgeon is not performing their duty, but rather the welfare of the patient is everyone's main concern (Figure 4.34).

Instrument Maintenance

In addition to understanding all the instrumentation and equipment and how it works, the assistant is responsible for maintaining that equipment during the procedure. Blood and other gross

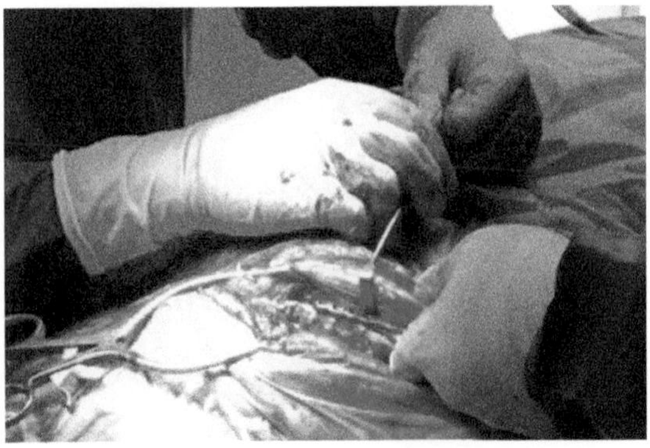

Figure 4.34 Assistant providing retraction.

material are very damaging to instruments if allowed to dry on the instrument. Not only does it instigate corrosion and pitting, but more importantly, it hinders the efficient function of the instrument. If a hemostatic forceps box lock and tip is covered in blood, it will neither open and close easily nor will it provide the 100% hemostasis and clamping pressure it was designed to provide. That could prove catastrophic in an emergency situation. Cleanliness of instrumentation is paramount in situations where the instrument will be repeatedly used such as drill bits and taps for screw placement or rasps or files in joint arthroplasty procedures. Instruments should never be allowed to soak in saline as that is very damaging. Surgical assistants must continually clean and wipe off instruments with sterile saline and gauze. Each time the surgeon uses an instrument during a procedure, it needs to function as well as the first time it was used.

Scalpel Blade/Handle Assembly

Loading the scalpel blade is the responsibility of the technician running the instrument table. Care should be taken to avoid injury while performing this seemingly easy yet dangerous task. First of all, using the correct instrument to seat the blade on the handle is paramount. The ONLY instrument that should be used is a needle holder. Never use a hemostatic forceps as the grooves in the tip can be damaged by the metal of the scalpel blade and cause the forceps to perform inadequately when it needs to clamp a vessel. Another common method of loading the blade onto the handle is using one's thumb and index finger. This is extremely dangerous and should never be done; one slip and a career-altering injury can result. To correctly load the blade, use the needle holder and grasp the non-cutting side of the blade above the space where the handle attaches (Figure 4.35). Holding the blade handle so the grooved edge on the tip of the handle is facing the ceiling. Starting at the tip of the handle, begin placing the blade on the groove of the tip (Figure 4.36). Advance the blade until it seats securely on the blade handle (Figure 4.37). There may be an audible "click" when the blade is firmly in place. A gentle tug should be done to ensure the blade is securely in place.

Sponge/Instrument Count

Performing a sponge count and instrument count before the incision is made and before the incision is closed also falls to the scrub assistant. Knowing the status of all sponges and instruments is a critical role of the assistant. Sponges (and less frequently, instruments) have been left

Figure 4.35 Holding the scalpel blade with the needle holder.

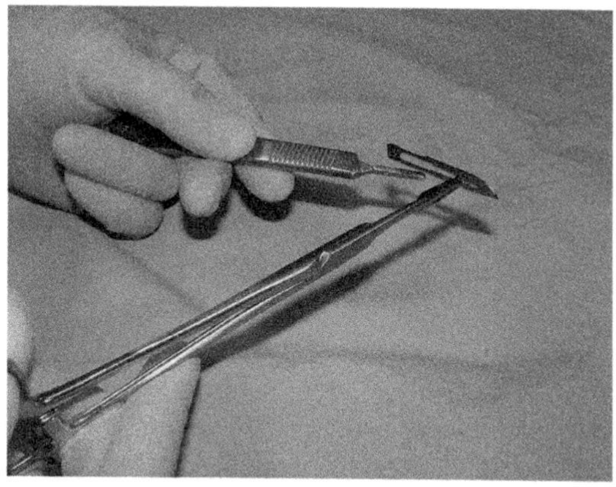

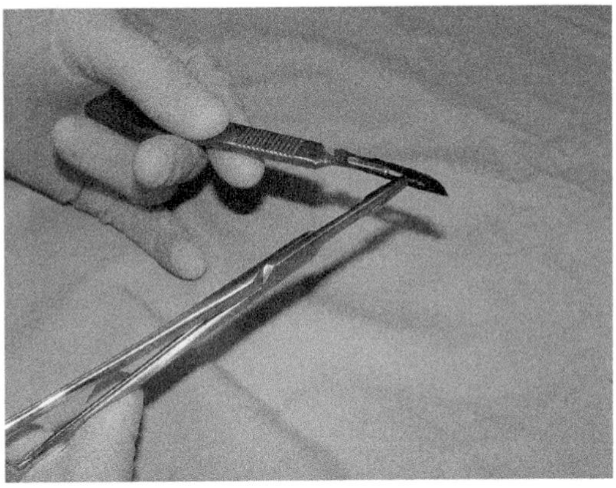

Figure 4.36 Begin placing the blade on the handle.

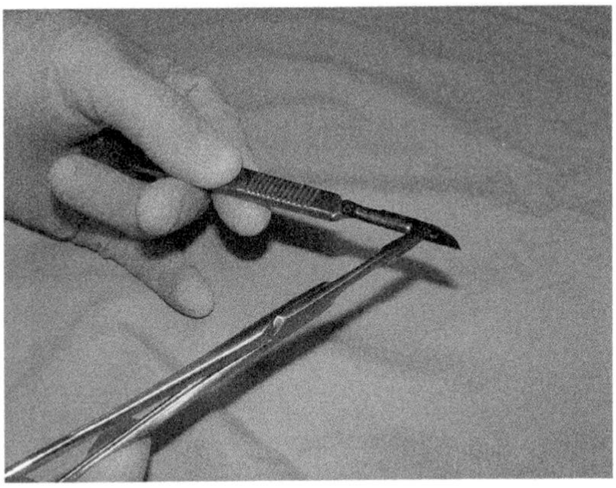

Figure 4.37 Fully seated blade.

in small animal patients. This incident is unacceptable as it is completely avoidable, especially when a technician is the surgical assistant. To perform a sponge count, all sponges on the sterile field are counted before the incision is made and reported to the circulating nurse. A note should be made on the operating room report form. As sponges are added, they should be counted, reported to the circulating nurse, and added to the OR report form. As sponges are used, they should only be discarded in a designated place, whether a specified sponge bowl off the sterile field or a designated kick bucket on the floor, which is the only area where dirty gauze from the surgical procedure should be found. Sponges that are on a surgical field should be in one of three places; on the instrument table, in the hand of the surgeon and/or assistant, or in the dirty sponge bucket located off the sterile field. NEVER leave a sponge just lying on the surgical field! Before the incision closure begins, the unused sponges on the instrument table should be counted by the assistant. The used sponges off the sterile field are counted by the circulating nurse. Both numbers are added together and should equal the total number of sponges opened and reported on the OR report form. If there is a discrepancy, the hunt must begin for the missing sponge(s). Sponges often hide under drape corners or are inadvertently thrown in the wrong kick bucket. Missing sponges must be accounted for before the wound is closed. Small 4″ × 4″ or 4″ × 8″ sponges should not be used to pack off organs in the abdomen or chest as they are too small and are easily forgotten or misplaced. Large radiopaque lap sponges (Figure 4.38) are the only item that should be packed into a body cavity. With a larger surface

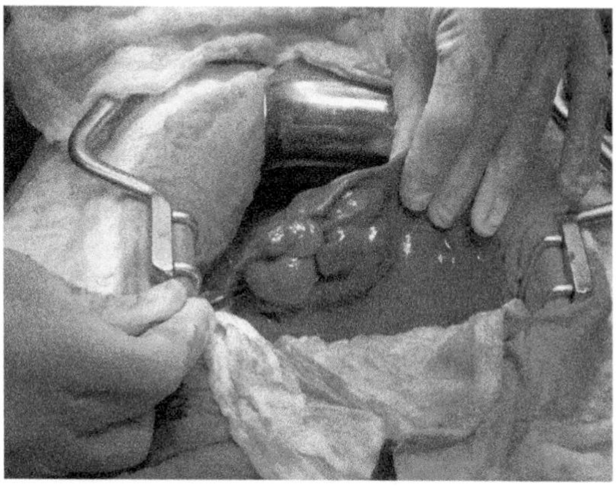

Figure 4.38 Moistened lap pad protecting tissues from Balfour retractor.

area and radiopaque indicator, they are more difficult to misplace or forget about. A lap sponge count should also be performed prior to closure of any body cavity.

Procedure Specific Duties

Depending on the procedure, there may be additional expectations of the assistant. During an arthroscopy, it is imperative that experienced hands are assisting the surgeon. Manipulating the limb for maximum visibility, monitoring the limb for fluid extravasation, and assisting with instrument manipulation are all talents the surgeon expects of the assistant. Knowing the assistant will step up and perform without being asked is invaluable to the surgeon. Other minimally invasive procedures have equally critical needs for the assistant. Having the monitor positioned properly for a laparoscopy and knowing which trocar and cannula are needed before the laparoscope is placed can make a procedure run effortlessly. Stifle surgeries and fracture repairs can benefit greatly from an efficient assistant being a member of the sterile team. Whether assisting with a tibial plateau leveling osteotomy (TPLO) (Figures 4.39 and 4.40) or a mid-humeral fracture repair with plates and screws, having an assistant who knows the order of the instruments needed for screw placement (drill guide, drill bit, depth gauge, screw, and screwdriver) and hands them as the surgeon needs them can save measurable time during a procedure.

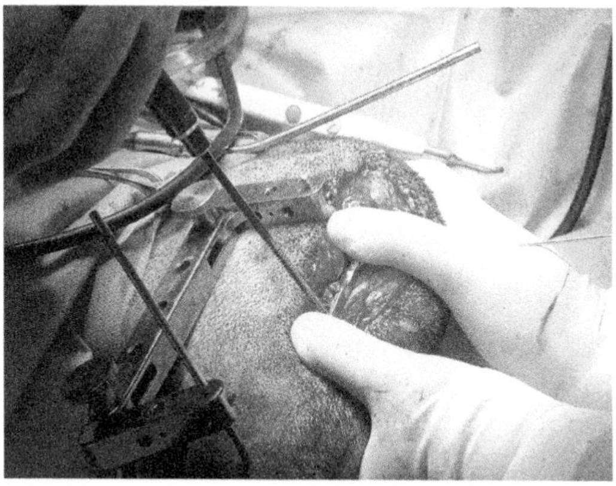

Figure 4.39 Assistant stabilizing limb for placement of a TPLO plate.

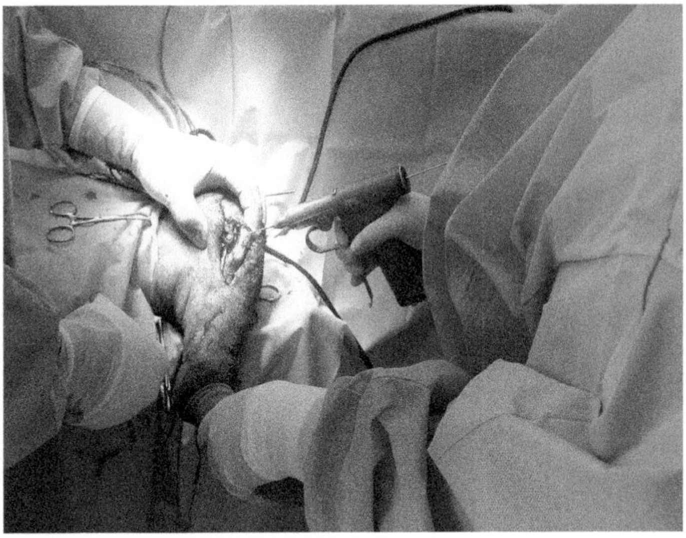

Figure 4.40 Assistant removing pins.

Suture Materials and Suture Patterns

Another skill required of the surgical assistant is the knowledge of suture materials, suture patterns, and stapling devices that may be utilized during the procedure. In addition, the surgical assistant must be familiar with specific characteristics of each suture type, indications for use, patterns chosen by the surgeon, and the stapling options available. If there were a perfect suture, it would have the following characteristics:

- pliability for easy handling
- low tissue drag
- minimal tissue reactivity
- little memory
- consistent uniform diameter
- high tensile strength
- predictable performance

Many of these characteristics are achieved by suture material currently available, but there is no ideal suture. Having said that, these characteristics as well as others will influence the decision regarding which suture is chosen. Often not only are the suture characteristics taken into consideration, but the surgeon's personal preference as well. Availability of product, area of the body being sutured, the patient's overall health, and the viability of the tissue being sutured also affect the decision (Table 4.1).

Characteristics

Pliability of the suture is an important factor to consider. The easier it is for the surgeon to handle and manipulate the suture, the faster the procedure will progress. In addition, ease of handling generally equates to better knot security. Most frequently multifilament sutures will be easier to handle.

Table 4.1 Suture characteristics.

Suture name	Generic name	Natural/ synthetic	Absorbable/ non-absorbable	Monofilament/ multifilament	Tensile strength	Absorption rate	Comments
Plain gut		Natural	Absorbable		Tensile strength loss affected by patient characteristics	Absorbed by enzymatic process	Available as yellowish tan and dyed blue
Chromic Catgut		Natural	Absorbable	Monofilament	Tensile strength loss affected by patient characteristics	Absorbed by enzymatic process	Available brown and dyed blue
PDS	Polidioxanone	Synthetic	Absorbable	Monofilament	70% remains at 2 wk 50% remains at 4 wk 25% remains at 6 wk	At 6 mo essentially complete	Available in clear, blue, and violet
Biosyn	Glycomer 631	Synthetic	Absorbable	Monofilament	75% at 2 wk; ~40% at 3 wk	Complete between 90 and 110 d	Excellent knot security, minimal memory
Maxon		Synthetic	Absorbable	Monofilament	75% at 2 wk; 65% at 3 wk; 50% at 4 wk	Minimal for first 60 d; complete within 6 mo	Excellent handling; minimal memory
Monocryl	Poliglecaprone 25	Synthetic	Absorbable	Monofilament	50–60% remains at 1 wk, 20–30% remains at 2 wk, and lost by 3 wk	91–119 d shows completion	Available undyed and violet. Also available with antimicrobial coating
Caprosyn	Polyglytone 6211	Synthetic	Absorbable	Monofilament	Lost by 21 d postimplantation	Complete in 56 d	Excellent handling; excellent know security
Vicryl	Polyglactin 910	Synthetic	Absorbable	Multifilament	75% remains at 2 wk, 50% remains at 3 wk, and 25% remains at 4 wk	56–70 d to completion	Available undyed and violet. Also available with antimicrobial coating
Dexon		Synthetic	Absorbable	Multifilament	65% at 2 wk and 35% at 3 wk	Complete between 60 and 90 d	Available dyed green or undyed
Ethilon	Nylon	Synthetic	Non-absorbable	Monofilament	Gradual loss over time due to hydrolysis	Gradual encapsulation over time	Available green, clear, and violet
Prolene	Polypropylene	Synthetic	Non-absorbable	Monofilament	No degradation	Non-absorbable	Available clear and in blue
Silk		Natural	Non-absorbable	Multifilament	Gradual loss over time due to progressive degradation	Gradual encapsulation over time	Available in violet and white
Mersilene	Polyester	Synthetic	Non-absorbable	Multifilament	No change known to occur	Gradual encapsulation over time	Available in white and green

Tissue drag means the suture moves easily through the tissues and therefore causes less irritation to the tissue. It is desirable for sutures to have this characteristic to minimize tissue irritation and stress, which could compromise wound healing. Monofilament and coated sutures often provide minimal tissue drag.

Memory is the act of the suture returning to its packaged coiled state, which provides challenges when working with it. Suture that coils tends to become knotted or tangled more easily. Multifilament sutures generally have less memory than other sutures.

Tensile strength is the amount of force, in pounds, that the suture can withstand before breaking. This characteristic is important to consider when suturing tissues that are under a lot of physical stress. Frequently, the tensile strength of a suture increases with the size (diameter) of the suture.

A uniform diameter size is critical for insuring quality knot security. If the suture is wider in one section of the strand than in others, the knots will not be equally formed and therefore will not have good security. This characteristic is controlled by quality assurance practices of the suture manufacturer. Suture of lesser quality may not have the stringent quality control measures of higher-grade materials.

Finally, predictable performance is important from the surgeon's perspective. Surgeon's preference often determines the suture chosen and if a surgeon has had a bad experience using a particular suture, it is unlikely to be chosen again.

Sizing

Suture material is sized according to United States Pharmacopeia (USP) standards. The easiest way to remember suture sizing is the following: The more the zeros, the smaller the suture, and the larger the whole number, the larger the suture. Suture sizes can be written one of two ways – 000 is three zeros so it is called three ought. This could also be written as 3-0. A suture that is 00000 is five zeros or five ought or 5-0 and is a smaller suture in diameter than the 3-0. Number 2 suture is a whole number and is, therefore, larger in diameter than 3-0. The size suture chosen by the surgeon has many factors influencing the decision including patient size and the tissue being worked with. Other criteria that are considered by the surgeon before selecting a size include intended purpose, tissue integrity, number of layers of closure to be used, and type of suture pattern placed. In general, surgeons will choose the smallest size possible to hold the tissue as it heals. This practice minimizes additional tissue trauma and results in the least amount of foreign material in the patient. Wounds over active joints (stifle and elbow) may need a larger-size suture to bear the additional stress on the wound. Incisions on non-weight-bearing areas (abdomen and medial limb) may be adequately closed with a smaller-sized suture.

Classification

Sutures are classified using three qualities: absorbable vs. non-absorbable; multifilament vs. monofilament; and synthetic vs. natural.

Absorbable vs. Non-absorbable

The quality of absorbable vs. non-absorbable is fairly self-explanatory. Absorbable sutures are broken down in the body by one of two different methods. Natural/organic absorbable suture is broken down by tissue enzymes that weaken the suture strand, which results in phagocytosis. Synthetic absorbable suture is hydrolyzed, which means water penetrates the strands and breaks down the polymers. This type of absorption causes much less tissue reaction than enzyme degradation. There is a rare instance of a non-absorbable *eventually* breaking down (i.e. silk), but it is safe to say non-absorbable suture will remain in the tissue for an indefinite time period following implantation. Non-absorbable sutures, when used internally, are encapsulated or walled off by fibrous tissue. Absorbable suture is almost exclusively used on internal tissue. Absorbable sutures are most often used in general surgery except for cardiovascular, ophthalmic, and neurologic procedures. The experienced circulating nurse will know what type of suture the surgeon is most likely to choose and the pattern of placement that will probably be employed. Although entirely the surgeon's decision/preference and case dependence, the technician can *anticipate* which material will be used, but will also be able to provide whatever the surgeon requests (Figure 4.41).

Monofilament vs. Multifilament

Monofilament sutures are one solid strand of material. This type of suture is often chosen when the risk of infection is present as it does not harbor bacteria, which can cause an infection later. Another advantage of this type of suture is that it glides more easily through the tissue (low tissue drag) thus causing less tissue trauma. Monofilament suture usually ties easily, but care must be taken to avoid kinking the material while making knots. Kinking can weaken the suture and lead to premature breakdown of the strand. Multifilament sutures are multiple strands twisted or braided together. This type of suture handles wonderfully, has little memory, and provides good knot security. The disadvantages include increased tissue resistance when passing through tissue, and increased risk of infection as it can "wick" or harbor harmful bacteria which can cause infections (Figure 4.42). Both monofilament and multifilament suture materials are available with an antibacterial coating to counteract the colonization of bacteria in the suture.

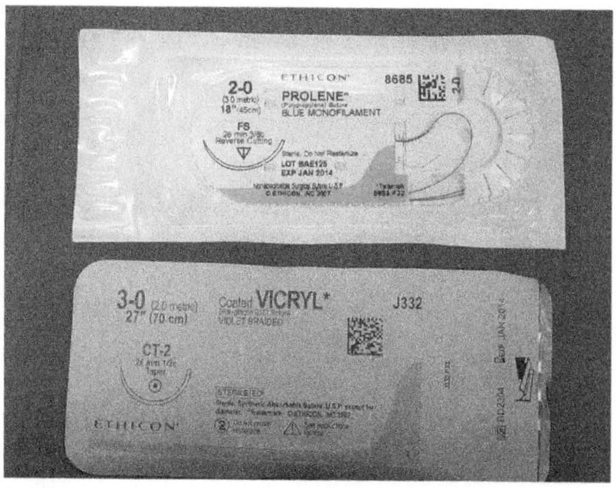

Figure 4.41 Absorbable (bottom) vs. nonabsorbable.

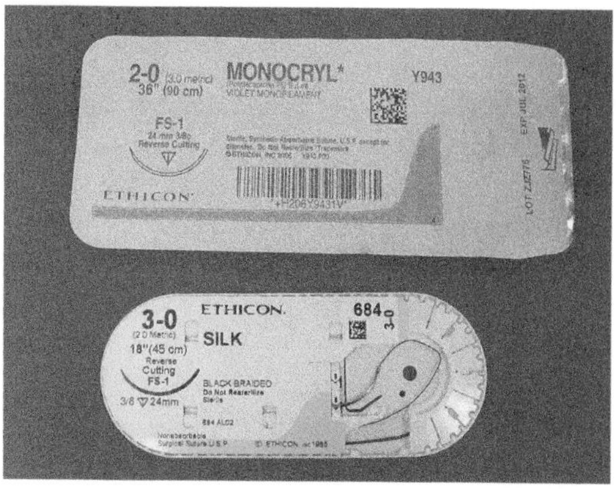

Figure 4.42 Monofilament (top) vs. multifilament (braided).

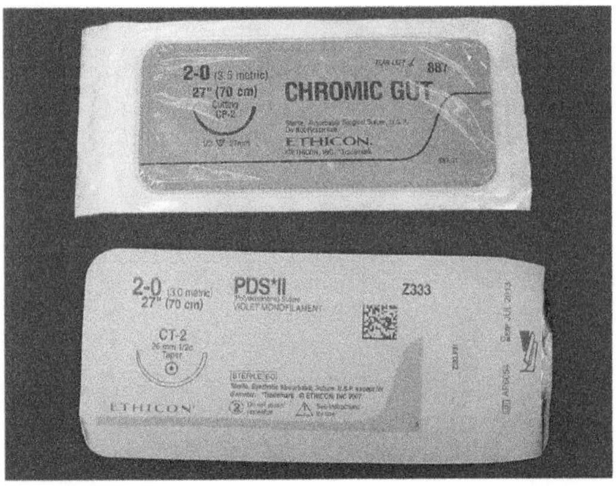

Figure 4.43 Natural (top) vs. synthetic.

Natural/Organic vs. Synthetic

Natura/organic sutures are made of materials found in nature, such as catgut and silk. Synthetic suture is that which is created as a product of man-made materials. Some examples of synthetic suture include those made of polypropylene or polymers (Figure 4.43).

Suture Material

Absorbable Sutures – Monofilament

Catgut is one of the most commonly used absorbable sutures. It is made of sheep intestine submucosa or beef intestinal serosa. It is 97–98% pure collagen that is spun into strands and then polished into a monofilament product. Both plain gut and chromic gut are available. Plain gut has a very rapid absorption time (completed by 70 days) but tensile strength is only maintained for 5–7 days. Plain gut has very limited use in veterinary surgery and is therefore not seen very often. Chromic catgut is plain gut that has been treated with chromium salts that resist enzymes and therefore extend the absorption time up to 90 days. With chromic gut tensile strength, duration is doubled to 10–14 days. The treatment with chromium salts will turn the whitish/yellow plain gut into a brownish/tan colored suture. Catgut has a notable inflammatory response in tissue which must be considered when used.

Other monofilament sutures that have been available for a while include polydioxanon (PDS®) and polyglyconate (Maxon®). Both are synthetic products that have varying absorption times from three to six months, yet are known for maintaining their tensile strength for >21 days. For gastrointestinal, respiratory, and urinary procedures, a monofilament absorbable suture will often be chosen. In a case where the tissues are more traumatized or diseased, this longer timeframe may be desirable. Despite their inert property and ability to move easily through tissue, they do present some difficulties when working with them. These sutures are fairly stiff, have excessive memory, and require additional throws for good knot security. These properties illustrate that these sutures are not the best choices for subcutaneous or intradermal suture patterns.

Newer monofilament absorbable sutures include poliglecaprone 25 (Monocryl®), glycomer 631 (Biosyn®), and polyglytone 6211 (Caprosyn®). These products may be a better choice for uncompromised tissue that will regain strength rapidly. Urinary bladder cases as well as certain gastric procedures would be good indications for choosing these sutures. One of the factors that surgeons consider when choosing a suture is to match the healing rate of the tissue with the degradation of the suture material. Other benefits of some of the newer monofilament absorbable products are increased ease of handling, significant tensile strength loss up to 14 days post-placement, minimal tissue reactions, and complete absorption as early as 56 days.

Absorbable – Multifilament

Multifilament absorbable sutures like polyglactin 910 (Vicryl®) and polyglycolic acid (Dexon®) are proven classics. These are also synthetic sutures that have absorption times from 42 to 70 days. As a multifilament, their use in visceral tissue is contraindicated, however, due to their ease of handling, they are often used as subcutaneous sutures. Some multifilament sutures are available with a coating of glycolide lactide and calcium stearate, which allows the suture to pass through tissues with much less resistance. Frequent cases of tissue reaction at the incision when polyglactin 910 (Vicryl) is used have created some hesitancy to use this suture. A new multifilament absorbable suture is Polysorb® and offers a new alternative to surgeons. Due to its tensile strength decreasing to 30% at 21 days and its complete absorption by 60 days postplacement, the opportunity for tissue reaction is lessened, thus resulting in fewer incisional issues.

Non-absorbable Suture – Monofilament

Monofilament non-absorbable sutures are used primarily for skin closure, tube security, or holding wound-covering devices in place. Occasionally non-absorbable suture material may be used internally, such as in stifle surgeries or in closure of the abdominal wall of a patient with adhesions or multiple surgery history where healing may be compromised. Cardiovascular procedures (graft placement, valve replacement, etc.) will use non-absorbable sutures to ensure that the integrity of the repair is not compromised by suture that can break down. Internal structures with limited blood supply (i.e. tendons and fascia) are often apposed with non-absorbable suture due to the slow healing of the tissue. When using non-absorbable suture for skin closure, the color of the suture should be taken into consideration based on the patient's hair coat color. For example, finding black nylon skin sutures on a black Labrador Retriever 14 days postimplantation is quite a challenge. However, blue polypropylene sutures on the same patient would be much easier to see and accomplish the same end result. The most commonly seen monofilament non-absorbable sutures are nylon (Ethilon®) and polypropylene (Prolene®). Available in a variety of sizes, either suture is suitable for feline to equine patients. Nylon is available in both black monofilament and braided styles. Polypropylene (Prolene) is a bright blue color and it is easily distinguishable with almost every color hair coat. Stainless steel is the final monofilament non-absorbable choice. Although not used frequently in veterinary patients, it is sometimes chosen to help deter licking of the incision by anxious patients.

Non-absorbable – Multifilament

Braided non-absorbable sutures include polyester (Mersilene®), silk, and Vetafil® or Fluorofil®. Polyester is a pliable braided suture indicated for internal use for all types of procedures including cardiovascular, ophthalmic, and neurologic cases. It is contraindicated as a skin suture due to its braided nature. Silk is another multifilament of non-absorbable suture that is frequently used for ligation or cardiovascular cases. Silk has long been regarded as the premier suture when it comes to ease of handling. The raw silk filament, which is produced by the silk worm, is degummed and then braided into strands. The naturally occurring gum on the suture enables the cocoon to hold together but is of no benefit in surgery. Although classified as a non-absorbable suture, silk is relatively non-detectable in tissue two years after implantation. Vetafil is a synthetic non-absorbable suture. It is basically a hollow suture that has multiple strands constructing the wall around a hollow middle. It is inexpensive compared to other non-absorbable choices and therefore is often used as a skin closure material. As with absorbable sutures, final selection of a non-absorbable suture is the decision of the surgeon; however, technicians can anticipate what will be requested. Circulating techs should refrain from opening any suture until either asked to do so or until they have checked with the surgeon.

Suture Patterns

Some states allow credentialed technicians to suture skin incisions of surgical patients. Although a wonderful use of a surgical assistant, it is fair to say these states are in the minority. Even if the technician will not be performing the suturing, it is important that they understand the placement process of the patterns. "Running" the suture during a continuous pattern and being ready to cut the sutures to the correct length during an interrupted pattern are very important skills for the assistant. Suture patterns are either continuous or interrupted. Continuous patterns are placed by the surgeon without ever cutting the suture until at the end of the pattern. Interrupted patterns have the suture cut after each stitch is placed. Continuous patterns are faster to place but bear the risk of incisional dehiscence if even one stitch breaks down. Interrupted patterns take longer to place and use more suture, but the entire incision is not compromised if one stitch has issues.

Suture patterns are also classified by the way they appose tissue. Appositional patterns mean the tissue edges just meet and healing occurs side to side. Everting patterns result in the skin edges turning out away from the patient. These patterns usually result in more scarring as well as slower healing. Inverting patterns turn the tissue edges inward, toward the patient, and are reserved for use on hollow organs such as intestines or the stomach.

Continuous Patterns

Simple Continuous

Probably the most commonly used continuous pattern is the simple continuous (Figure 4.44). It is used to close muscle layers, body cavities, and even skin closures. It is placed by taking a

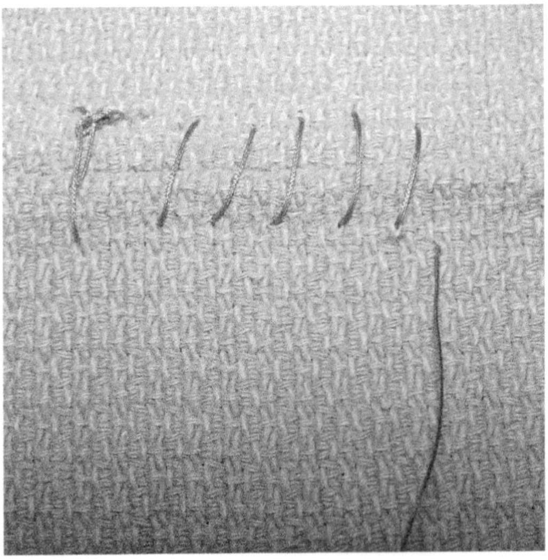

Figure 4.44 Simple continuous.

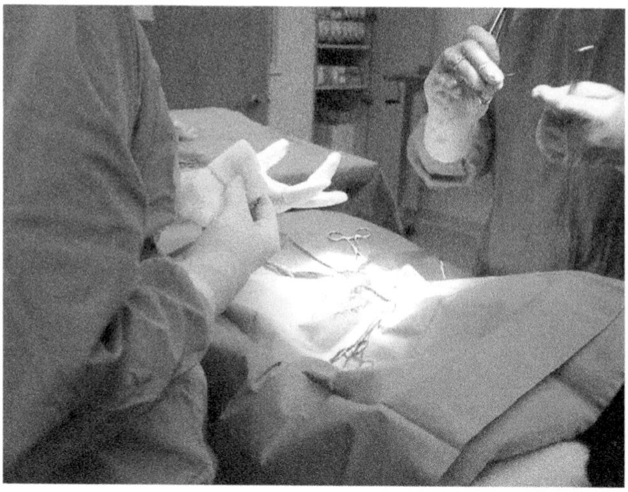

Figure 4.45 Assistant running suture for surgeon.

bite on one side of the tissue gap, passing the needle under the tissue gap, and then the needle comes up on the other side, an equal distance from the gap as the initial bite. The next bite starts on the same side as the first bite, passes under the tissue, and comes up on the opposite side – following the same process as the first stitch. The suture is pulled to appose the edges and the pattern continues to the end of the wound. As the surgeon progresses through the wound closure, the assistant is responsible for holding the suture or "running" the suture (Figure 4.45). Holding the suture out of the way for the surgeon will greatly assist in the speed with which the pattern can be placed. Maintaining enough tension, but not too much, on the suture also is the responsibility of the assistant. Ending the pattern can be accomplished by not pulling the suture tight with the last stitch. Leaving a loop provides a method of creating the knot to end the pattern. Depending on where the pattern is being placed, some people choose to bury the knot. This can be done by only cutting the loop strands of the knot. This leaves the long end of the suture still intact. The needle is passed under the tissue beyond the end of the suture line, and the needle re-surfaces ~½″ to 1″ beyond the end of the suture line and is pulled tight. This results in the knot being pulled under the tissue. The suture is cut close to the tissue so the suture end disappears once cut.

Ford Interlocking

The Ford interlocking continuous pattern is used less frequently in small animal surgery than in large animal surgery. This suture pattern resembles a "blanket stitch" for anyone familiar with sewing patterns (Figure 4.46). The benefit of a Ford interlocking pattern is its strength and it is primarily used as a skin closure pattern. Having an assistant who can effectively run the suture with this pattern is especially helpful for the veterinary surgeon. When beginning the pattern, the first bite is the needle starting approximately ½″ lateral to the incision, passing the needle under the tissue gap, and then having the needle exit an equal distance from the incision on the opposite side. The suture strand is held parallel to the incision and the needle passes over the long strand. The stitch is repeated in the same fashion, passing over the long strand each time to create the pattern.

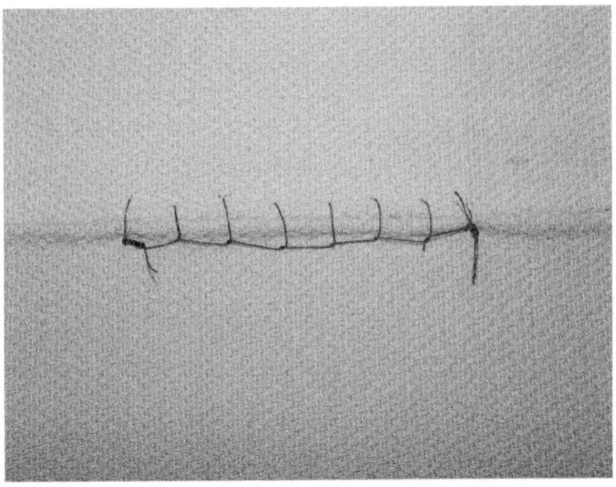

Figure 4.46 Ford interlocking.

Lembert, Cushing, and Connell Patterns

These three patterns are inverting continuous patterns used to close hollow organs. Surgical assistants are less frequently called upon to assist with organ closure, but may still need to run the suture for the surgeon placing one of these patterns.

Interrupted Patterns

Simple Interrupted

This is the most frequently used interrupted pattern (Figure 4.47). This pattern can be used internally, subcutaneously, or externally. To create this pattern, the needle is passed through the tissue ~½″ from the wound edge, under the incision or tissue gap, and exiting on the opposite side, an equal distance from the wound. The suture is then tied with the knot off to one side so it is not on the incision. If internal, this stitch should have the suture ends cut close to the knot, without cutting the knot. If placed externally, the suture strands should be cut ~½″ to ¾″ in length so they can be found and held during suture removal.

Horizontal Mattress

This suture pattern is often used in areas where there is a lot of tension. It is, therefore, rarely seen as a skin suture, unless tension is present (Figure 4.48). To place this suture pattern, the needle is driven through the skin, ~½″ from the wound edge, on the far side, and under the incision. The

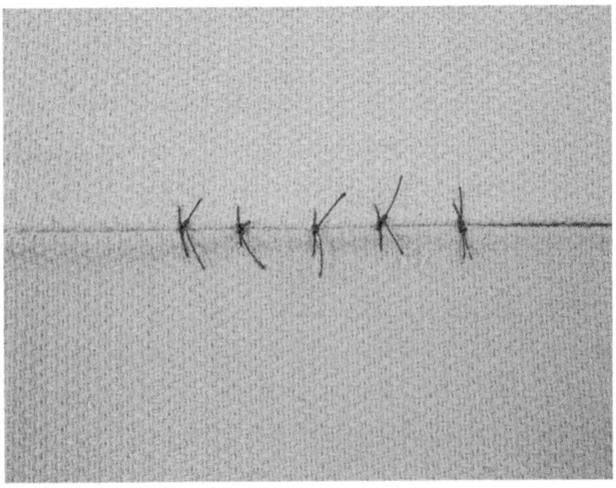

Figure 4.47 Simple interrupted.

Figure 4.48 Horizontal mattress.

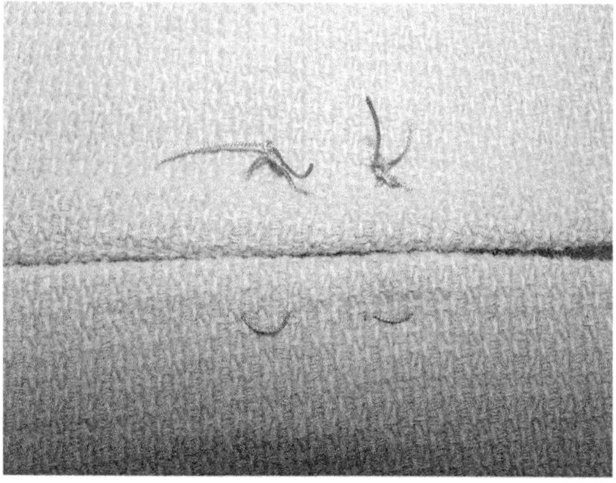

Figure 4.49 Cruciate.

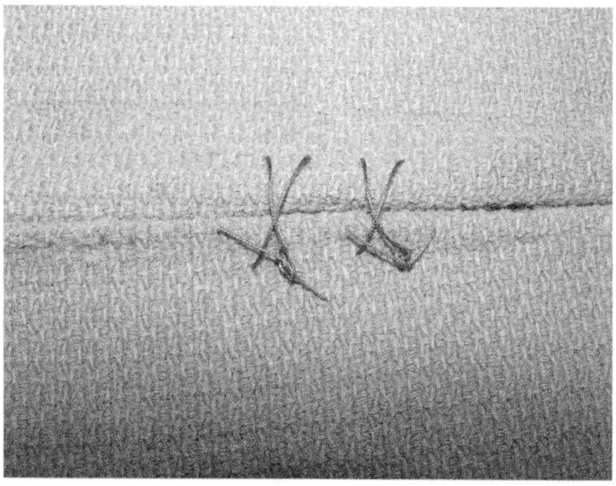

needle exits on the near side of the wound, ~½″ from the wound edge. The needle is then moved ~4 mm down the incision line and introduced from the near side. The needle passes under the wound and exits on the far side, ~½″ from the wound edge. The suture is then tied and the knot rests on the skin parallel to the wound. It is easy to evert this pattern, so if assistants are involved with the placement, care must be taken to avoid over-pulling the suture and creating the eversion.

Cruciate Pattern

This pattern is a variation of the horizontal mattress pattern and can be used internally as well as externally (Figure 4.49). This pattern starts exactly the same way as the horizontal mattress. In the Cruciate pattern, the needle is introduced through the tissue on the far side of the wound with the needle placement ~½″ from the wound edge. The needle is passed under the tissue gap and exits ~½″ from the edge of the wound on the opposite side. Now to make it different from the horizontal mattress, the needle is moved about 4 mm down the wound and passed through the tissue, starting on the far side. The suture is now tied and an "X" appears created from the suture over the wound. As with the simple interrupted pattern, the knot is usually placed off the wound line.

Vertical Mattress

The vertical mattress pattern may be placed where there is a lot of tension, as with the horizontal mattress. Known to be stronger than the horizontal mattress, it takes more time to place this pattern (Figure 4.50). The needle is introduced ~8 mm from the wound edge on the far side of the

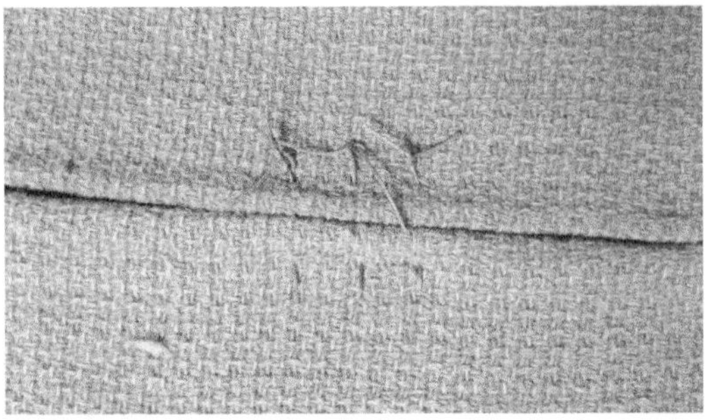

Figure 4.50 Vertical mattress.

wound. The needle passes under the tissue gap and exits on the opposite side, again 8 mm from the wound edge. The needle is then re-introduced on the same side it just exited, half way between the exit site and the wound edge. The needle passes under the tissue gap and exits on the opposite side, again halfway between the wound edge and the first puncture. The suture is then tied and the knot is on the side of the wound.

Cutting Suture

In addition to being knowledgeable about the pattern being placed and the characteristics of the suture, the surgical assistant must know how long or short to leave the suture ends when they are asked to cut the suture. The surgeon may give some indication of the length desired, but a great assistant will already know. Assistants must also know if they are cutting just one strand of the suture or both. Frequently, the surgeon will indicate "just one or both," but there is nothing more frustrating than to have both strands cut when a continuous pattern was to be used.

Internal Sutures

When cutting internally placed suture material, the assistant must know that the suture ends need to be short, but not so short that the knot is compromised or even cut. Internal sutures are generally cut short to decrease the amount of foreign material in the body that can potentially lead to inflammation and infection. To accomplish just the right consistent length, the blades of the operating scissors can be opened ~½″ and slid down the suture until the knot is reached. The scissor blades are then turned 45° and the suture is cut. This will provide for a short suture end without being too close to the knot (Figure 4.51).

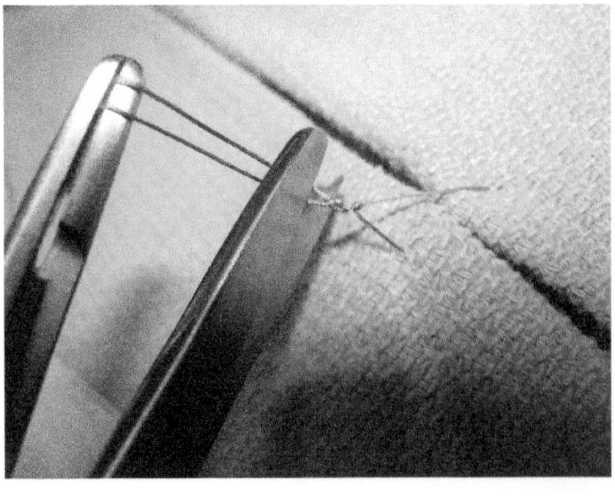

Figure 4.51 Scissor position for cutting internal sutures.

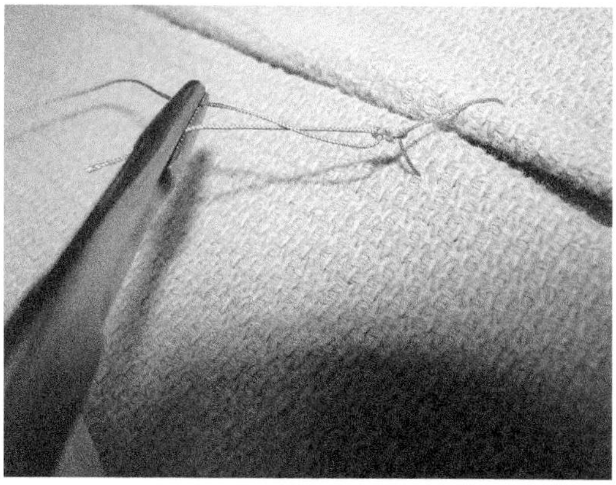

Figure 4.52 Suture strands crossed to indicate where to cut external sutures.

External Sutures

External sutures may vary in size depending on several factors. The surgeon must consider the number of layers of tissue already closed. When more layers are closed with suture, the dependency on the skin for strength with healing decreases. In addition, the surgeon must be considerate of the personality of the patient. This is where the technician can provide valuable information. If the patient has the type of personality that will lead to increased licking or chewing of the incision and sutures, then that information should be shared as it will affect what the surgeon chooses to use. Finally, the surgeon must think about the anatomic location of the wound. If it is a very tense skin closure (i.e. mastectomy) or an incision that will be exposed to a lot of motion due to the fact that it is over a joint, the surgeon will adjust the suture type and pattern. Externally placed sutures, whether to secure drains, close an orifice (i.e. purse string suture), or skin incision sutures, must have suture "tails" or ends left long enough so they can easily be found when it is time to remove the sutures. Usually drain sutures or orifice sutures are removed shortly after they are placed (hours to two to three days). Skin sutures are generally removed 7–14 days postplacement. Patient healing status as well as other factors (medications such as corticosteroids, environment, and patient tolerance) may affect that timeframe. When cutting external sutures, generally a ½″–¾″ suture end is left. Often times, the surgeon may cross the two strands of suture, and where the two meet is an indication of where to cut the suture (Figure 4.52).

Staples

External (Skin) Staples

External skin staples may be used to close the skin instead of conventional sutures. The benefits of skin staples include shorter anesthesia time, faster wound closure, increased integrity due to the fact that staples can withstand more patient licking than sutures, and relative ease of removal. Disadvantages include expense, poor performance in incisions with increased tension, and tendency for rotation, which makes removal more challenging. Skin staples also easily evert the wound edges, which in turn makes the healing much less cosmetic. Skin staples are metal implants that are enclosed within a gun-like apparatus (Figure 4.53). After the wound edges are apposed with a thumb tissue forceps, the stapler trigger is squeezed and a staple is placed. Staples are not as secure as skin sutures and should be placed ~6 mm apart from one another. As with skin sutures,

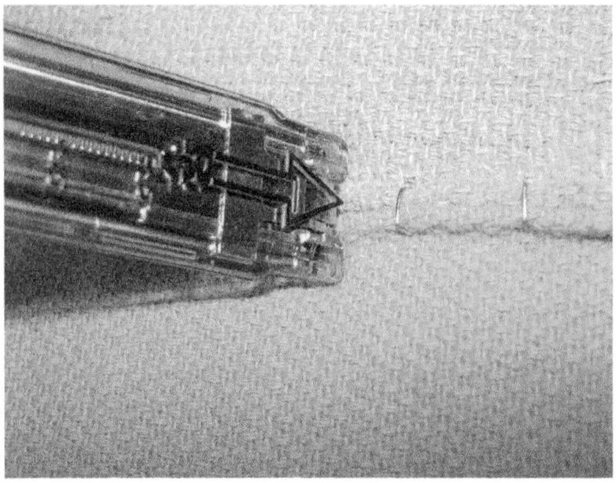

Figure 4.53 Proper approach for skin staple placement.

the number of staples placed should be recorded in the patient's medical record so that at the time of removal no staples or stitches are accidentally left in the animal.

Internal Staples

Internal stapling devices are intended to be used instead of sutures. Although expensive, the benefit of shaving critical minutes off the procedure is overwhelmingly beneficial. Staples and the accompanying stapling devices are named for their function. For example, a TA™ stapler is intended for thoracoabdominal cases. TA staplers also have a number in the name, which indicates the number of "B"-shaped staples that will be placed. All of the internal stapling devices discharge the entire cartridge when activated. Careful attention to loading and handling the loaded device is critical to avoid a costly accidental discharge. TA staples are used for lung lobectomies, tumor resections, or other situations where a straight line of staples is needed. This stapling device is available in three sizes, namely 30, 55, and 90 mm, which indicates the length of the staple line when discharged (Figure 4.54). Intestinal surgical cases have three different options for staplers, should the case warrant it. The GIA™ (gastrointestinal anastomosis) stapler is a linear device that has two double rows of staggered B-shaped staples and then cuts in between the two rows (Figure 4.55). The GIA is available in 50, 60, 80, and

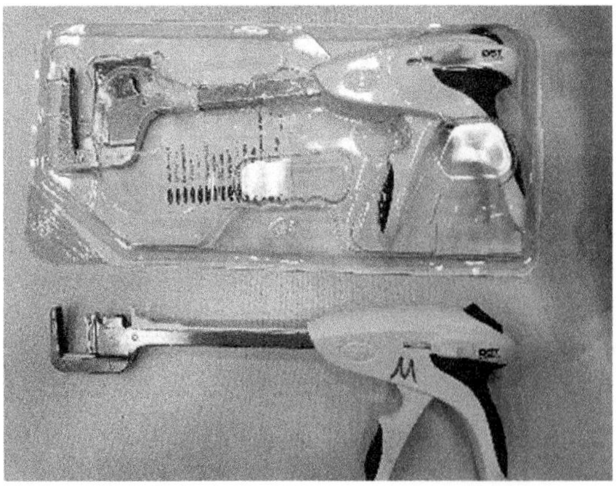

Figure 4.54 TA stapling device.

Figure 4.55 GIA stapling device.

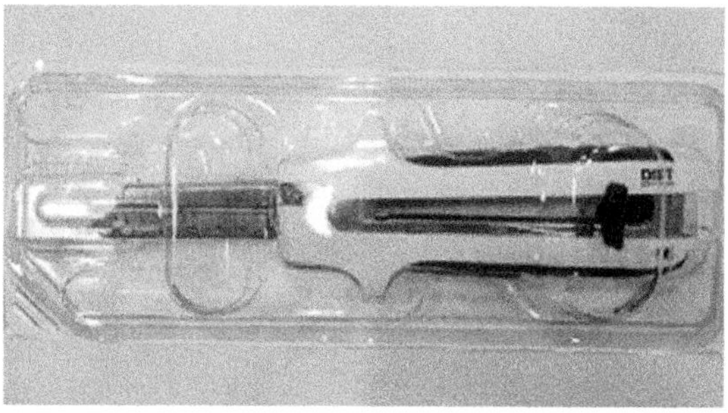

90 mm lengths. The intestinal linear anastomosis (ILA) stapler places the same rows of staples as the GIA, however, the ILA staples are of a different size. The EEA™ (end-to-end anastomosis) places a circular double row of staples. The circular blade within the cartridge removes the excess inverted tissue, thus creating a new lumen. Staples can be especially beneficial when performing an anastomosis due to the increased time required for the extensive suturing that is required.

Circulating Nurse

Another very important role of the technician within the surgical suite is that of the circulating nurse. The responsibilities of the circulator include setting up and preparing the operating room for the procedure, aseptically opening all needed equipment, anticipating the needs of the surgeon, retrieving any equipment or supply requested, and most importantly, monitoring the asepsis of the procedure.

Setting Up the Room

Before any surgical case begins, the surgical suite needs to be prepared. All surfaces including tables, shelves, light fixtures, etc. must be wiped free of dust that may have settled. Using a cloth and 70% isopropyl alcohol is sufficient to accomplish this task. Next, the equipment necessary for the case must be placed in the room. Especially in a multi-doctor facility, it is helpful for the circulating nurse to have "case sheets" for each surgeon/case. For instance, if Dr. Smith likes his patients positioned a certain way for a procedure, that information could be on the sheet as well as all the special equipment he wants for that procedure. Dr. Johnson, however, likes her patients positioned a different way for the same procedure and she uses different equipment. The case sheets will help ensure that the room is ready with that surgeon's particular needs. Placing the packs and equipment in the proper location for ease of opening and flow of getting the procedure started is very important (Figure 4.56). Placing the electrosurgery ground plate on the table should also be the responsibility of the circulating nurse. Some electrosurgery ground pads are designed to adhere to the patient. Others are metal/vinyl plates and must be covered with a saline or water-soaked sponge to ensure proper grounding. Electrode gel is another option that often works better as it does not dry out. Alcohol must NEVER be used as it is flammable (Figure 4.57). Setting up the suction machine and ensuring antifatigue mats are in place are additional steps in setting up the room.

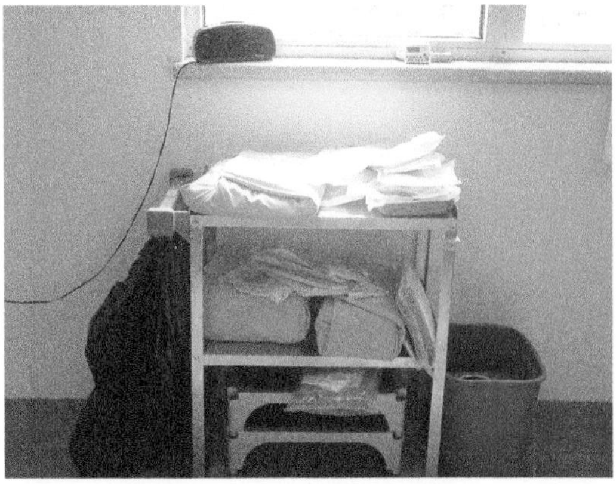

Figure 4.56 Equipment needed for procedure on cart in room.

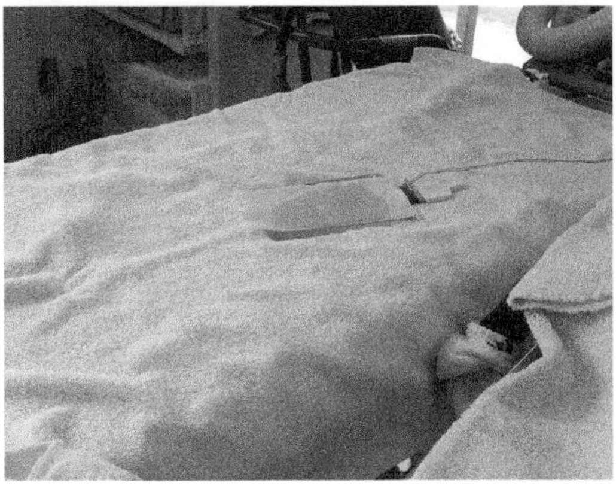

Figure 4.57 Electrosurgery ground plate on surgery table prior to the arrival of the patient.

Determining that all needed equipment and suture is available is something that must be attended to by the circulating nurse prior to the beginning of the procedure.

Opening Packs

Aseptically opening all the equipment and supplies used for a procedure is a very important task for the circulating nurse. Depending on the type of pack to be opened, the method of opening the pack can be different. For instance, if it is a gown pack, there is no sterile person to take the pack after the first wrapper is opened, so the circulating nurse must open both wrappers. To avoid dropping any of the contents of a gown pack as well as providing a sterile field for the person gowning, the pack should be sitting on a flat surface as it is opened. When opening any pack, the first step is to determine that it is in fact the pack that is desired. Reading the tape label and a quick check to ensure the pack has been through a sterilizing cycle is very important. Remove the tape and if the pack was wrapped in an envelope fashion, the tab that is facing the opener should be pulled and unfolded AWAY from the opener (Figure 4.58). Then, either side is grasped at the corner of the wrapper and unfolded (Figure 4.59). Next, the other side of the wrapper at the corner is grasped and unfolded (Figure 4.60). If at any time the wrapper is wrinkled or not lying flat, the circulating nurse is not allowed to touch the wrapper! Leave the wrinkle in the wrapper and the surgeon will work around it. The last tab should be grasped at the corner and pulled/unfolded toward the opener (Figure 4.61). The inner wrap is unfolded in exactly the same fashion (Video 4.2). This

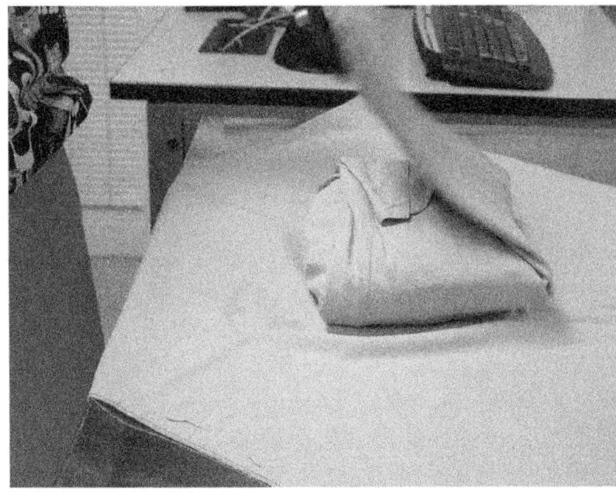

Figure 4.58 Opening first flap of wrapped pack.

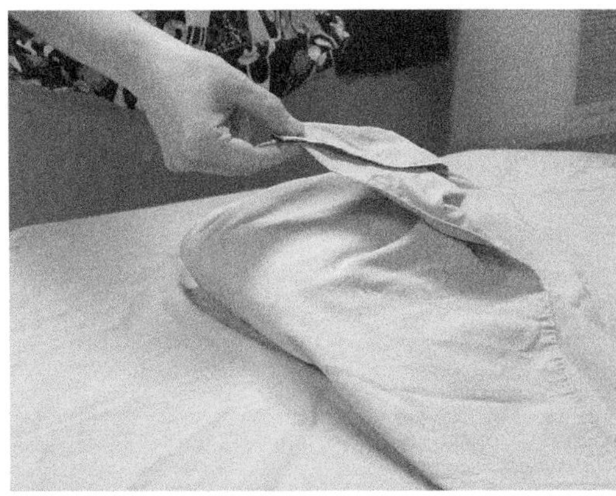

Figure 4.59 Opening second flap of wrapped pack.

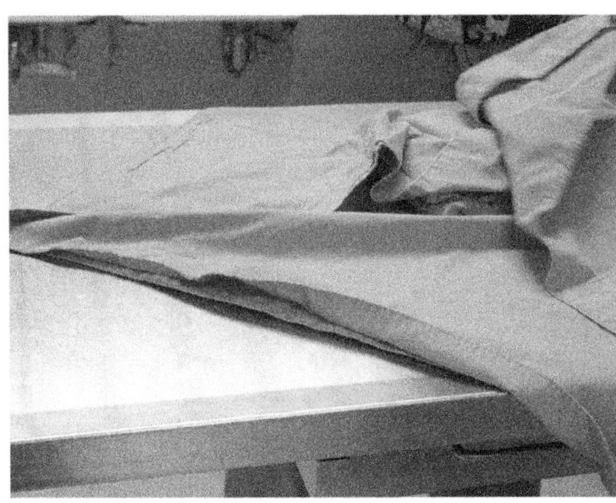

Figure 4.60 Opening third flap of wrapped pack.

method of opening encourages reduced opportunity for contamination of the pack contents. Once the gown is opened, the circulating nurse can open the gloves onto the sterile field created by the pack wrappers. Opening the glove wrapper should be done in a very controlled fashion in order to avoid contaminating the gloves within the pack. First of all, position the hands opposite one another grasping a flap of the wrapper in each hand (Figure 4.62). By slightly opening the sealed seam on either side of the wrapper first, the risk of the glove wrapper tearing down the middle is

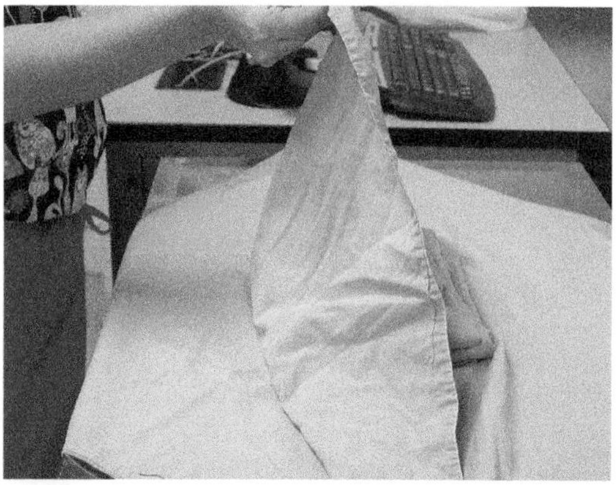

Figure 4.61 Opening final flap of wrapped pack.

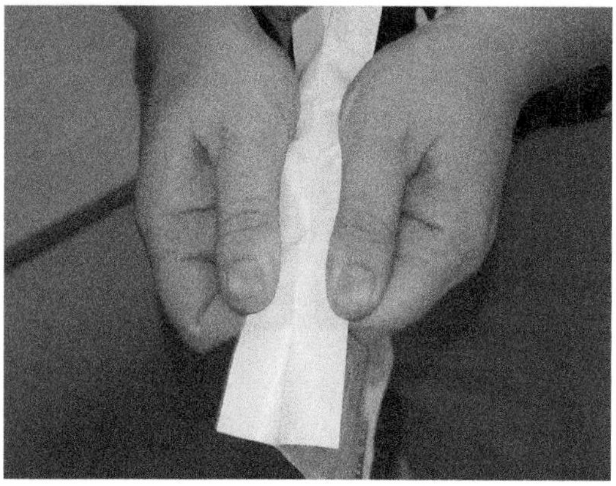

Figure 4.62 Proper placement of hands on the glove wrapper to open the pack.

reduced. With the hands holding the opening flaps, slowly pull the hands apart so the side seams of the wrapper unpeel. Continue opening the wrapper until the gloves are lying in a horizontal position in front of the opener (Figure 4.63). Now by simply rotating the wrists, the gloves will "fly" onto the sterile field (Figure 4.64). There is no need to throw the gloves. Now the surgeon can gown and glove while the circulating nurse is performing other duties. While the surgeon or assistant is gowning and gloving, the circulating nurse should be opening the instrument pack. With the pack sitting on the instrument table, the outer wrap, if an envelope-style wrap, is opened using the same method as described for the gown pack. If it is a horizontal style wrap, the first side wrap is unfolded. Then, the second side wrap is unfolded. The next flap should be unfolded AWAY from the circulating nurse. This is an important step because there should still be one flap covering the sterile inner pack protecting it from contamination. The final flap is unfolded toward the opener. The inner pack is sterile and should be left for the sterile person to unfold. Now that there is sterile person available to take other equipment from the circulating nurse, the remaining packs can be opened with a different method. Holding the pack in the hand with the fingers and thumb firmly holding the pack, the tape is removed after verification that it is the correct item to be opened. The tab of the outer wrap should be facing the opener. The tab is gently pulled toward the opener, and the flap is unfolded away from the opener. The next visible side flap should be opened with the corresponding hand to avoid crossing arms over the pack. The second side flap is then opened. If necessary to avoid crossing arms over the pack, the hand holding the pack should be switched. The wrapper that is hanging below the pack should be gathered into one hand by the circulating nurse.

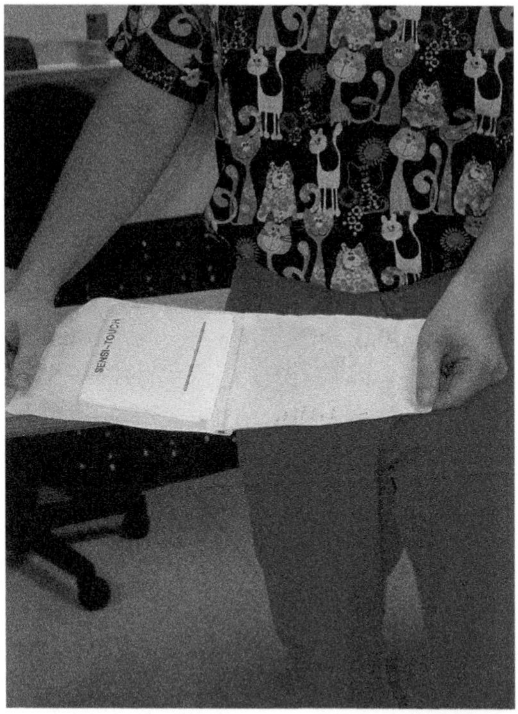

Figure 4.63 Opened glove wrapper in a horizontal fashion.

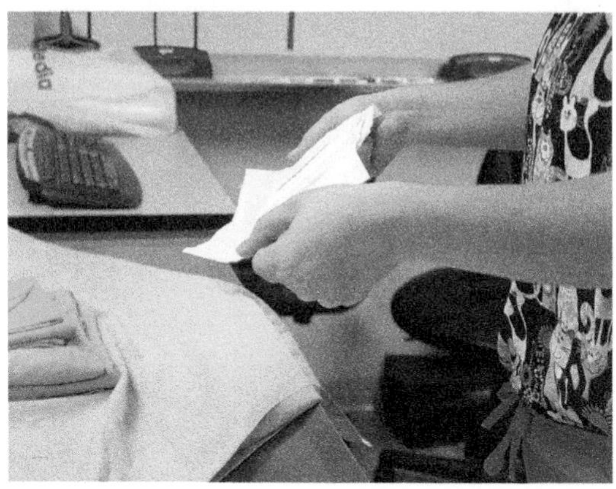

Figure 4.64 Turning wrists to flip the gloves onto the sterile field.

The sterile inner pack can then be offered to the sterile member of the team (Figure 4.65; Videos 4.3 and 4.4). The circulating nurse may then continue to open items for the surgeon. Anything packed in a peel pack (suture, separate instruments, etc.) should be opened using the method described for opening gloves (Figures 4.66 and 4.67). Items opened for the surgical team may be handed to the team member or they may be flipped up onto the instrument table. Heavy instruments or delicate instruments are best handled by having the sterile member take the item from the circulating nurse (Videos 4.5 and 4.6). Lighter items such as suture, scalpel blades, and sponges may be deposited on the instrument table. Care MUST be taken to adhere to strict asepsis when opening items. At no time can the arms of the circulating nurse extend over the sterile field, as this is a break in aseptic technique and could compromise the patient.

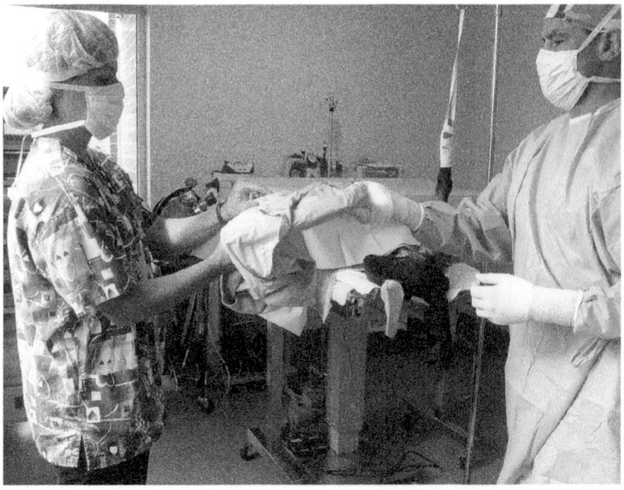

Figure 4.65 Circulating nurse offering sterile inner wrapped pack to surgeon.

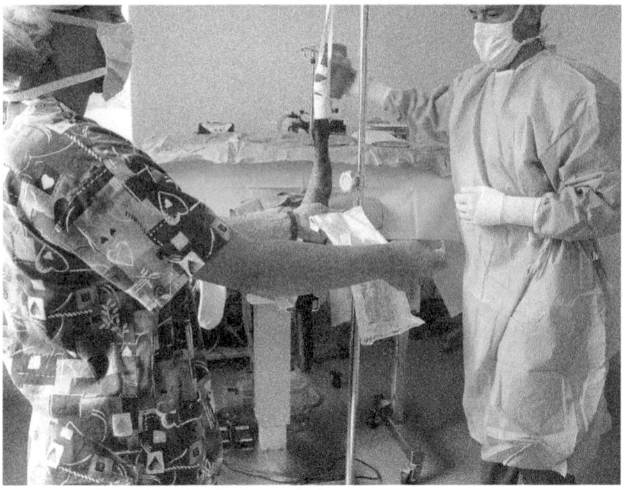

Figure 4.66 Circulating nurse opening peel pack item for surgeon.

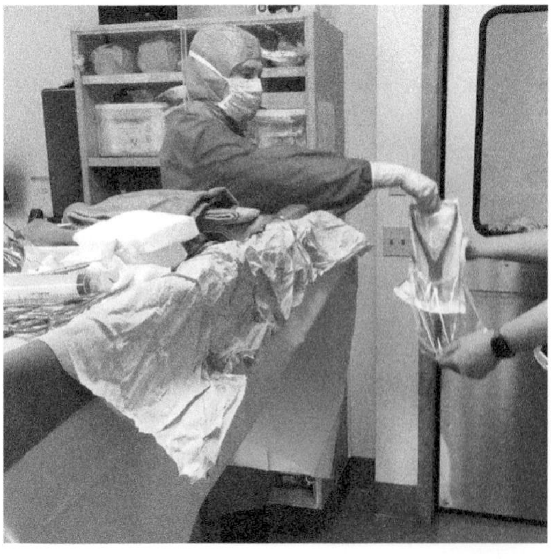

Figure 4.67 Sterile person taking item from opened peel pack.

Monitoring Aseptic Technique

It is imperative that the surgical area be kept as microorganism free as possible. The risk to the patient from other uncontrollable factors is high enough, therefore every effort must be made to control those measures that pose a risk of infection for the patient. Not only do the patient's health status, immune system strength, age, and nutritional state affect healing but also so do factors outside of the patient. The length of surgery, the surgical site (GI vs. bone), and the inadvertent introduction of pathogens to the surgical wound can affect healing. It is the primary responsibility of the circulating nurse to act as the patient's advocate and monitor the surgical procedure and the people involved for breaks in aseptic technique. Often times, sterile personnel do not realize they have inadvertently contaminated themselves and it is the responsibility of the circulating nurse to report such incidents. The patient's welfare and surgical healing are at stake, so the circulating nurses should not be shy about reporting observed breaks. Sterile members, being informed they have broken technique, must not argue or debate the report, but merely take measures to correct the situation. Often changing gloves is all that is needed, but changing gowns or entire instrument packs may also be necessary, depending on the severity of the break-in technique. The rules of aseptic technique are found in Table 4.2.

Monitoring the Room During the Surgery

In addition to vigilant monitoring of aseptic technique, there are other things that may occur during a surgical case for which the circulating nurse is responsible. As items are opened, the cloth

Table 4.2 Rules of aseptic technique.

Rule	Reason/example
Sterile personnel only touch sterile items; non-sterile members only touch non-sterile items	Sterile members touching non-sterile items would result in cross-contamination; non-sterile personnel touching sterile items would result in contamination
Talking is minimal	Aerosolized particles could contaminate instruments or the wound
Sterile members should pass each other back to back if passing one another is necessary	Any other orientation to each other would result in contamination of the sterile area of the gown/gloves
Air space over the surgical field is considered sterile and should not be invaded by non-sterile personnel	Shedding skin cells from arms of a non-sterile person, dust, lint, or other particles may fall when reaching over a sterile field and contaminate the field
Anything below surgery table level is considered non-sterile	Movement of items below the table cannot be controlled and are at risk of contamination
Sterile personnel may not cross their arms and place gloved hands in auxiliary regions	Moisture from sweat in the auxiliary region may contaminate gloves
Sterile members should face the sterile field at all times	The back of the gown is not considered sterile even if wearing a wraparound gown
If the sterility of an item is in question, it should be considered non-sterile	Contamination of an item can occur and not be visible to the eye
If a sterile member sits down during a procedure, they must remain seated for the entire procedure	Items are considered sterile only if above the surgery table. Moving from sitting to standing would result in contamination of the field

Source: Adapted from Fossom [2].

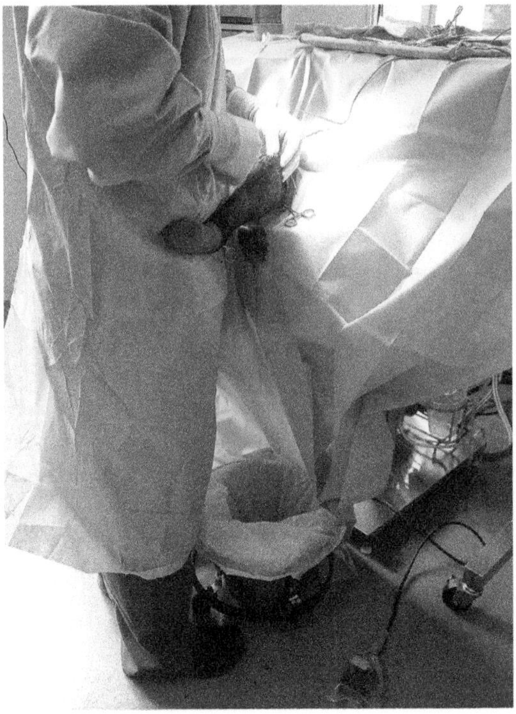

Figure 4.68 Kick bucket positioned to catch runoff of fluid from a stifle surgery.

wrappers should be thrown in the laundry bag. The paper wrappers should be thrown in the trash. Ideally, there would be a large trash bag in the surgery room for collecting the large volume of disposable items that will be generated to avoid overflowing the kick buckets in the room. Any trash from the sterile field that misses the kick bucket should be picked up right away and placed in the trash. Litter should not be allowed to accumulate on the floor of the operating room.

If the potential exists for fluid to fall from the sterile field, a kick buck should be positioned to catch as much of the runoff as possible (Figure 4.68). A towel can be placed on the floor to collect fluid if the kick bucket will be in the way of the surgeon. Keeping the surgery room as clean and neat as possible during the procedure will permit a speedier cleanup.

Connecting various pieces of equipment and accessories also falls to the circulating nurse. Plugging in the electrosurgery ground plate to the unit as well as plugging in the handpiece once that end is thrown off the sterile field should be done as soon as possible. Connecting the suction hose to the suction bottle is important to do as soon as possible, especially if the procedure may have lots of fluid early in the procedure (i.e. evacuation of an abdomen before completing the approach). Other duties may include attaching a nitrogen-powered tool to the nitrogen tank, plugging in arthroscopic or laparoscopic cables, or even talking a surgeon through the setup or use of a piece of equipment they may not be familiar with. Another situation that arises too often in the operating room is troubleshooting equipment when it does not function as expected. Surgeons need to have the equipment ready for use, and if that is not the case, the circulating nurse needs to be able to figure out how to fix it.

Finally, but certainly equally important is the recordkeeping responsibilities of the circulating nurse. Either the anesthetist or the circulating nurse should ensure the completion of the surgery checklist prior to the incision being made. A cessation of activity should happen to allow for a verbal conversation with all members of the team in the room. The name of the patient, the procedure being done (including limb if an orthopedic procedure), the anesthetic status of the patient, and any other concerns anyone may have about the patient or procedure should be discussed. Recording supplies used for accurate billing, making notes in the medical record, or completing discharge instructions as the surgeon is closing are all examples of documentation that fall to the circulating nurse.

References

1 Beale, B.S. (2010) How to Make Yourself Indispensable as a Surgical Assistant. *Proceedings from ACVS Symposium*, Chicago, IL.

2 Fossum, T. (2007) *Small Animal Surgery*, 3rd edn. Mosby Elsevier, St. Louis, MO.

Additional Resources

Further Reading

Randall Thompson, R. (2022) Suture materials and patterns small animal. Lincoln Memorial University College of Veterinary Medicine. Microsoft Power Point presentation.

https://www.medtronic.com/covidien/en-us/products/vessel-sealing/ligasure-technology.html [accessed on 3 March 2023].

https://www.sciencedirect.com/topics/nursing-and-health-professions/anastomotic-device [accessed on 4 March 2023].

5

Surgical Procedures

Teri Raffel Kleist, JoAnne Mead[1], and Gerianne Holzman[2]*

[1] *North Carolina State University, College of Veterinary Medicine, Raleigh, NC, USA*
[2] *University of Wisconsin, School of Veterinary Medicine, Emerita, Madison, WI, USA*

Veterinary technicians play major roles during surgical procedures as surgical assistants and circulating nurses. Important knowledge includes instrument identification, anatomical structures, and special needs of individual surgeries and surgeons. Surgeon's preference will dictate specific information such as patient positioning and special instrumentation. This chapter outlines many **advanced and some common surgical** procedures based on their anatomical location. It includes conditions, causes, clinical signs, corrective procedures, positioning, special instrumentation, the surgical assistant's role, and postoperative care. All patients require postsurgical monitoring, incision care, pain control, and perhaps some form of wound protection. Patients should be fed as tolerated.

Abdominal

Digestive

GDV Gastric Dilatation Volvulus (Bloat)

a) *Definition*: Stomach is twisted causing enlargement (may have simple dilatation without volvulus (twisting) (Figure 5.1) [1].
b) *Cause*: Gastric outflow is blocked causing gas and fluid to accumulate in stomach, etiology unknown, although may be related to overeating and anatomic conditions, most common in large, deep-chested dogs
c) *Clinical signs*: Abdominal tympany, abdominal distention, splenomegaly may be palpated, weak peripheral pulses, tachycardia, prolonged CRT, pale MM, dyspnea, unproductive vomiting
d) *Diagnosis*: Obvious distended abdomen on palpation and radiographs
e) *Surgery*: Ventral midline approach to the cranial abdomen, reduction of dilation and/or volvulus of stomach, resection of necrotic gastric tissue if necessary, possible gastropexy, routine closure (Figure 5.2).

* Madison College, Madison, WI, USA.

Surgical Patient Care for Veterinary Technicians and Nurses, Second Edition.
Edited by Gerianne Holzman and Teri Raffel Kleist.

Companion website: www.wiley.com/go/holzman/patient

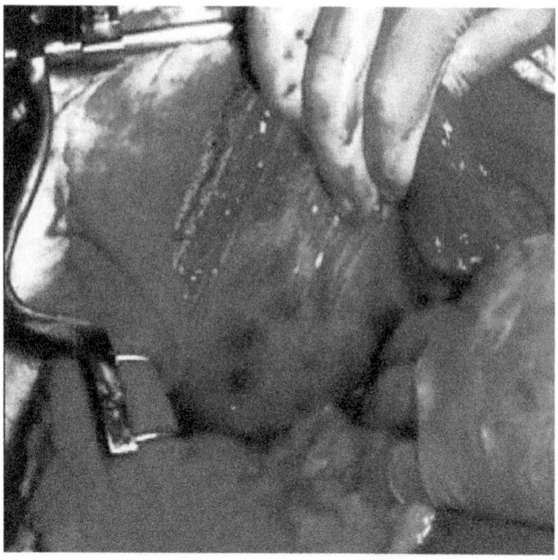

Figure 5.1 Distended stomach with spotty necrosis. *Source:* Dale Bjorling, University of Wisconsin, Madison, WI. Reproduced with permission of Dale Bjorling.

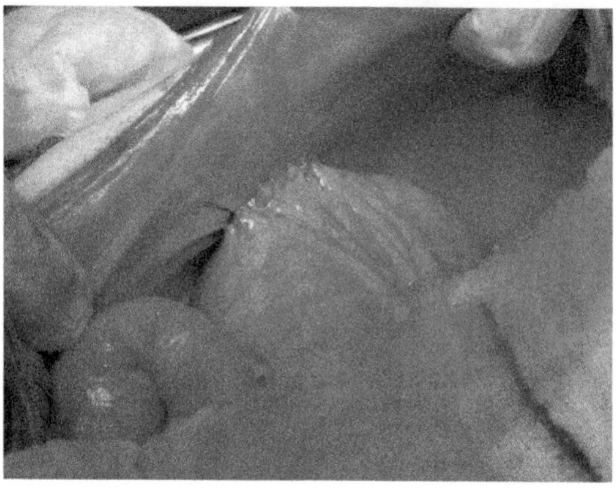

Figure 5.2 Gastropexy. *Source:* Dale Bjorling, University of Wisconsin, Madison, WI. Reproduced with permission of Dale Bjorling.

f) *Positioning*: Dorsal recumbency
g) *Special instrumentation*: Lap pads, suction, cautery, lavage, non-absorbable, monofilament suture if performing gastropexy, internal stapling device if partial gastrectomy performed
h) *Assistant's role*: Moisten tissue, suction, tissue retraction, cut sutures
i) *Postoperative care*: Monitor electrolytes and acid–base balance, especially potassium as patients tend to become hypokalemic, feed small amounts of water, and soft low-fat diet during first few days postop, incisional care as with celiotomy.

Gastric Foreign Body

a) *Definition*: Ingestion of anything that cannot be digested such as plastic, clothing, string, yarn, ribbon, and may include bones and rawhide chews
b) *Cause*: Dogs will eat anything, cats enjoy playing with yarn, etc.
c) *Clinical signs*: Vomiting, known ingestion of foreign material, unproductive vomiting
d) *Diagnosis*: Possible abdominal pain, may see string attached to tongue, endoscopy, radiographs, ultrasound (US)
e) *Surgery*: None if retrievable by endoscopy, ventral midline approach to the abdomen, placement of stay sutures to elevate stomach, incise stomach, and remove foreign body. Inspect

stomach for compromised tissue, lavage abdomen after closure of stomach. Change to second set of instruments, gloves, and drapes for closure to avoid contamination from stomach contents.

f) *Positioning*: Dorsal recumbency
g) *Special instrumentation*: Lap pads, Balfour retractor, lavage, second set of drapes and instruments
h) *Assistant's role*: Hold stay sutures to elevate stomach, suction, cut sutures, hydrate tissues on field
i) *Postoperative care*: Monitor for vomiting, provide food and water as tolerated, feeding tube may be indicated, incisional care as with celiotomy

Intestinal Foreign Body

a) *Definition*: Ingestion of anything that cannot be digested such as plastic, clothing, string, yarn, ribbon, and may include bones and rawhide chews, may be partial or complete obstruction, can lead to intestinal necrosis and perforation
b) *Cause*: Items may be small enough to pass through the esophagus and stomach but become trapped in the smaller diameter of the intestine
c) *Clinical signs*: Anorexia, constipation and vomiting, abdominal pain, possible known foreign body ingestion, cats are more prone to linear foreign bodies
d) *Diagnosis*: Physical exam findings of abdominal pain, bunched intestines may be evident with linear objects, radiographs, contrast imaging, US, known ingestion of foreign object
e) *Surgery*: Ventral midline approach to the abdomen, evaluation of entire intestinal tract, enterotomy for simple foreign body, resection and anastomosis for linear foreign body (Figures 5.3 and 5.4).
f) *Positioning*: Dorsal recumbency
g) *Special instrumentation*: Balfour retractor, intestinal clamps, internal staplers, second set of drapes, gowns, gloves, instruments, lavage, suction, electrosurgery, camera
h) *Assistant's role*: Occlude intestine with index finger and third finger of each hand if resection and anastomosis performed, load internal stapler if used, moisten tissue, suction, cut sutures
i) *Postoperative care*: Monitor for vomiting and peritonitis, correct fluid and electrolyte imbalances if present, provide food and water as tolerated, incisional care as with celiotomy

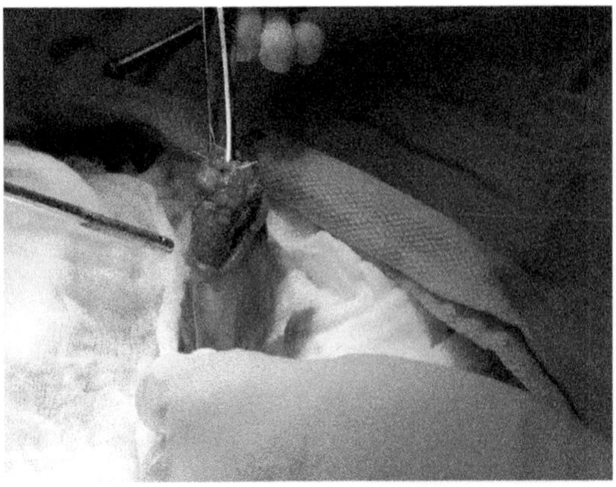

Figure 5.3 Intestinal foreign body. *Source:* Robert Hardie, University of Wisconsin Veterinary Care. Madison, WI. Reproduced with permission from Robert Hardie.

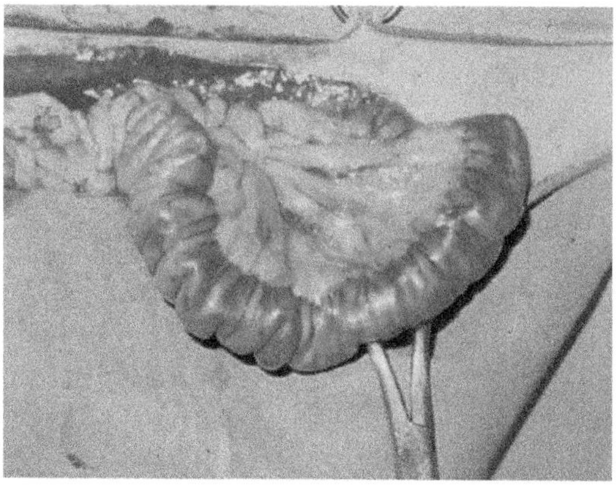

Figure 5.4 Plication of intestine from a linear foreign body. *Source:* Dale Bjorling, University of Wisconsin, Madison, WI. Reproduced with permission of Dale Bjorling.

Exploratory Laparotomy

a) *Definition*: A variety of conditions may require surgical exploration of the abdomen
b) *Cause*: Varies based on diagnosis – neoplasia, chronic disease (i.e. porto-systemic shunt), or emergency conditions (i.e. gastric torsion, foreign body, trauma)
c) *Clinical signs*: Dependent upon condition being treated, most commonly vomiting, diarrhea, anorexic, lethargy
d) *Diagnosis*: Abdominal palpation, laboratory tests, radiographs, dependent upon assumed disease or injury
e) *Surgery*: Abdominal exploratory (celiotomy) [2] – Surgical incision into the abdominal cavity, ventral midline approach to the abdomen, exploration of entire abdomen, biopsy or excision of affected organ (Figures 5.5 and 5.6).
f) *Positioning*: Dorsal recumbency
g) *Special instrumentation*: Balfour retractor, lap pads, biopsy instruments if indicated, internal staplers if indicated, suction, electrosurgery, formalin jars for samples, lavage fluid
h) *Assistant's role*: Lavage tissue, suction, provide hemostasis, hand biopsy instruments, cut sutures, occlude intestine if resection and anastomosis are performed (Figures 5.7 and 5.8).
i) *Postoperative care*: Monitor incision for redness, swelling, drainage, dehiscence, E-Collar or body stocking to protect the surgical site, exercise restrictions until sutures are removed

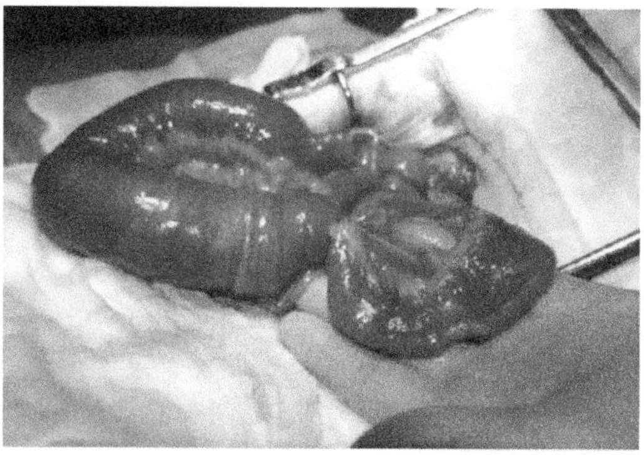

Figure 5.5 Intestinal intussusception before reduction. *Source:* Dale Bjorling, University of Wisconsin, Madison, WI. Reproduced with permission of Dale Bjorling.

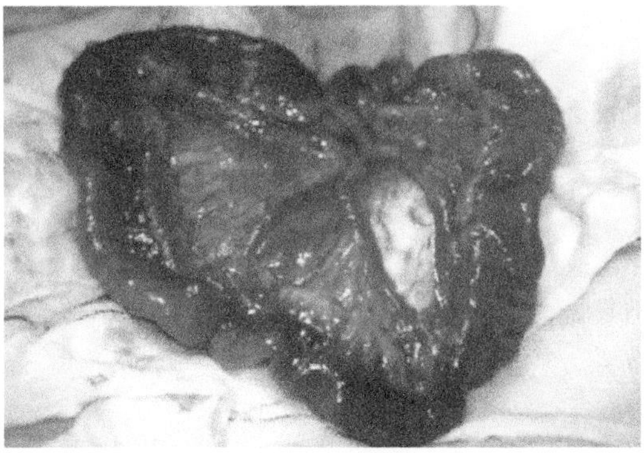

Figure 5.6 Intestinal intussusception after reduction – note compromised vascularity. *Source:* Dale Bjorling, University of Wisconsin, Madison, WI. Reproduced with permission of Dale Bjorling.

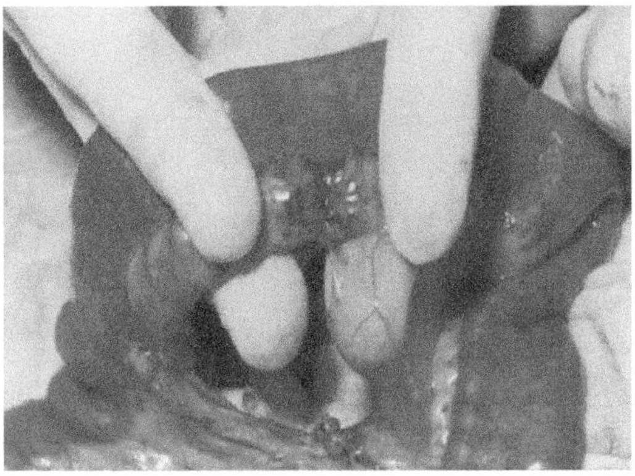

Figure 5.7 Assistant occluding intestine prior to resection.

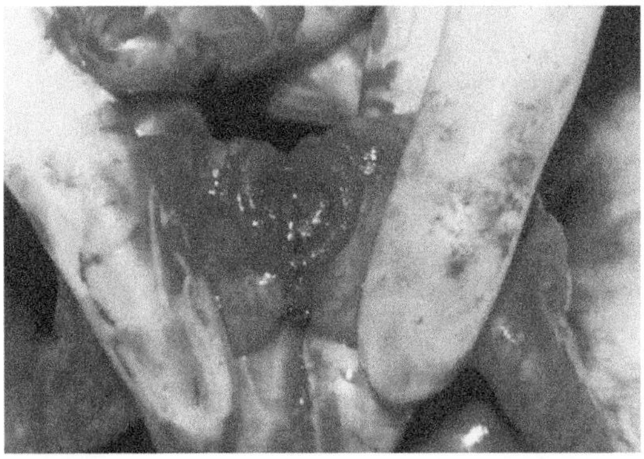

Figure 5.8 Assistant occluding intestine for anastomosis.

Gallbladder

Cholecystectomy

a) *Definition*: A variety of conditions may affect the gallbladder.
b) *Causes*: Trauma, severe cholecystitis, neoplasia, and damage to the cystic duct.
c) *Clinical signs*: Abdominal pain, vomiting, diarrhea, dehydration, serum electrolyte imbalances.
d) *Diagnosis*: Coagulopathy may be present because of decreased absorption of vitamin K, US, radiographs.
e) *Surgery*: Cholecystectomy, the removal of the gallbladder, to avoid damage to the remainder biliary duct system and prevent leakage to the peritoneal cavity.

f) *Positioning*: Dorsal recumbency.
g) *Special instruments*: General pack, Balfour, right-angle forceps, malleable retractors, hemoclips, bipolar electrosurgery, 7 fr Frazier suction tip, different sizes of red rubber and Pezzer catheters, may need a Jackson Pratt drain and G-tube placed, culture bile
h) *Assistant role*: Load hemoclips, retract tissue, cut suture, moisten tissues.
i) *Postoperative care*: Maintain IV fluid until eating, monitor for evidence of bile peritonitis, pancreatitis, and incision infection. Recheck every three to six months for recurrence of biliary obstruction

Liver

Liver Lobectomy

a) *Definition*: Surgical resection of a liver lobe or part of a lobe (Figures 5.9 and 5.10).
b) *Cause*: Hepatic masses or nodules
c) *Clinical signs*: Hepatomegaly, hyperbilirubinemia, persistent increase in liver enzymes
d) *Diagnosis*: X-ray, US, serum chemistry to check for increase in liver enzymes
e) *Surgery*: Ventral midline incision should start caudal to the xiphoid. Monopolar electrosurgery is used. To improve exposure, a moistened lap sponge is placed between the diaphragm and the liver lobes. A TA stapler is used to staple the liver lobe and then a scalpel blade is used to cut

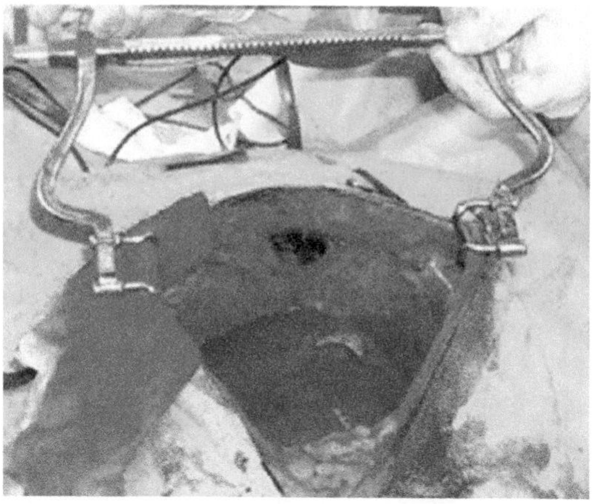

Figure 5.9 Liver lobe mass. *Source:* Courtesy of Dr. Mathews NCSU-CVM.

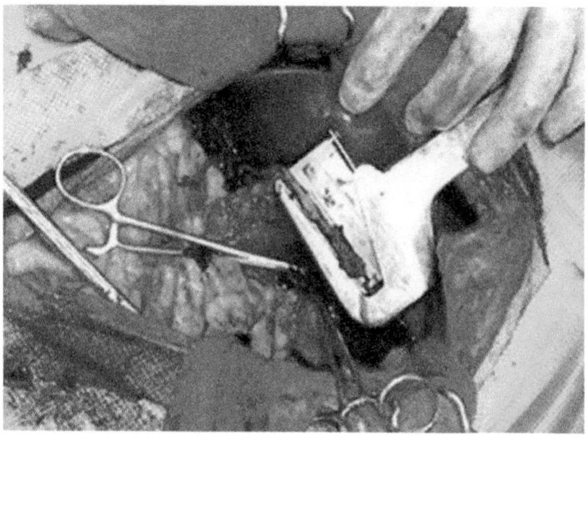

Figure 5.10 Liver lobectomy with TA stapler. *Source:* Courtesy of Dr. Mathews NCSU-CVM.

the lobe. A monofilament suture or hemoclips are used to tie off any vessels. Ways to obtain a liver biopsy: guillotine, box suture, skin punch, keyhole incision

f) *Positioning*: Dorsal recumbency

g) *Special instruments*: Abdominal pack, Balfour, right-angle forceps, harmonic scalpel, TA staples, Surgicel, Argon cautery, hemoclips, vessel loops, Gelfoam (Figures 5.11 and 5.12).

h) *Assistant's role*: Retract tissue, cut suture, load staples or hemoclips, moisten tissue, cauterize any vessels that are hemorrhaging

i) *Postoperative care*: Check for hemorrhaging, measure hematocrit immediately after surgery and then several hours later to evaluate for progressive anemia

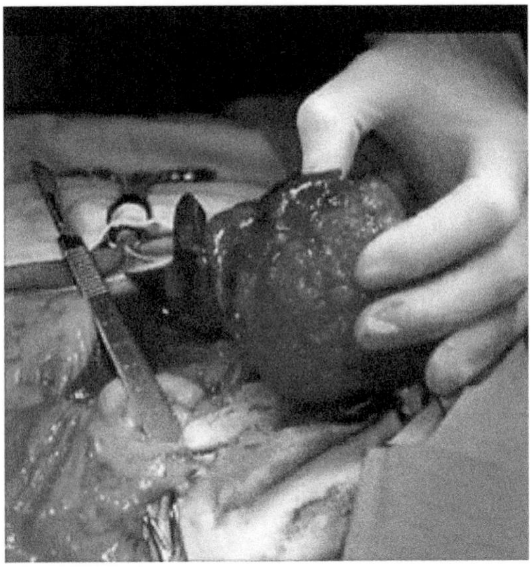

Figure 5.11 Liver tumor. *Source:* Dale Bjorling, University of Wisconsin, Madison, WI. Reproduced with permission of Dale Bjorling.

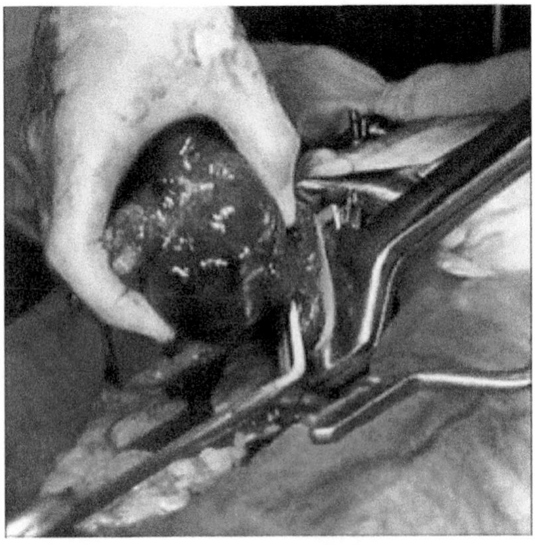

Figure 5.12 Use of TA stapler to excise a liver tumor. *Source:* Dale Bjorling, University of Wisconsin, Madison, WI. Reproduced with permission of Dale Bjorling.

Portosystemic Shunt (PSS)

a) *Definition*: Blood vessels bypass the liver and drain from the stomach, intestines, spleen, and pancreas directly into the circulatory system thus partially eliminating the liver's filtering properties – may be intrahepatic or extrahepatic [3, 4]
b) *Cause*: **Congenital** (intrahepatic) when ductus venosus does not close at birth, **congenital** (extrahepatic) when an anomalous vessel allows blood to flow directly from the portal vein to the general circulatory system, **acquired** (extrahepatic) from portal hypertension in patients with liver disease, most common in young, pure bred dogs and shorthair cats, hereditary in Yorkshire Terriers
c) *Clinical signs*: Small size for breed, vomiting, seizures, behavioral changes
d) *Diagnosis*: Radiographs, positive contrast portography, US, laboratory tests including liver function, and pre-/postprandial bile acids
e) *Surgery*:
   i) Extrahepatic: A ventral midline incision is made. Dissection occurs to identify the shunt. Placement of a constrictor or cellophane band occurs (Figure 5.13). Occasionally ligation is performed. Routine closure.
   ii) *Intrahepatic*: Caudal sternebrae/cranial abdominal ventral midline incision. The shunt is identified and ligated.
f) *Positioning*: Dorsal recumbency
g) *Special instrumentation*:
   i) *Extrahepatic*: Ameroid constrictor, Balfour retractor, lap pads, suction, electrosurgery, cellophane band if ameroid constrictor not used, right-angle forceps.
   ii) *Intrahepatic*: Umbilical tape, 3½ or 5 fr. Polypropylene catheter, right-angle forceps, silk ligature, or suture requested by surgeon
h) *Assistant's role*: Lavage, tissue retraction, cut sutures
i) *Postoperative care*: Critical care monitoring for portal hypertension (painful abdomen) and seizures, low protein diet for two to three months until recheck liver values show return-to-normal function.

Reproductive

Cesarean Section

a) *Definition*: Removal of fetuses may be performed with an ovariohysterectomy (OHE) [5]
b) *Cause*: Fetuses are not able to be delivered without intervention; may be performed for dystocia or elective procedures for specific breeds or patients with a decreased pelvic canal opening, e.g. following pelvic fracture

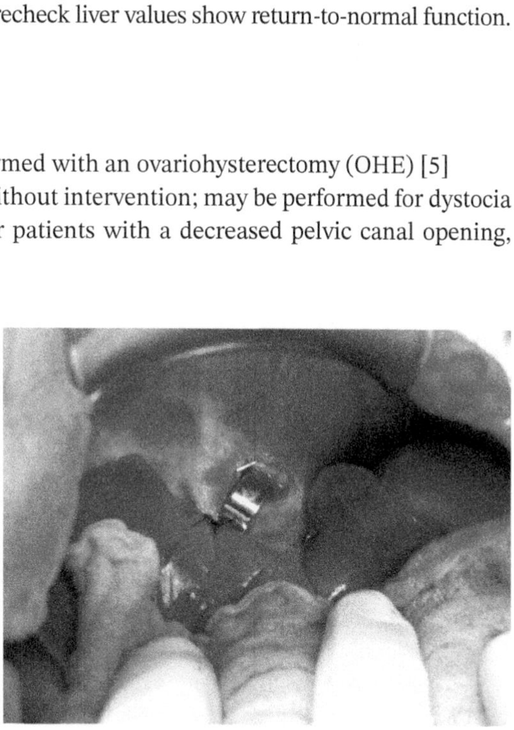

Figure 5.13 Ameroid constrictor placed on an extra-hepatic portosystemic shunt. *Source:* Robert Hardie, University of Wisconsin Veterinary Care. Madison, WI. Reproduced with permission from Robert Hardie.

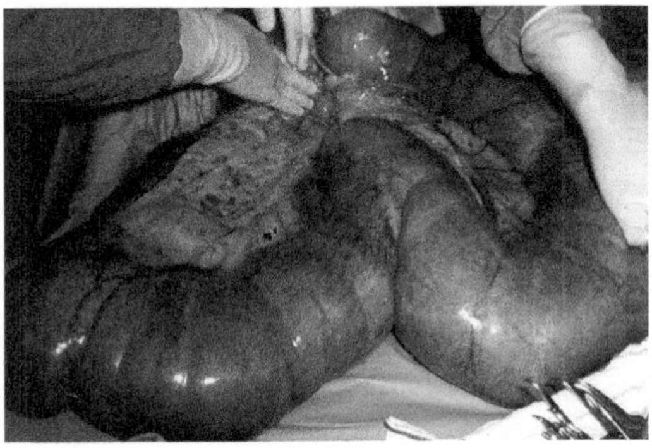

Figure 5.14 Gravid uterus exteriorized from abdomen. *Source:* Jonathan McAnulty, University of Wisconsin-Madison, Madison, WI. Reproduced with permission from Jonathan McAnulty.

c) *Clinical signs*: Difficulty giving birth (dystocia), end-term pregnancy (elective)
d) *Diagnosis*: Palpation +/− radiographs
e) *Surgery*: Cesarean section (C-section) – incision into the uterus (hysterotomy) to remove fetuses, may be performed with an OHE, ventral midline approach to the abdomen, exteriorize gravid uterus (Figure 5.14). Incise uterus for removal of fetuses. Clamp and transect umbilical cord of each fetus prior to handing them off the sterile field to an assistant, close uterus, lavage abdomen, re-drape, change gloves, and open new instruments for closure to avoid contamination
f) *Positioning*: Dorsal recumbency. **Note: Much of the prep of the patient is performed prior to anesthesia to decrease anesthetic effects on the fetuses.**
g) *Special instrumentation*:
   i) *Bitch/queen*: Lap pads, suction, cautery, oxytocin in room, lavage fluids, extra hemostats
   ii) *Newborns*: Warm environment, suture to ligate umbilicus, bulb syringe for suctioning nares, dry towels, intubation supplies (small endotracheal tubes [ET] – 18 ga × 2″ IV catheters may be used for ET tube), oxygen source (Figure 5.15).
h) *Assistant's role*: Assist with elevation of gravid uterus out of abdomen, suction, hand instruments quickly as newborns are removed, hand off newborns to waiting circulating tech or another non-sterile assistant
i) *Postoperative care*:
   i) Newborn care includes suctioning nares, briskly rubbing and drying to stimulate respiration, keep warm.
   ii) *Bitch or queen*: Monitor incision for redness, swelling, drainage, dehiscence, E-Collar or body stocking to protect the surgical site as needed, exercise restrictions until sutures are removed, encourage lactation (Figure 5.16).

Orchiectomy (Neuter/Castration)

a) *Definition*: Sterilizing a male dog/cat to prevent breeding, decrease aggressive behavior, and prevent hormone-related diseases such as prostate conditions and perineal hernias
b) *Cause*: Intact male animal, testicular condition such as tumor
c) *Clinical signs*: Generally normal physical exam, intact male animal
d) *Diagnosis*: Determine if both testes are descended, evaluate prostate
e) *Surgery*:
   i) *Canine*: A prescrotal incision is made and testicles are squeezed out of incision one at a time. Ligation and transaction of testicular structures, closure of scrotum may or may not include skin sutures (Figure 5.17).
   ii) *Feline*: A scrotal incision is made over each testicle. The testicle is removed and ligated or self-tied, no scrotal closure (Figure 5.18).

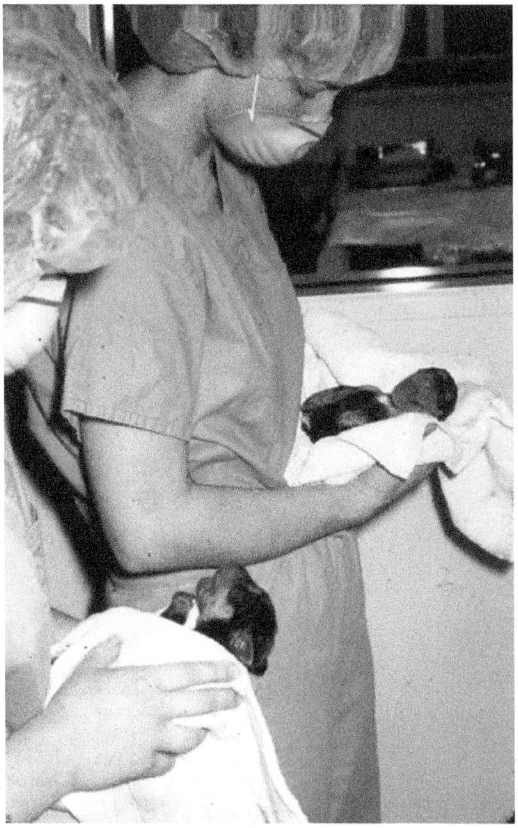

Figure 5.15 Resuscitation of newborn. *Source:* Jonathan McAnulty, University of Wisconsin-Madison, Madison, WI. Reproduced with permission from Jonathan McAnulty.

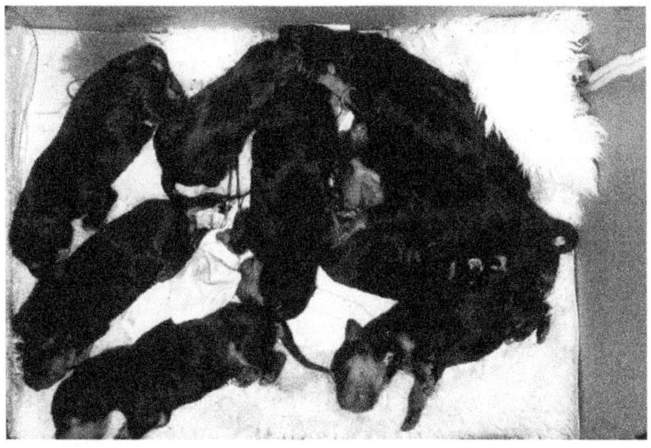

Figure 5.16 Happy ending! *Source:* Jonathan McAnulty, University of Wisconsin-Madison, Madison, WI. Reproduced with permission from Jonathan McAnulty.

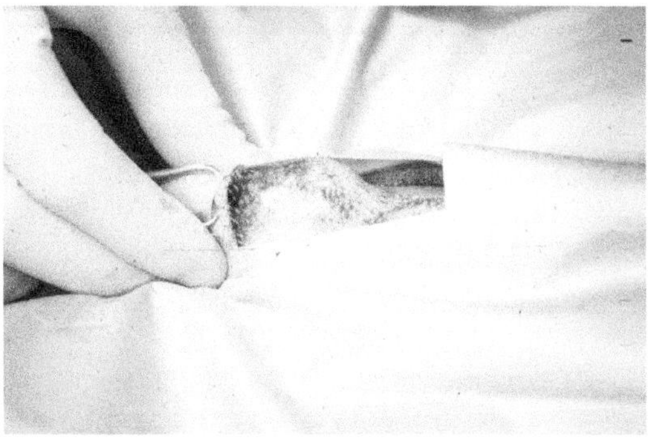

Figure 5.17 Draped area for canine castration. *Source:* Jonathan McAnulty, University of Wisconsin-Madison, Madison, WI. Reproduced with permission from Jonathan McAnulty.

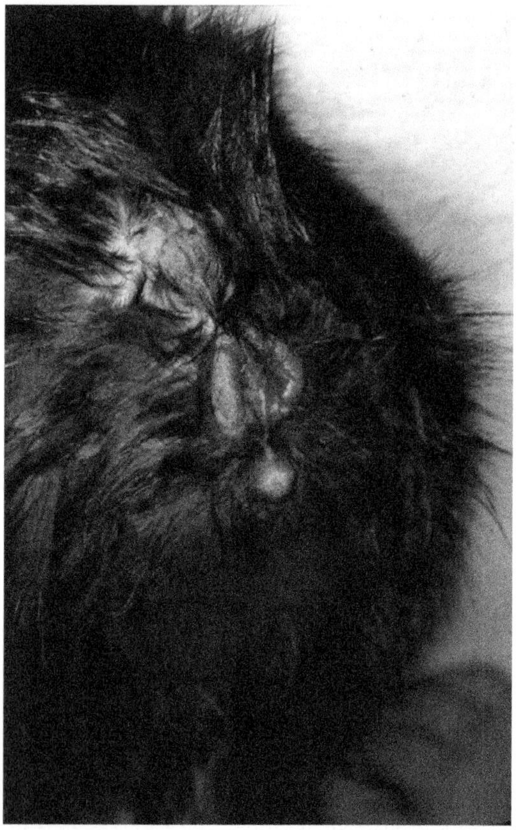

Figure 5.18 Postoperative incisions from feline neuter. *Source:* Jonathan McAnulty, University of Wisconsin-Madison, Madison, WI. Reproduced with permission from Jonathan McAnulty.

f) *Positioning*: Dorsal recumbency; lateral recumbency may be used for felines
g) *Special instrumentation*: None needed
h) *Assistant's role*: Not usually present
i) *Postoperative care*: Monitor incision for redness, swelling, drainage, dehiscence, E-Collar to protect the surgical site as needed, exercise restrictions until sutures are removed

Ovariohysterectomy (OHE/Neuter/Spay)

a) *Definition*: Sterilizing a female dog/cat to prevent breeding and prevent hormone-related diseases such as mammary tumors and pyometra
b) *Cause*: Intact female, uterine conditions such as pyometra
c) *Clinical signs*: Generally normal but may have enlarged uterus, purulent or bloody vaginal discharge indicating estrus or infection
d) *Diagnosis*: Check for vaginal discharge, enlarged vulva
e) *Surgery*:
   i) *Routine*: Ventral midline abdominal approach, identification of ovaries, uterine horn and uterus, ligation and removal of ovaries, uterine horns and uterus, routine closure
   ii) *Laparoscopic*: Minimally invasive procedure for the removal of ovaries, uterine horns, and uterus, ligation or electrosurgical sealing of transected tissue (Figures 5.19 and 5.20).
f) *Positioning*:
   i) *Routine*: Dorsal recumbency
   ii) *Laparoscopic*: Dorsal or lateral recumbency

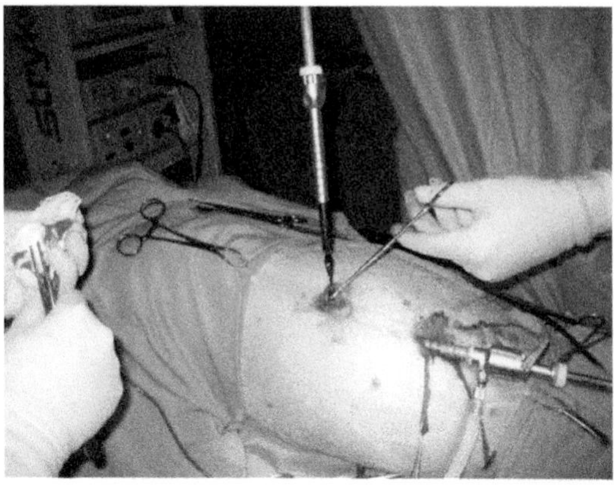

Figure 5.19 Set up for laparoscopic OHE. *Source:* Robert Hardie, University of Wisconsin Veterinary Care. Madison, WI. Reproduced with permission from Robert Hardie.

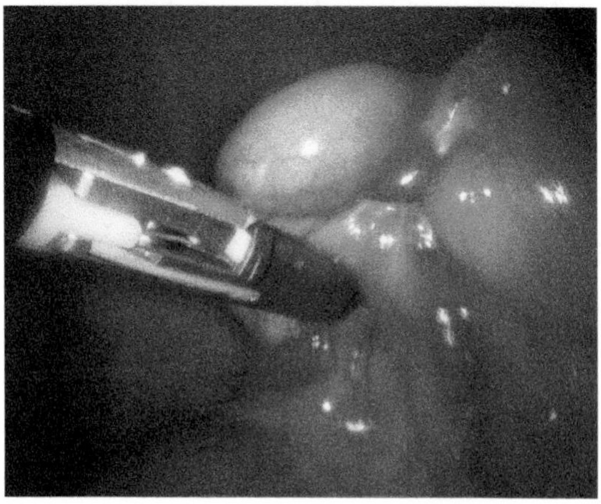

Figure 5.20 Ovariectomy via laparoscope. *Source:* Robert Hardie, University of Wisconsin Veterinary Care. Madison, WI. Reproduced with permission from Robert Hardie.

g) *Special instrumentation*:
  i) *Routine*: None needed
  ii) *Laparoscopic*: Laparoscope, laparoscopic instrument set, CO_2 insufflator
h) *Assistant's role*:
  i) *Routine*: Usually not present
  ii) *Laparoscopic*: Monitor insufflation pressure, manipulate scope as needed, cut sutures
i) *Postoperative care*: Monitor incision for redness, swelling, drainage, dehiscence, E-Collar to protect the surgical site as needed, exercise restrictions until sutures are removed

Spleen

Splenectomy

a) *Definition*: A variety of conditions may affect the spleen
b) *Cause*: Trauma, tumor, or torsion
c) *Clinical signs*: Enlarged spleen, possibly anemia
d) *Diagnosis*: Palpation, radiographs, laboratory tests
e) *Surgery*: Splenectomy [6] – partial or total removal of the spleen, ventral midline approach to the abdomen with visualization of spleen, careful exteriorization of the spleen, double ligation or stapling of all splenic vessels, routine closure (Figures 5.21 and 5.22).

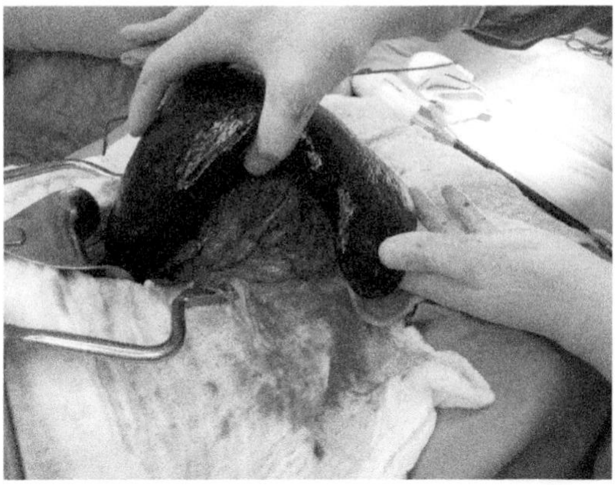

Figure 5.21 Spleen being exteriorized. *Source:* Robert Hardie, University of Wisconsin Veterinary Care. Madison, WI. Reproduced with permission from Robert Hardie.

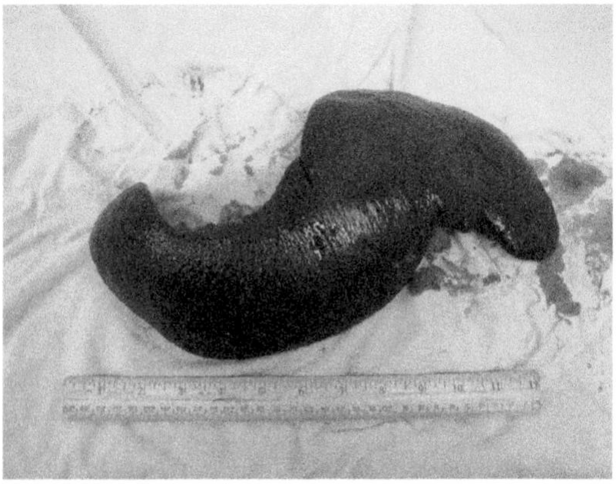

Figure 5.22 Spleen following excision from abdominal cavity. *Source:* Robert Hardie, University of Wisconsin Veterinary Care. Madison, WI. Reproduced with permission from Robert Hardie.

f) *Positioning*: Dorsal recumbency
g) *Special instrumentation*: Lap pads, +/− Balfour retractor, internal stapler (usually LDS), lavage fluid, ligature suture if stapler not used, suction, electrosurgery, specimen container, comparative measure device (ruler), camera
h) *Assistant's role*: Load stapler if used, run suture, cut suture if ligatures used, moisten tissues
i) *Postoperative care*: Monitor closely for postoperative hemorrhage and disseminated intravascular coagulation (DIC), blood transfusions if indicated for anemic patients

Urinary

Cystotomy

a) *Definition*: The surgical incision into the urinary bladder to create an opening to remove cystic and ureteral calculi, repair trauma, correct congenital abnormalities, or place a tube
b) *Cause*: Cystolithialities, neoplasia, or rupture (Figure 5.23).
c) *Clinical signs*: Obstruction of urinary flow, uroabdomen, abdominal distension, postrenal azotemia, hyperkalemia
d) *Diagnosis*: Physical exam, X-ray, US, serum chemistry
e) *Surgery*: A ventral abdominal incision is made. The bladder is isolated and a longitudinal incision on the ventral or dorsal surface of the urinary bladder body is made. Neoplasia or debris is removed, and then the bladder is flushed to check for any obstruction. A monofilament suture is used to close the bladder (Figure 5.24).

Figure 5.23 Urolith. *Source:* Courtesy of Dr. Mathews NCSU-CVM.

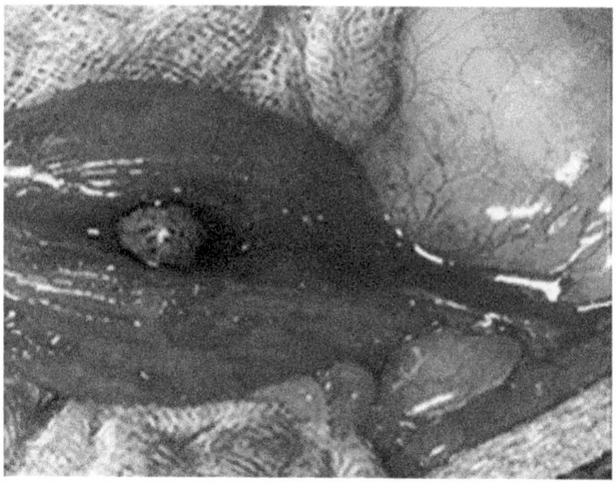

Figure 5.24 Urinary bladder isolated during cystotomy. *Source:* Courtesy of Dr. Mathews NCSU-CVM.

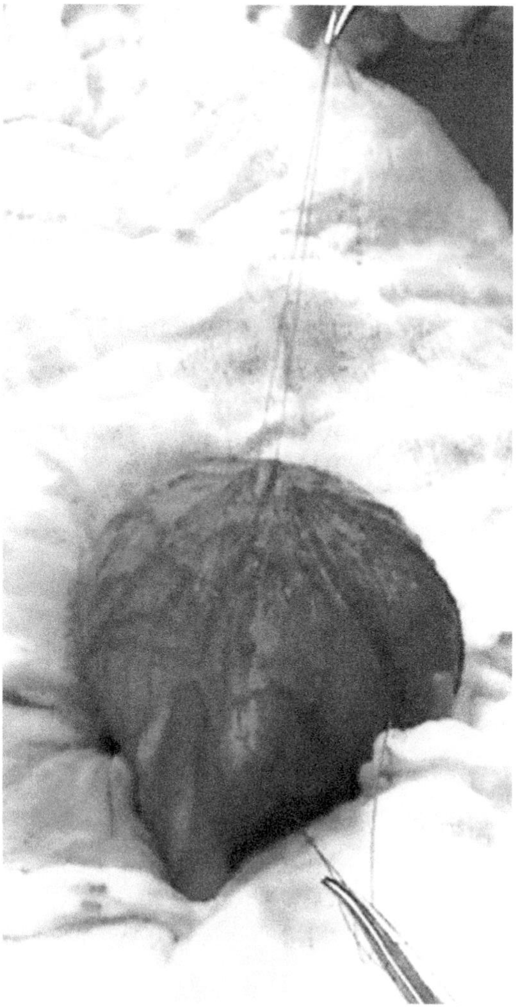

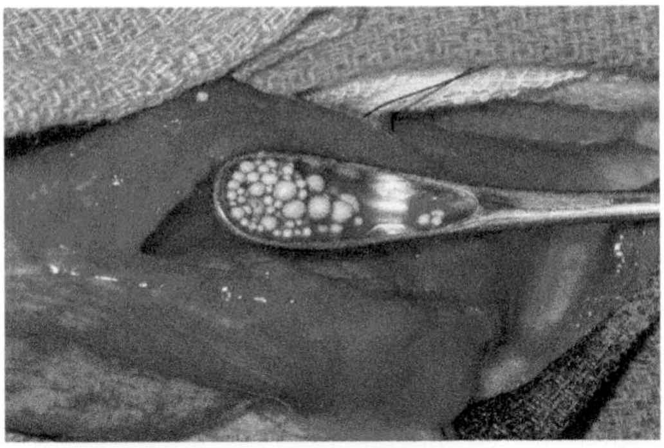

Figure 5.25 Bladder spoon with numerous urinary calculi.

f) *Positioning*: Dorsal recumbency
g) *Special instruments*: General pack, stone scoop, red rubber catheter, suction, electrosurgery (Figure 5.25).
h) *Assistant's role*: Gently holding the bladder, retract tissue, cut suture, and moisten tissue
i) *Postoperative care*: Monitor urination to detect obstructions, IV fluids until postobstructive diuresis ceases, monitor blood work and pain, bladder should be decompressed with a catheter until the patient can urinate normally, an E-collar should be placed if an indwelling urinary catheter is placed to prevent early catheter removal or self-mutilation, antibiotics should be started depending on the culture if calculi were present

Nephrectomy

a) *Definition*: The removal of the kidney
b) *Cause*: Renal neoplasia, uncontrollable bleeding, persistent urine leakage, pyelonephritis, hydronephrosis, urethral abnormalities
c) *Clinical signs*: Chronic kidney disease (CKD), acute renal failure (ARF), acute renal injury (AKI), azotemia, dehydration, polyuria, uroabdomen
d) *Diagnosis*: X-ray, US, blood work (hyperkalemia and hypokalemia), EKG
e) *Surgery*: The removal of the kidney and its associate ureter. A ventral abdominal incision is performed. The affected kidney and ureter are ligated with non-absorbable monofilament suture (Figure 5.26).
f) *Positioning*: Dorsal recumbency
g) *Special instruments*: Abdominal pack, ENSEAL™ vessel sealer, Balfour, bipolar electrosurgery with small forceps, right-angle forceps, Debakey forceps, hemoclips, malleable retractors
h) *Assistant's role*: Retract tissue, load hemoclips, cut suture, and moisten tissue

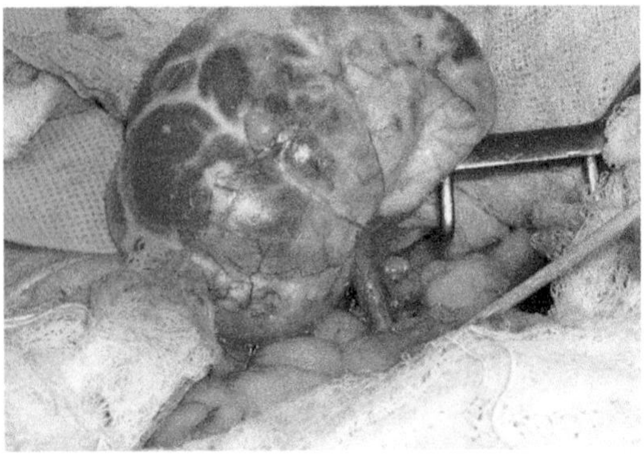

Figure 5.26 Kidney prior to nephrectomy. *Source:* Courtesy of Dr. Mathews NCSU-CVM.

i) *Postoperative care*: Monitor PCV for abdominal bleeding, placement of an abdominal drain to monitor any fluid, central venous pressure (CVP), and urine outflow to monitor dehydration, patient may need a urinary catheter if an obstruction develops, monitor blood work for increased or decreased electrolytes, analgesics should be given as needed

Perineal Urethrostomy – Male Cats

a) *Definition*: Inability to urinate
b) *Cause*: Feline lower urinary tract disease (FLUTD), urethral calculi, tumor, trauma, more common in overweight, middle-aged, indoor cats, less commonly found in dogs,
c) *Clinical signs*: Inappropriate urination, hematuria, anuria, anxious, anorexia, vomiting
d) *Diagnosis*: Palpable large bladder that cannot be expressed, radiographs
e) *Surgery*: Perineal urethrostomy (PU) [7] (penile amputation to alleviate chronic urethral obstruction if not relievable by other means), dissection and release of caudal urethra, extension of urethra allows suturing of pelvic urethra to the skin to allow a wider path for the passage of urine, increased urethral width decreases risk of re-obstruction, caudal urethra and penis are removed/amputated (Figure 5.27).
f) *Positioning*: Ventral recumbency with hind limbs hanging over the end of the surgery table, rolled up towel underneath hips to prevent pressure/nerve damage, tail taped up to allow access to perineal area, purse-string suture placed in anus
g) *Special instrumentation*: Head loops, tom cat catheter, ophthalmic instruments (baby Metzenbaum scissors, delicate thumb tissue forceps), surgical spears for hemostasis, small needle holder (Derf, short Mayo/Olsen-Hegar)
h) *Assistant's role*: Hemostasis, manipulation of urinary catheter, cut sutures
i) *Postoperative care*: Shredded paper or commercially available paper source litter, E-Collar to prevent licking until sutures are removed, gentle cleaning of surgical site with damp cotton swab, Vaseline® around urethral opening if needed for urine scald, sedation required for suture removal, intermittent monitoring for urinary tract infection

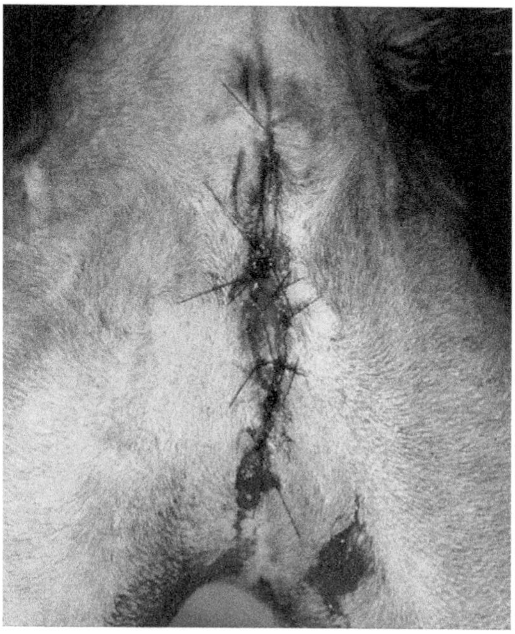

Figure 5.27 Postoperative perineal urethrostomy site. *Source:* Dale Bjorling, University of Wisconsin, Madison, WI. Reproduced with permission of Dale Bjorling.

Subcutaneous Ureteral Bypass (SUB)

a) *Definition*: A subcutaneous ureteral bypass (SUB) device is a device to maintain the flow of urine from the kidney to the bladder. It consists of a nephrostomy catheter and a cystostomy catheter joined subcutaneously by an injection port.
b) *Cause*: Obstruction of the ureters; causes of obstruction include: ureteral stones, trauma, strictures (scarring or narrowing), cancer, infection
c) *Clinical signs*: Obstruction of the ureters, straining to urinate
d) *Diagnosis*: Radiographs, CT, US, MRI
e) *Surgery*: A ventral incision is made into abdomen, the affected kidney is isolated, fluoroscopic imaging is used for guidance to place the SUB into the kidney, sterilely glue device to the kidney and bladder, placement of SUB port laterally, subcutaneously, and to the left of the incision in order to flush and remove urine, monofilament suture is used for closure of all layers of the skin.
f) *Positioning*: Dorsal recumbency
g) *Special instruments*: General pack, Balfour, right-angle forceps, small Frazier suction tip, C-arm and covers, iohexol contrast, malleable retractors, Babcock forceps
h) *Assistant's role*: Retract tissue, cut suture, cauterize vessels, help place and glue SUB device in place
i) *Postoperative care*: Pain management, fluid therapy, and antibiotic therapy are continued for a period of two to four weeks based on culture and sensitivity results; complications include: urine leakage, dislodgement, obstruction, and recurrent urinary tract infection

Head and Neck

Auditory

External Ear Canal and Pinna

a) *Definition*: Surgery is considered if medical treatment for otitis externa fails.
b) *Causes*: Tumors, otitis (discharge), congenital or malformation, head shaking for aural hematoma
c) *Clinical signs*: Pain, severe thickness, and firm ear canal, tilting of the head, loss of hearing, otitis (Figure 5.28).
d) *Diagnosis*: Radiographs of the skull, otoscopic examination, CT scan, MRI.
e) *Surgery*: The severity of the disease depends on which surgery is performed: (i) lateral ear canal resection (LECR) or Zepps modification to expose the medial portion of the vertical and horizontal ear canal. (ii) Vertical ear canal ablation (VECA) to remove the vertical canal and preserve the horizontal canal. (iii) Total ear canal ablation (TECA) to remove the entire ear canal without causing trauma to the facial nerve.
f) *Positioning*: Lateral recumbency with the front legs pulled back and a towel placed under the head. The affected ear is hung from an IV pole during draping but let down for surgery.
g) *Special instruments*: General pack, curettes, Kerrison rongeurs, medium or small Gelpi self-retaining retractor, Surgairtome, Lone Star retractor, bipolar electrosurgery, needle-tip monopolar electrosurgery, culture ear canal surgery after flushing with saline, collect tissue samples (Figures 5.29 and 5.30).
h) *Assistant's role*: Help drape the ear, retract tissue, moisten tissue, cut suture.
i) *Postoperative care*: Systemic antibiotics based on cultures, remove sutures/staples in 14 days, and place an E-Collar (Figure 5.31).

Figure 5.28 External pinna – aural hematoma.
Source: Courtesy of Dr. Mathews NCSU-CVM.

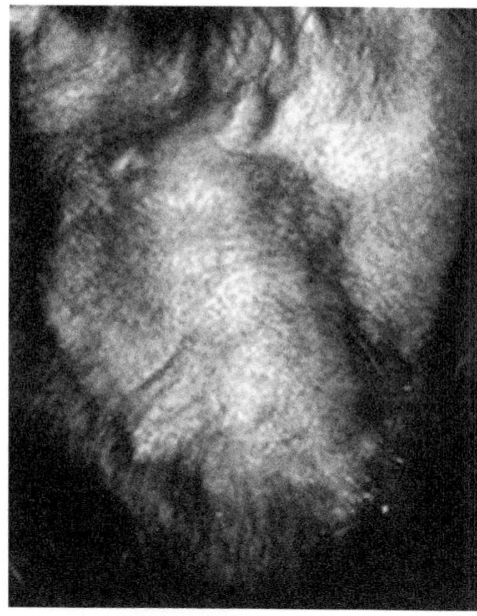

Figure 5.29 Total ear canal ablation – approach.
Source: Courtesy of Dr. Mathews NCSU-CVM.

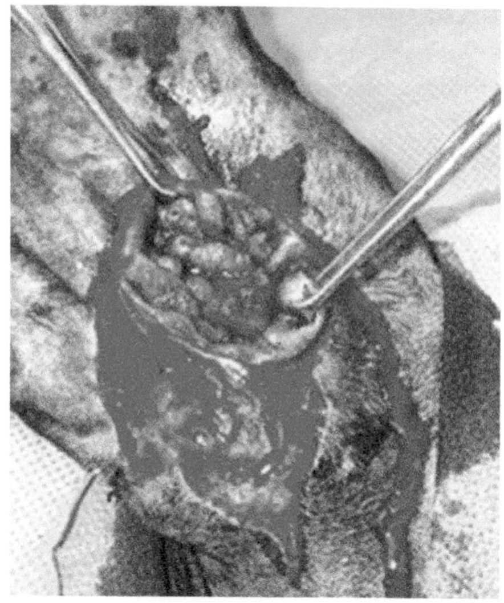

Figure 5.30 Total ear canal ablation – dissection.
Source: Courtesy of Dr. Mathews NCSU-CVM.

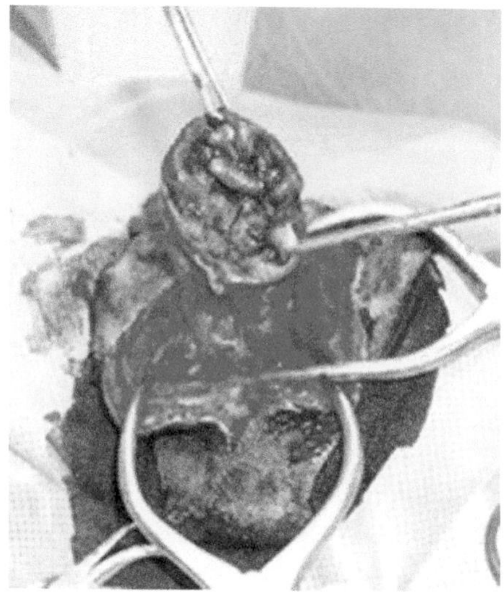

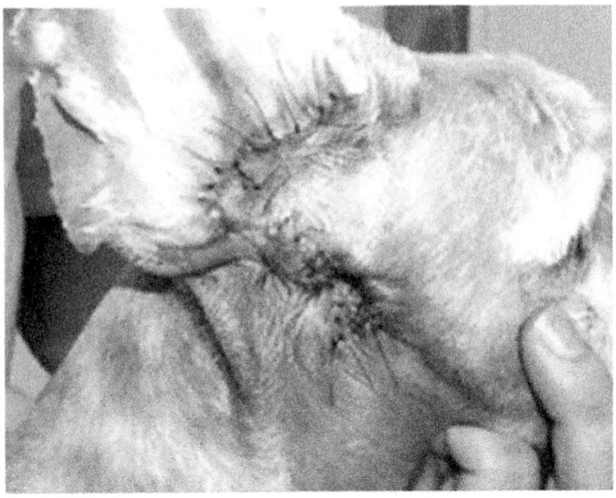

Figure 5.31 Total ear canal ablation – closure. *Source:* Courtesy of Dr. Mathews NCSU-CVM.

Otitis Media and Otitis Interna

a) *Definition*: Surgery is considered if medical treatment for otitis fails.
b) *Causes*: Tumors, otitis (discharge), congenital, or malformation.
c) *Clinical signs*: Pain, severe thickness and firm ear canal, tilting of the head, loss of hearing, otitis.
d) *Diagnosis*: Radiographs of the skull, otoscopic examination, CT scan, MRI.
e) *Surgery*: (i) Lateral bulla osteotomy (LBO) to provide access to the tympanic cavity and middle ear; a TECA is often performed with it. (ii) Ventral bulla osteotomy (VBO) to provide ventral drainage of the middle ear cavity.
f) *Position*: (i) LBO – the patient is placed in lateral recumbency with a towel under the neck with the legs pulled back. The ear is hung until draped for surgery. (ii) VBO – the patient is placed in dorsal recumbency with a towel under the neck with the legs pulled back (Figure 5.32).
g) *Special instruments*: General pack, curettes, Kerrison rongeurs, medium or small Gelpi self-retaining retractor, Surgairtome, Lone Star retractor, periosteal elevator, Steinmann pin, hand chuck and key, bipolar electrosurgery, needle-tip monopolar cautery, culture ear canal surgery after flushing with saline, collect tissue samples (Figure 5.33).
h) *Assistant's role*: Help drape the ear, retract tissue, moisten tissue, cut suture.
i) *Postoperative care*: Systemic antibiotics based on cultures, remove sutures/staples in 14 days, and place an E-Collar.

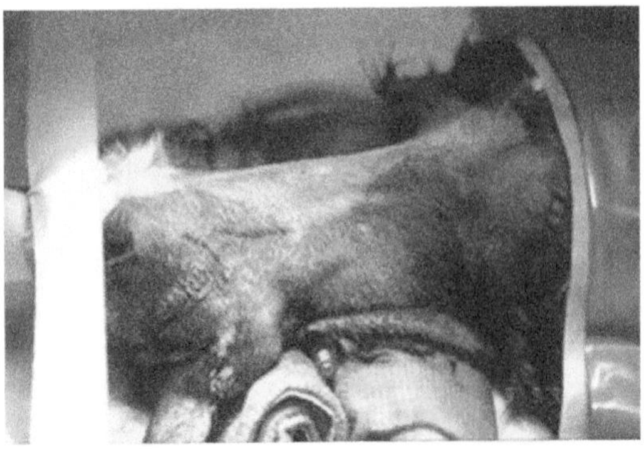

Figure 5.32 Ventral bulla osteotomy positioning. *Source:* Courtesy of Dr. Mathews NCSU-CVM.

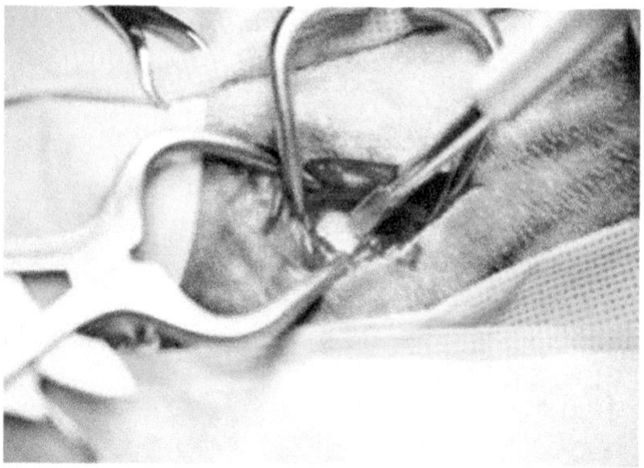

Figure 5.33 Ventral bulla osteotomy – intra-operative. *Source:* Courtesy of Dr. Mathews NCSU-CVM.

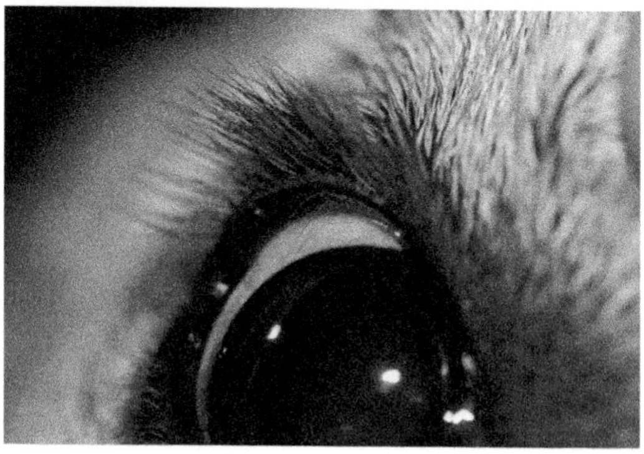

Figure 5.34 Distichiasis in upper eyelid. *Source:* Courtesy of Erin Barr NCSU-CVM.

Ophthalmic

Distichiasis

a) *Definition*: Hairs that originate from the meibomian glands come in contact with the cornea and cause irritation (Figure 5.34).
b) *Cause*: Rolling inward of the eyelid is commonly seen in Cocker Spaniels, Golden Retrievers, and Shih Tzu breeds.
c) *Clinical signs*: Vary from conjunctivitis with mild serous discharge to severe blepharospasm with corneal ulceration and purulent discharge.
d) *Diagnosis*: Examination of the eyelids; when the eye is rolled inward, the hairs often touch the cornea.
e) *Surgery*: Cryoepilation – evert and stabilize the eyelid, freeze a 3 mm band along the base of the meibomian gland on the palpebral surface of the lid below each abnormal cilia (Figure 5.35).
f) *Positioning*: Dorsal recumbency.
g) *Special instruments*: Liquid nitrogen, Jaeger lid plate, chalazion clamp.
h) *Assistant's role*: No assistant is needed.
i) *Postoperative care*: To minimize swelling, give a systemic anti-inflammatory prior to surgery. Most common complication is a recurrence three to five months postoperatively. Place an E-Collar

Entropion

a) *Definition*: Eyelid rolls inward
b) *Cause*: Genetics – usually seen in young dogs and is common in the Chow Chow, Shar Pei, and hunting breeds. It can also occur in cats

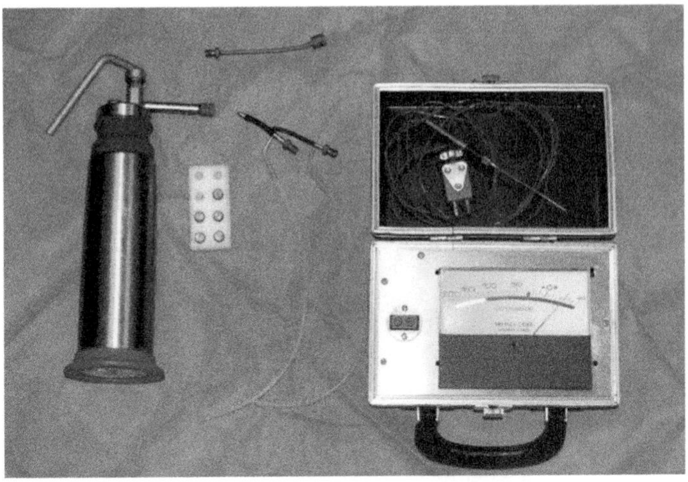

Figure 5.35 Ophthalmic cryogenic equipment. *Source:* Courtesy of Erin Barr NCSU-CVM.

c) *Clinical signs*: Vary from conjunctivitis with mild serous discharge to severe blepharospasm with corneal ulceration and purulent discharge
d) *Diagnosis*: Examination of the eyelids; when the eye is rolled inward, the hairs often touch the cornea
e) *Surgery*: (i) Eyelid tacking – temporarily everts the skin to prevent rolling on the eye. (ii) Removal of skin 2–3 mm from the lid margin and closing with a monofilament nylon suture
f) *Positioning*: Lateral recumbency with a towel under the patient's head
g) *Special instruments*: General extraocular pack, tenotomy scissors, Bishop Harmon tissue forceps, Barraquer eye speculum, Jaeger lid blade, Jameson Strabismus hook, colibri corneal forceps, 23 ga lacrimal cannula
h) *Assistant's role*: Retract tissue, moisten tissue, cut suture
i) *Postoperative care*: Place an E-Collar around the neck to prevent trauma. Apply antibiotics topically four times a day for 14 days. Apply warm and cold compresses to reduce eyelid swelling. Remove sutures in 14 days.

Enucleation

a) *Definition*: The removal of the eye
b) *Cause*: Cause may be injury, neoplasia, severe proptosis, or uncontrolled disease of the eye
c) *Clinical signs*: Pain, eye swelling, tachycardia
d) *Diagnosis*: Examination
e) *Surgery*: (i) Transconjunctival – most common procedure; reduces orbital tissue loss and reduces bleeding. (ii) Lateral – better visualization of the tissue before the eye is removed but increases tissue loss and bleeding. (iii) Transpalpebral superior confinement of the ocular surface from the surgery site which is good for infection and neoplasia
f) *Positioning*: Sternal recumbency with towel under the head; use of vacuum-assisted positioning aid
g) *Special instruments*: General extraocular pack, curved enucleation scissors, tenotomy scissors, Bishop Harmon tissue forceps, Barraquer eye speculum, Jaeger lid plate, Jameson Strabismus hook, colibri corneal forceps, 23 ga lacrimal cannula
h) *Assistant's role*: Retract tissue, moisten tissue, cut suture

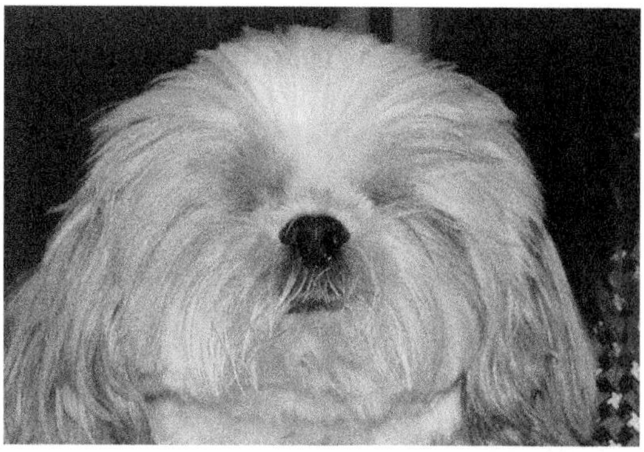

Figure 5.36 Healed patient following bilateral enucleation. *Source:* Courtesy of Erin Barr NCSU-CVM.

i) *Postoperative care*: Place an E-Collar around the neck, apply cold compresses to reduce eyelid swelling, may need to bandage/cover front feet to protect incision from scratching, remove sutures in 14 days (Figure 5.36).

Neoplasia of the Eye

a) *Definition*: Neoplastic tissue present on eyelid.
b) *Cause*: Common in dogs. Most masses are benign, 20–30% are malignant, with sebaceous adenoma being the most common.
c) *Clinical signs*: Discomfort/pain, may interfere with the eyelid function, and may cause keratitis.
d) *Diagnosis*: Examination with a description of the history. Cytology and histopathology with a fine needle aspirate and punch biopsy of the mass may differentiate inflammatory from neoplastic lesions.
e) *Surgery*: Eyelid mass resection by making a V wedge, or advanced skin flaps to oppose the edges of the defect. Eyelid mass resection then cryotherapy with the use of liquid nitrogen. Surgical removal of eyelid margin masses with a CO_2 laser.
f) *Positioning*: Sternal or lateral recumbency with a towel under the head
g) *Special instruments*: General extraocular pack, tenotomy scissors, Bishop Harmon tissue forceps, Barraquer eye speculum, Jaeger lid blade, Jameson Strabismus hook, colibri corneal forceps, 23 ga lacrimal cannula.
h) *Assistant's role*: Retract tissue, moisten tissue, cut suture
i) *Postoperative care*: Place an Elizabethan collar around the neck to prevent trauma. Apply antibiotics topically four times a day for 14 days. Apply warm and cold compresses to reduce eyelid swelling. Remove sutures in 14 days.

Thyroidectomy

a) *Definition*: Surgical removal of the thyroid gland
b) *Cause*: Hyperthyroidism, thyroid adenocarcinoma
c) *Clinical signs*: Weight loss, polyphagia, behavior changes, poor hair coat, hyperactivity, polydipsia, vomiting, neck swelling
d) *Diagnosis*: Echocardiography to check heart function, scintigraphy (CT) to determine if the condition is unilateral or bilateral, serum chemistry to evaluate for hypokalemia and renal dysfunction
e) *Surgery*: Unilateral/bilateral surgical removal of the thyroid glands; a ventral incision is made over the thyroid glands, monopolar and bipolar cautery are used to control hemorrhage. Hemoclips also may be used to control hemorrhage. Monofilament suture is used for closure (Figures 5.37 and 5.38).

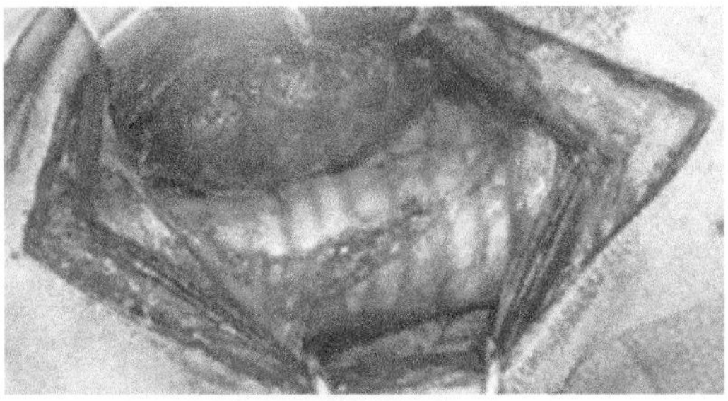

Figure 5.37 Thyroidectomy dissection intra-op. *Source:* Courtesy of Dr. Mathews NCSU-CVM.

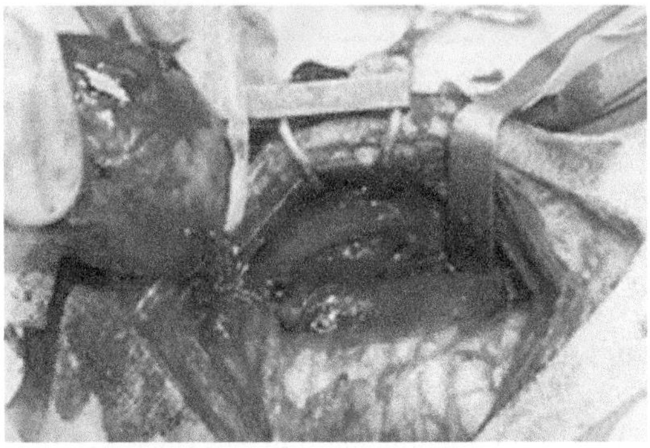

Figure 5.38 Excision of thyroid. *Source:* Courtesy of Dr. Mathews NCSU-CVM.

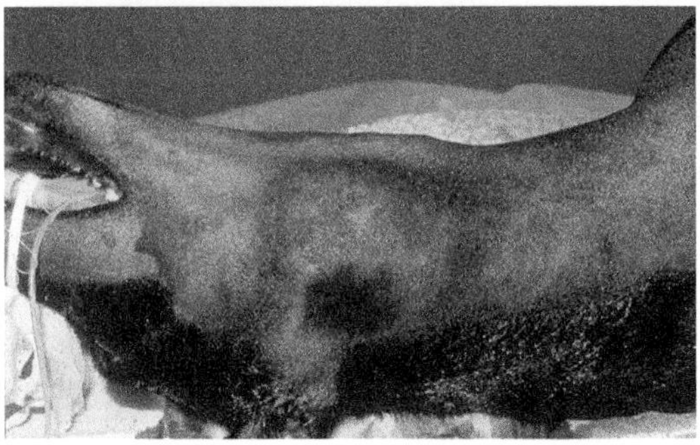

Figure 5.39 Thyroidectomy positioning. *Source:* Courtesy of Dr. Mathews NCSU-CVM.

f) *Positioning*: Dorsal recumbency with the front legs pulled caudally, elevate the neck with towels, vacuum-assisted positioner, or beanbag (Figure 5.39).
g) *Special instruments*: General and delicate pack, monopolar and bipolar electrosurgery, hemoclips, small Frazier suction tip, small and medium Gelpi, small/medium blunt Weitlaner retractor, vessel loops
h) *Assistant's role*: Retract tissue, cut suture, hemostasis, moisten tissue
i) *Postoperative care*: Monitor for hemorrhage, arrhythmias, laryngeal dysfunction, and hypokalemia

Upper Respiratory System

Elongated Soft Palate

a) *Definition*: Soft palate extends 1–3 mm caudal to the epiglottis (Figure 5.40) [8].
b) *Cause*: Congenital condition in brachycephalic breeds
c) *Clinical signs*: Noisy breathing, exercise intolerance, increased respiratory effort

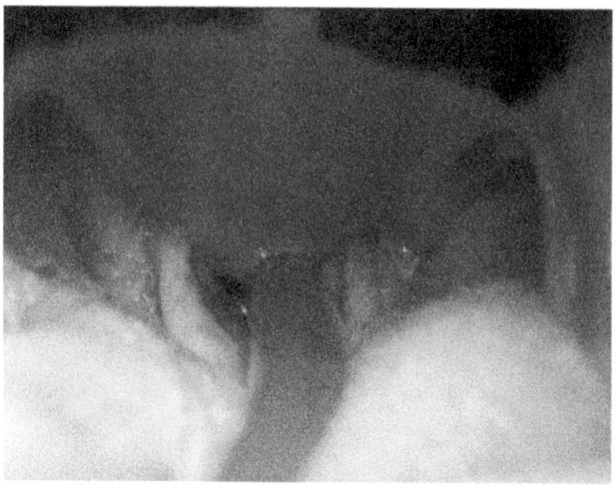

Figure 5.40 Pre-operative view of an elongated soft palate in an English Bulldog. *Source:* Robert Hardie, University of Wisconsin. Madison, WI. Reproduced with permission from Robert Hardie.

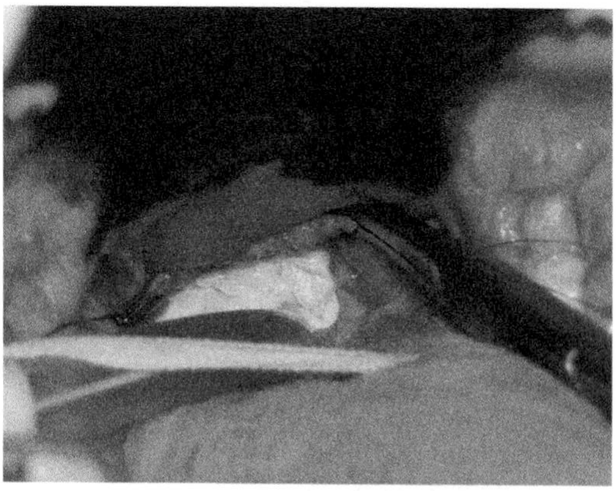

Figure 5.41 Right-angle clamp on transected palatal tissue. *Source:* Robert Hardie, University of Wisconsin Veterinary Care. Madison, WI. Reproduced with permission from Robert Hardie.

d) *Diagnosis*: Pharyngoscopy exam, radiographs to determine if any other underlying cardiac or thoracic abnormalities
e) *Surgery*: Following evaluation of the soft palate, the surgeon places stay sutures along the intended line of resection. Minimal handling of the soft palate is encouraged. Metzenbaum scissors are used to transect small amounts of excessive tissue. Closure of the wound with a simple continuous pattern of monofilament absorbable suture following each small resection. This alternating pattern of cut/suture continues until all tissue is removed (Figure 5.41).
f) *Positioning*: Sternal recumbency with a piece of roll gauze through mouth, just caudal to canine teeth, used to suspend maxilla from IV pole. Roll gauze is passed just caudal to the mandibular canines and taped to the table to keep the mouth open (Figure 5.42).
g) *Special instrumentation*: Long instruments if available, light source, electrosurgery
h) *Assistant's role*: Provide lateral retraction of tissue by holding hemostats attached to stay sutures.
i) *Postoperative care*: Close monitoring for respiratory distress, prolonged intubation in immediate postop period +/− oxygen therapy, provide small amounts of water when fully awake, delay feeding for 18–24 hours postop, slowly feed soft food formed into meatballs for 5–7 days to slow ingestion, use harness instead of neck collar for 2–4 weeks to avoid trauma to the surgery site

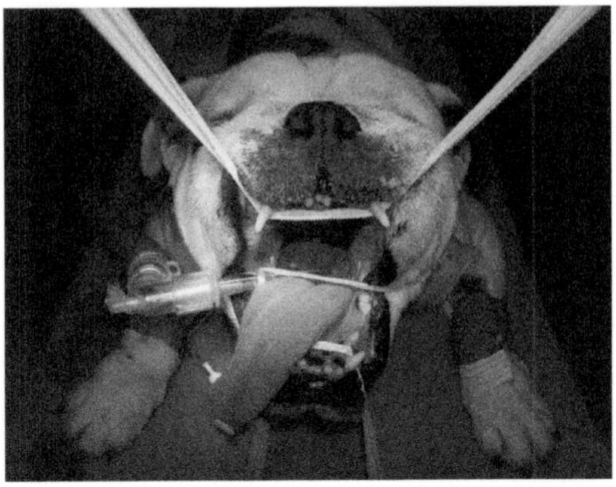

Figure 5.42 Positioning for elongated soft palate reduction. *Source:* Robert Hardie, University of Wisconsin Veterinary Care. Madison, WI. Reproduced with permission from Robert Hardie.

Laryngeal Paralysis

a) *Definition*: Failure of the arytenoid cartilages to open through inspiration and close during swallowing; they remain stationary
b) *Cause*: Muscles and nerves that cause abduction of the arytenoid cartilage to cease function may be idiopathic or congenital, more common in large breed, male dogs
c) *Clinical signs*: Hoarse barking, exercise intolerance, inspiratory stridor
d) *Diagnosis*: Laryngoscopy, radiographs to determine if any other underlying cardiac or thoracic abnormalities and to assess aspiration pneumonia and esophageal function
e) *Surgery*:
   i) *Arytenoid lateralization*: Approach to larynx is through a lateral incision, transection of the inter-arytenoid ligament, monofilament suture is used to abduct the arytenoid cartilage moderately lateral.
   ii) *Partial laryngectomy*: Oral approach – a long-handled scalpel or Metzenbaum scissors is used to resect the corniculate process and the proximal half and base of the cuneiform process. Hemostasis is provided with gauze sponges or electrosurgery.
   iii) *Partial laryngectomy*: Ventral approach – a ventral approach is made to expose the larynx. Excision of the corniculate, cuneiform, and vocal processes over the arytenoid cartilage is performed. Vocal folds are also excised. Defect is closed with small monofilament absorbable suture, routine muscle, and skin closure.
f) *Positioning*:
   i) *Arytenoid cartilage lateralization*: Lateral or dorsal recumbency, rolled towel placed under neck to elevate ipsilateral mandible. Tape head to table.
   ii) *Partial laryngectomy*: Oral approach – sternal recumbency with the maxilla elevated via roll gauze placed caudal to the maxillary canines. Mandible can be held open by assistant, taped to table, or place roll gauze just caudal to the mandibular canines and tape gauze to table.
   iii) *Partial laryngectomy*: Ventral approach – dorsal recumbency with head extended and taped to table.
g) *Special instrumentation*:
   i) *Arytenoid cartilage lateralization*: Electrosurgery, suction
   ii) *Partial laryngectomy*: Oral approach – long instruments
   iii) *Partial laryngectomy*: Ventral approach – Gelpi, small (4-0 to 6-0) monofilament suture

h) *Assistant's role*: Visualize larynx through mouth at surgeon's request for the ventral approach, suction, cut sutures, tissue retraction
i) *Postoperative care*: Close monitoring for respiratory distress, provide small amounts of water when fully awake, delay feeding for 18–24 hours postop, slowly feed soft food formed into meatballs for 5–7 days to slow ingestion, use harness instead of neck collar for 2–4 weeks to avoid trauma to the surgery site, restrict exercise for 6–8 weeks, minimize barking, monitor closely for aspiration, may need elevated feedings

Stenotic Nares

a) *Definition*: Nostrils with very narrow openings
b) *Cause*: Congenital condition in brachycephalic breeds
c) *Clinical signs*: Dyspnea, exercise intolerance, collapse
d) *Diagnosis*: Physical exam: medial deviation of nares +/− respiratory distress, radiographs to determine if any other underlying cardiac or thoracic abnormalities
e) *Surgery*: This procedure may or may not be performed in a surgical suite. Resection of some dorsolateral cartilage or horizontal or lateral tissue wedge resections of the nares will result in widened nares (Figures 5.43 and 5.44).
f) *Positioning*: Sternal recumbency, head taped to table for stability
g) *Special instrumentation*: #11 blade, electrosurgery
h) *Assistant's role*: Not usually present
i) *Postoperative care*: Close monitoring for respiratory distress, prolonged intubation in immediate postop period, E-Collar to protect surgery site, weight reduction if indicated

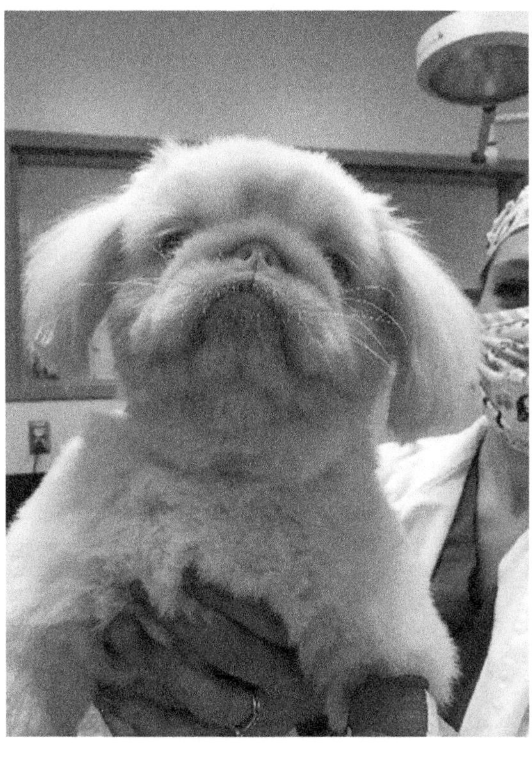

Figure 5.43 Stenotic nares – before correction.

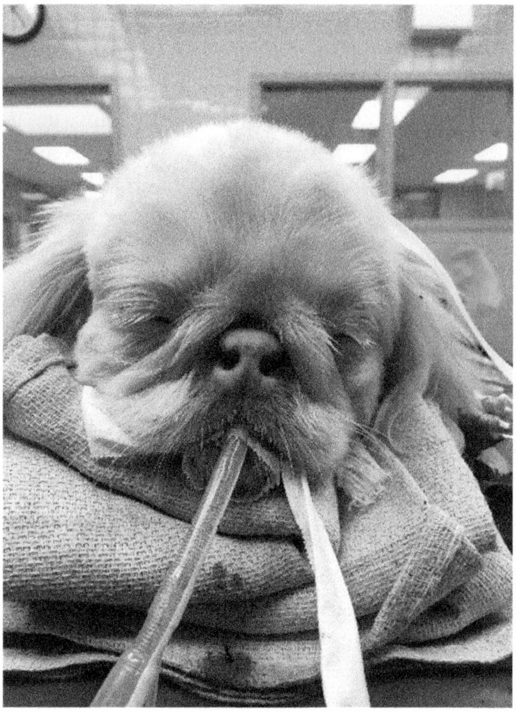

Figure 5.44 Stenotic nares – after correction.

Minimally Invasive

Arthroscopy

a) *Definition*: Internal visualization of a joint through a camera and employing instruments through ports to perform intra-articular surgery or for diagnosis; less invasive than an arthrotomy
b) *Cause*: Joints may be explored for a variety of conditions, including inspection of the internal structures (cruciate ligaments, menisci) during stabilization of a CCL injury. Other reasons include septic joints for flushing and for elbow dysplasia and shoulder conditions.
c) *Clinical signs*: Varies with reason for surgery; lameness, joint effusion, drainage from open wound
d) *Diagnosis*: Varies with condition; may include imaging, arthrocentesis, physical exam
e) *Surgery*: The cannula and arthroscope are placed along with a fluid inflow line. A fluid outflow portal is placed as well as a portal for hand instruments. Evaluation and repair of the joint occur if possible. Evaluation of the joint may also result in performing an arthrotomy (Figure 5.45).
f) *Positioning*: Depends entirely on procedure and joint having arthroscopic evaluation. Refer to surgeon preference.
g) *Special instrumentation*: Arthroscope, camera, arthroscopic instrumentation, monitor tower, extra fluids (Figure 5.46)
h) *Assistant's role*: Monitor fluid flow during procedure to avoid extravasation
i) *Postoperative care*: Varies with disease, generally exercise restrictions for two to four weeks, rehabilitation

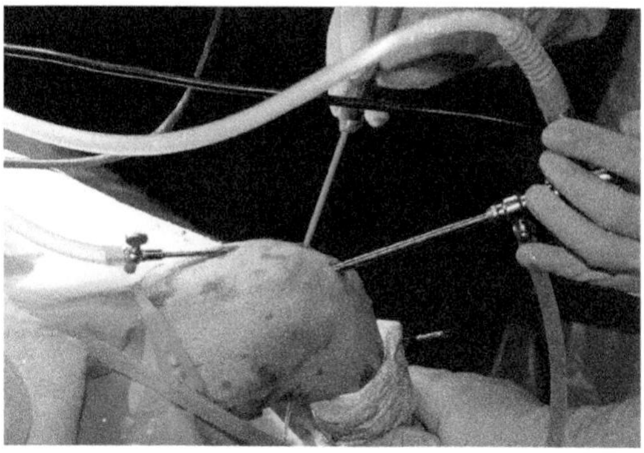

Figure 5.45 Triangulation of arthroscope, hand instrument, and outflow portal. *Source:* Paul Manley, University of Wisconsin, Madison, WI. Reproduced with permission from Paul Manley.

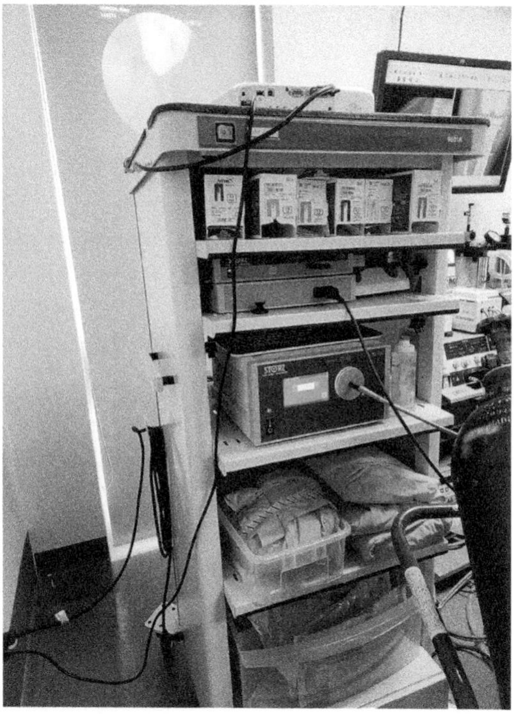

Figure 5.46 Arthroscopy tower with projector, shaver accessories, camera box, light source, instrument packs.

Laparoscopy

a) *Definition*: The minimally invasive procedure that has the same maneuvers as a laparotomy
b) *Cause*: To treat diseases by taking biopsies and performing surgeries with reduced time and trauma
c) *Clinical signs*: To treat diseases by taking biopsies and performing surgeries with reduced time and trauma which include: ovariectomy, gastropexy, cryptorchid surgery, adrenalectomy, cholecystectomy, liver biopsy, nephrectomy
d) *Diagnosis*: X-ray and US. Examination and biopsies in surgery of liver, kidney, prostate, pancreas, lymph node, spleen, reproductive tract, masses, and intestines; cholecystocentesis
e) *Surgery*: Performed in 2–4 incisions of 0.5–1 cm located in various places in the abdominal wall with the insufflation of CO_2. Once the peritoneal cavity is distended, a scope is placed through

a cannula for visualization and another cannula is placed for instruments to pass through. Monofilament suture used to close the incisions, and non-absorbable monofilament suture is used to close the skin

f) *Positioning*: Dorsal recumbency, may have to tilt the patient from left to right or may be in a Trendelenburg position; lateral recumbency
g) *Special instruments*: General pack, 5 or 10 mm laparoscopic pack (palpating probe, dissecting scissors, biopsy cup forceps, punch biopsy forceps, Babcock forceps, 10 mm Duval forceps, suture scissors, fan retractor, right-angle dissection forceps, suction/irrigation system, curved unipolar electrode and cord), spiral and smooth cannulas and trocars, scope, camera, and light source, harmonic/ENSEAL™ vessel sealer, insufflation tubing, endoclips, SILS port, endo peanuts, Lonestar retractor, anti-fog solution for the scope (Figures 5.47 and 5.48).
h) *Assistant's role*: Hold scope and/or instruments, retract tissue, cut suture, and moisten tissue
i) *Postoperative care*: Removal of the CO_2 from the body cavity, analgesia management, IV fluids and possibly antibiotics, restriction of activity should be for at least three weeks

Thoracoscopy

a) *Definition*: The minimally invasive procedure that provides opportunity for exploration and surgical treatment within the chest
b) *Cause*: Obtaining a diagnosis or treating intrathoracic conditions: pleural effusion, pericardial effusion, pulmonary disease, mediastinal lesions, lymphadenopathy, chylothorax, persistent right aortic arch (PRAA), pulmonary mass lesions, occlusion of patent ductus

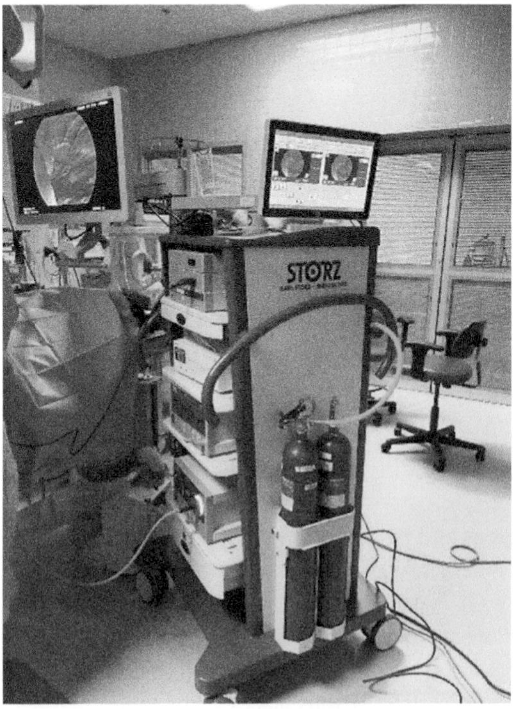

Figure 5.47 Tower used for thoracoscopic and laparoscopic procedures.

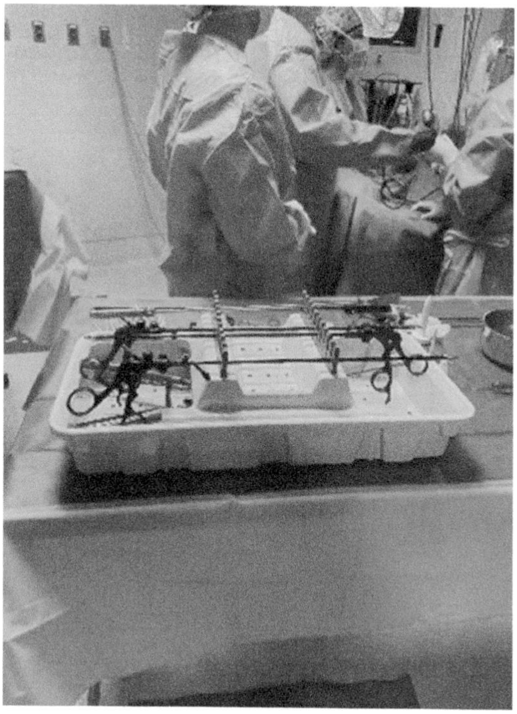

Figure 5.48 Instruments used for thoracoscopic and laparoscopic procedures.

arteriosus (PDA), spontaneous pneumothorax, pericardiocentesis, pericardiectomy, thoracic duct occlusion, lung lobectomy

c) *Clinical signs*: Having trouble breathing, neoplasia - CS dependent on condition
d) *Diagnosis*: Chest radiographs, US, CT
e) *Surgery*: Performed in 2–4 incisions of 0.5–1 cm located in various places in the chest wall without the use of CO_2. A scope and laparoscopic instruments are placed through thoraports. Monofilament suture is used to close the incisions, and non-absorbable monofilament suture is used to close the skin. The use of rigid scopes to magnify organs and spaces is normally approached by lateral thoracotomy or median sternotomy (Figures 5.49 and 5.50).
f) *Positioning*: Dorsal recumbency
g) *Special instruments*: Cardiothoracic pack, 5 or 10 mm laparoscopic pack (palpating probe, dissecting scissors, biopsy cup forceps, punch biopsy forceps, Babcock forceps, 10 mm Duval forceps, suture scissors, fan retractor, right-angle dissection forceps, suction/irrigation system, curved unipolar electrode and cord), spiral cannulas and trocars, scope, camera, and light source, harmonic/ENSEAL™ vessel sealer, thoraports, Mila chest tube, anti-fog solution for scope, thoracostomy tube
h) *Assistant's role*: Hold scope and/or instruments, retract tissue, cut suture, and moisten tissue
i) *Postoperative care*: ICU, removal of air from the chest with the placement of a thoracostomy tube, assessment of hemorrhaging, monitoring for any air leaks, monitoring for hypoxemia, the use of nasal oxygen tube may be needed and then removed after 12 hours, pain assessment

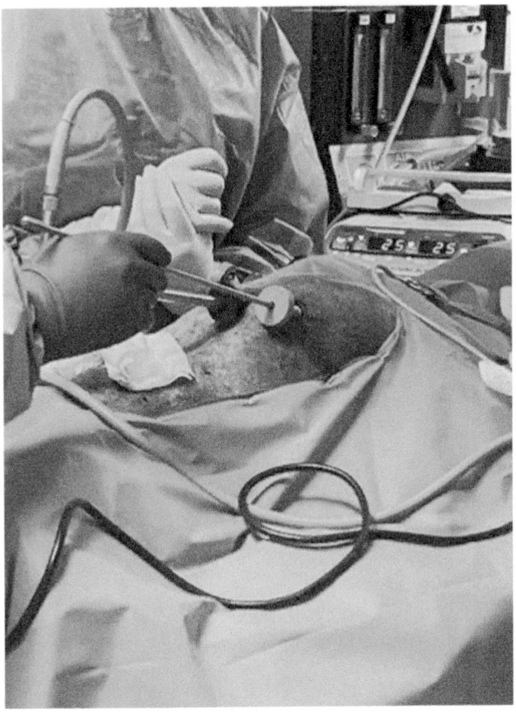

Figure 5.49 Thoracoscopy set up with scope, instruments, personnel.

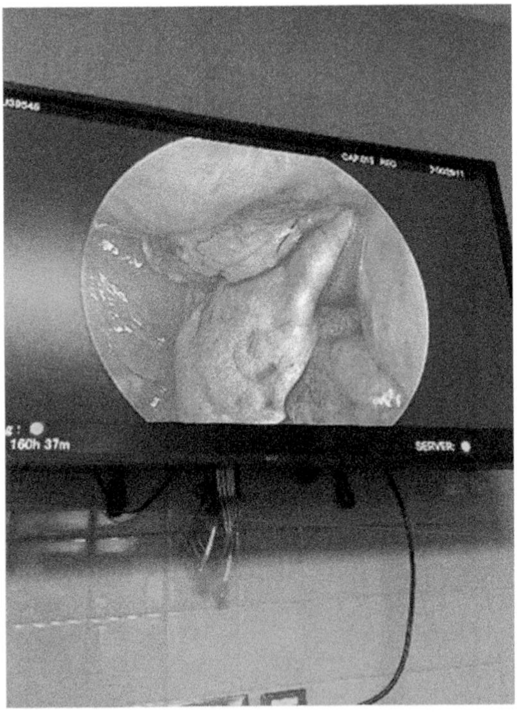

Figure 5.50 Thoracoscopic image of lung tissue.

Neurosurgery

Spine

Cervical

Ventral Slot

a) *Definition*: Degeneration and protrusion of intervertebral disc material into the spinal canal may cause compression of the spinal canal [9]
b) *Cause*: Genetics: most common in chondrodystrophic (abnormal cartilage) breeds such as Dachshund, Pekinese, Beagle, Basset Hound, and American Cocker Spaniel; Wobbler Syndrome most common in larger breed dogs particularly Doberman Pinschers and Great Danes. Trauma may also cause a sudden protrusion of an intervertebral disc
c) *Clinical signs*: Painful neck, paresis or paralysis of all four limbs
d) *Diagnosis*: Neurological exam checking proprioception, reflexes, pain response; radiographs, myelogram, CT, MRI +/− contrast
e) *Surgery*: Ventral slot – decompression of the cervical spinal cord via removal of a portion of a vertebral body to relieve pressure, provide access for removal of extruded intervertebral disc material. A ventral cervical incision is made. Dissection and muscle retraction proceed until the affected vertebral body/bodies are reached. A ronguer removes the ventral spinous processes. An air drill is used to create a window and allow removal of herniated disc material. No graft is used to fill the deficit. Routine closure follows the procedure.
f) *Positioning*: Dorsal recumbency with forelimbs extending caudally toward chest; head in hyperextension with a rolled-up towel under the neck; mandible taped to table
g) *Special instrumentation*: Pneumatic drill and burrs, electrosurgery, suction, Gelfoam®, #11 blade, ronguers, periosteal elevator, bone wax, dental spatula, dural hooks, 3-0/4-0 bone curettes.
h) *Assistant's role*: Irrigate wound during and following drilling, suction, lavage field, muscle retraction, hand instruments, cut sutures
i) *Postoperative care*: Intensive care, bladder expression if needed, maintaining spine in an even plane, rehabilitation, sling walking (front and rear) to encourage walking, quadriplegic cart if limb function doesn't return

Thoracolumbar

Laminectomy/Hemi-laminectomy

a) *Definition*: Degeneration and protrusion of intervertebral disc material into the spinal canal, may cause compression of the spinal canal
b) *Cause*: Genetics: most common in chondrodystrophic (abnormal cartilage) breeds such as Dachshund, Pekinese, Beagle, Basset Hound, and American Cocker Spaniel; trauma may also cause a sudden protrusion of an intervertebral disc
c) *Clinical signs*: Paresis or paralysis of the rear limbs, knuckling or dragging of the feet, inability to urinate, back pain, weakness, reluctance to rise, collapse, trembling
d) *Diagnosis*: Neurological exam checking proprioception, reflexes, pain response; radiographs, myelogram, CT, MRI +/− contrast (Figure 5.51).
e) *Surgery*: Hemilaminectomy – decompression of the spinal cord via removal of a portion of a vertebral body to relieve pressure, provides access for removal of extruded intervertebral disc material. Following a dorsal midline incision, dissection continues until vertebral bodies are reached. Ronguers and a drill are used to remove the dorsal lamina until an appropriate

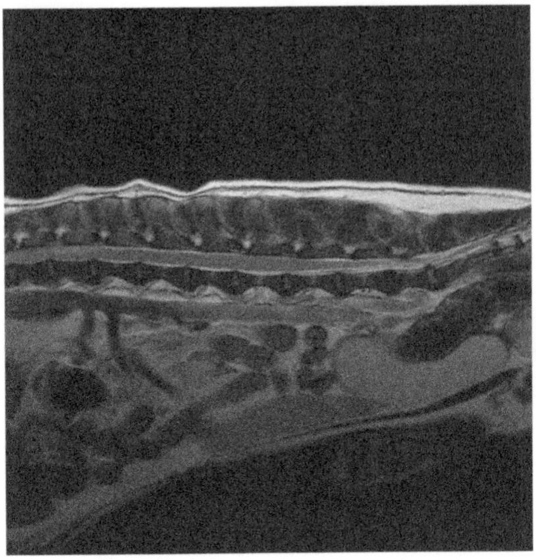

Figure 5.51 MRI performed on patient needing a hemi-laminectomy.

"window" is created to allow decompression. A fat graft is harvested and placed over the defect prior to closure

f) *Positioning*: Sternal recumbency with spine perfectly straight, positioning aids are often required
g) *Special instrumentation*: Hall air drill, neuro instruments (dural hooks, dental spatula, delicate thumb tissue forceps), Frazier suction tip, suction, electrosurgery, single-action rongeurs, double-action rongeurs, Kerrison rongeur, laminectomy retractor, Gelpi self-retaining retractor, periosteal elevator, Gelfoam, bone wax
h) *Assistant's role*: Hold stay sutures to elevate dura, drip saline as burring of vertebral roof is occurring, suction, cut sutures, lavage field, elevate dorsal spinous processes with towel clamp
i) *Postoperative care*: Intensive care, bladder expression, maintaining spine in an even plane, rehabilitation, sling walking to encourage walking, cart if never regains function of rear limbs

Orthopedic

Fractures

a) *Definition*: Fractures may occur in any bone. They are classified as transverse (defect from cortex to cortex), oblique (defect runs diagonally to the long axis of the bone), spiral (defect wraps around the long axis of the long bone), comminuted reducible (no more than two large fragments), comminuted non-reducible (multiple small fragments), and open (any break in the skin whether from the bone moving outward or foreign object moving inward) Grade I, II, or III(Figures 5.52–5.55). Physeal fractures: Salter-Harris I (runs through the physis), Salter-Harris II (through physis and portion of metaphysis), Salter-Harris III (runs through physis, epiphysis, and generally are articular), Salter-Harris IV (articular fractures that run through the epiphysis, physis, and metaphysis), Salter-Harris V (crushing injuries of the physis)
b) *Cause*: Trauma, neoplasia, osteoporosis, osteomyelitis
c) *Clinical signs*: Lameness, pain, swelling, redness, bone protruding through skin
d) *Diagnosis*: Known trauma, palpation, radiographs, CT (Figure 5.56).

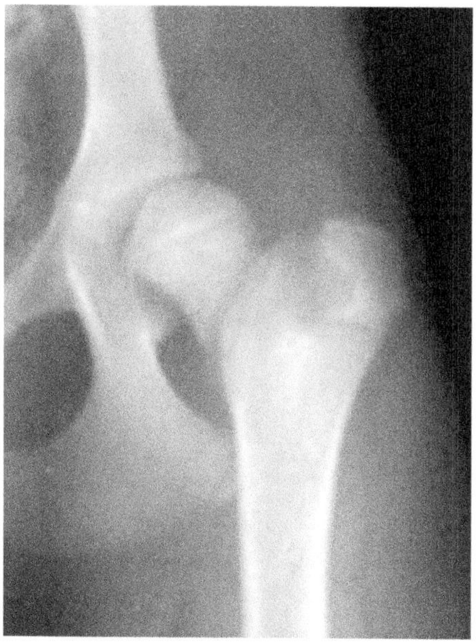

Figure 5.52 Transverse fracture of femoral neck. *Source:* Courtesy of Paul Manley University of Wisconsin retired.

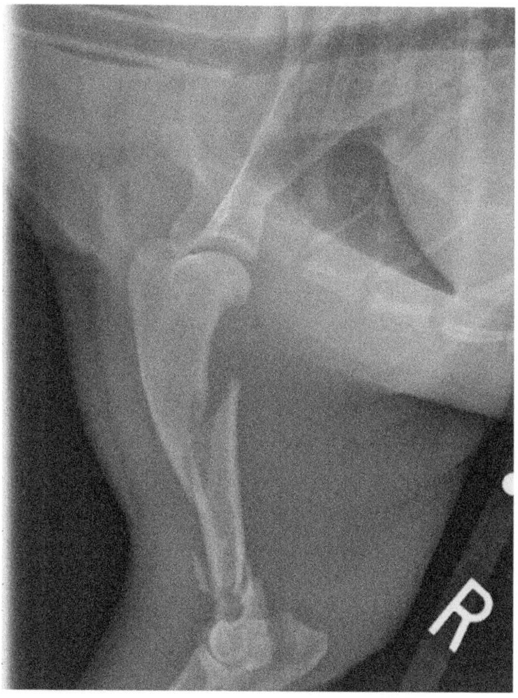

Figure 5.53 Mid-shaft spiral fracture of humerus. *Source:* Courtesy of Paul Manley University of Wisconsin retired.

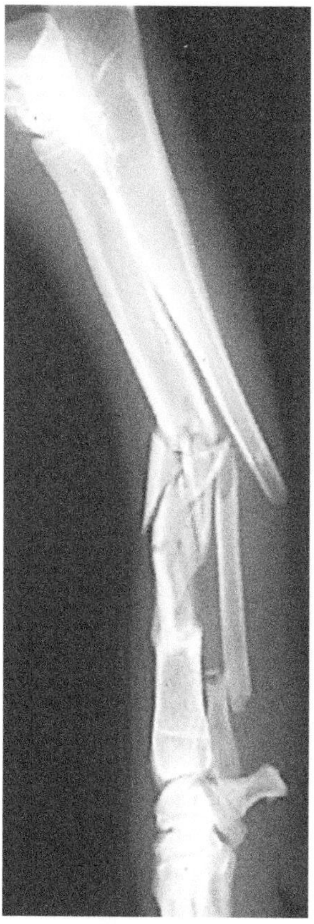

Figure 5.54 Comminuted non-reducible radius/ulna fracture. *Source:* Courtesy of Paul Manley University of Wisconsin retired.

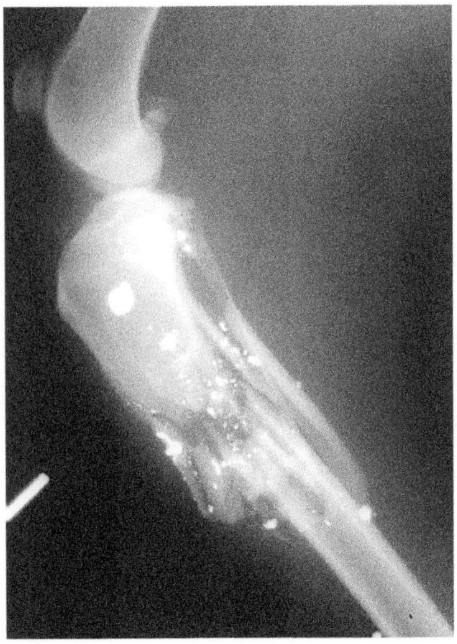

Figure 5.55 High-velocity bullet, open comminuted non-reducible fracture of tibia/fibula. *Source:* Courtesy of Paul Manley University of Wisconsin retired.

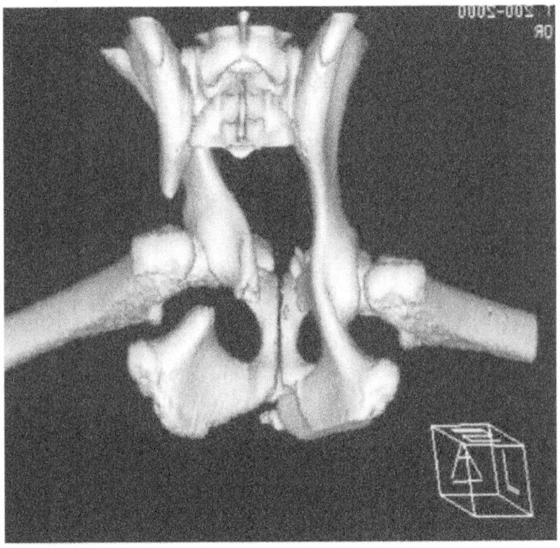

Figure 5.56 VD view of three-dimensional CT fractured pelvis. *Source:* Paul Manley, University of Wisconsin, Madison, WI. Reproduced with permission from Paul Manley.

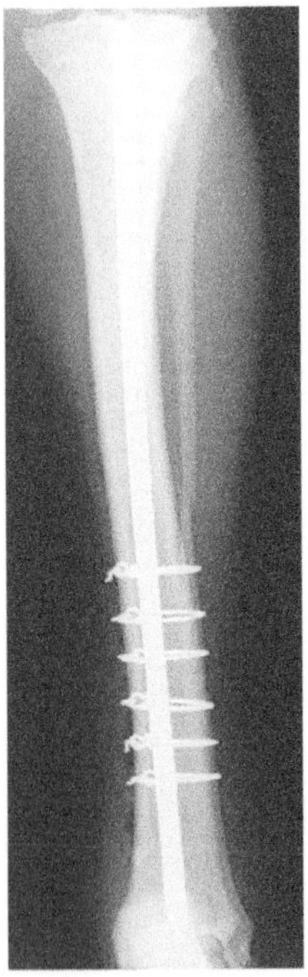

Figure 5.57 Post-op radiograph of repaired fractured tibia using pin and wire. *Source:* Paul Manley, University of Wisconsin, Madison, WI. Reproduced with permission from Paul Manley.

e) *Surgery*: Internal fixation (plate, pin, interlocking nail, wires, screws) or external fixation (external skeletal fixator – bars, ring fixators) – approach and dissection to reveal fractured bone (Figures 5.57–5.59). Reduction of fracture and stabilization with bone-holding forceps, implants of choice are placed, bone graft may/may not be harvested and implanted. Grafts may be autografts (from the same patient) or allografts (commercially available bones from the same species, chips, or granules). Grafts can be of cortical, cancellous, or corticocancellous bone. Autografts can be collected from various sites on the patient (proximal femur, proximal humerus, iliac crest, ribs, or pulverized bone pieces in non-reducible comminuted fractures) (Figures 5.60 and 5.61). Closure follows.
f) *Positioning*: Depends entirely on bone fractured and approach being used, however, often the repair will be done with the animal in lateral recumbency with the affected limb up
g) *Special instrumentation*: Power drill, battery, or nitrogen tank for drill, self-retaining retractors, bone-holding forceps, suction, electrosurgery, periosteal elevators, curette (if bone graft is harvested), plate benders (Figure 5.62).

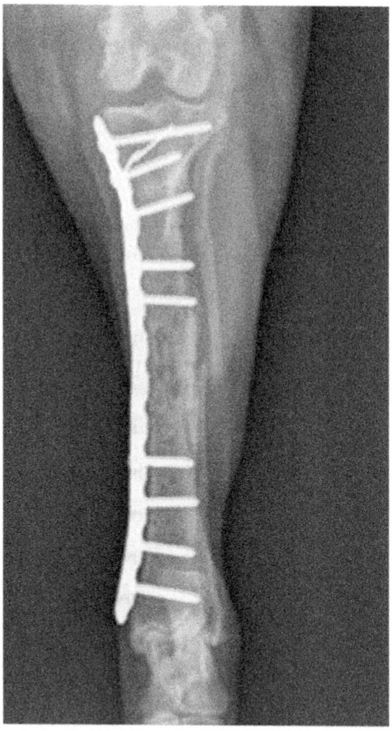

Figure 5.58 Tibial fracture stabilized with locking plate and screws. *Source:* Courtesy of Paul Manley University of Wisconsin retired.

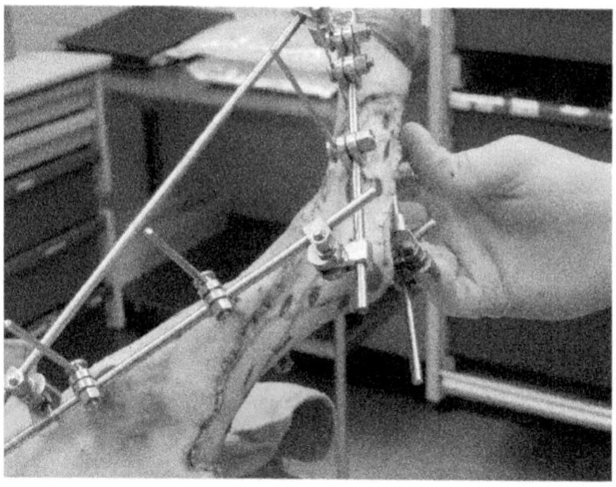

Figure 5.59 External fixator. *Source:* Paul Manley, University of Wisconsin, Madison, WI. Reproduced with permission from Paul Manley.

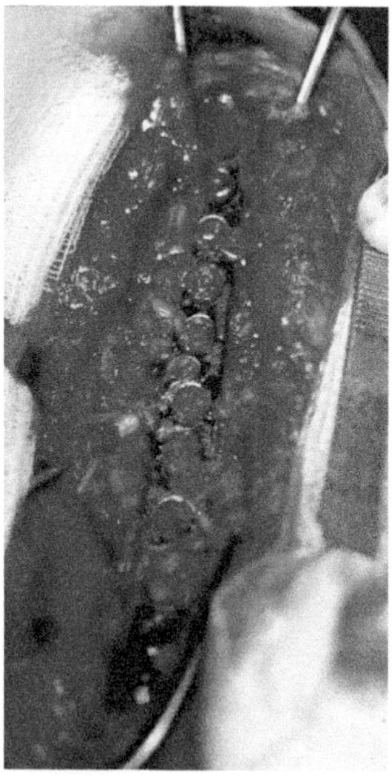

Figure 5.60 Autogenous bone graft packed around repaired fracture. *Source:* Courtesy of Paul Manley University of Wisconsin retired.

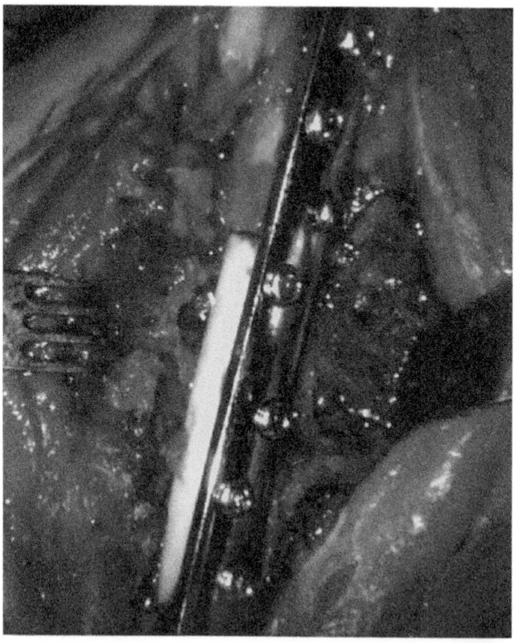

Figure 5.61 Allograft in place. *Source:* Paul Manley, University of Wisconsin, Madison, WI. Reproduced with permission from Paul Manley.

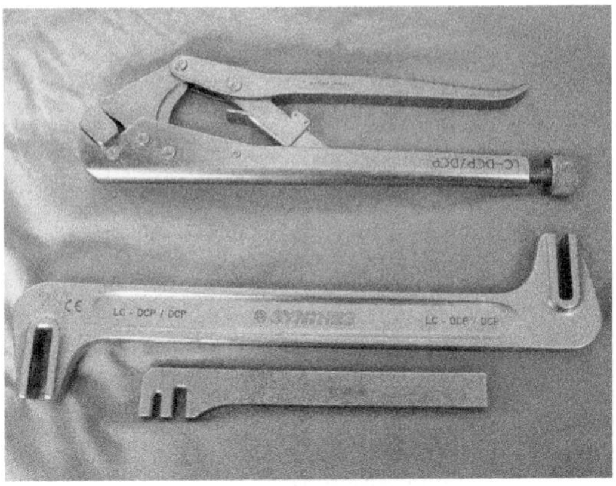

Figure 5.62 Plate benders used to manipulate bone plate to better conform to recipient bone. *Source:* Paul Manley, University of Wisconsin, Madison, WI. Reproduced with permission from Paul Manley.

h) *Assistant's role*: Hand instruments for screw placement in proper order (drill bit, drill guide, depth gauge, [tap, tap sleeve if tapping needed], screw, screwdriver), keep drill bit/tap clean between uses, moisten tissues, guard harvested bone graft to avoid accidental disposal, retraction, run suture, cut suture, potentially drilling screw holes, reduce fracture at direction of surgeon
i) *Postoperative care*: Dependent on fracture and fixation. Generally, exercise restrictions, physical rehabilitation, wound care +/− external coaptation

Forelimb

Shoulder

Osteochondritis Dissecans (OCD) of Proximal Humerus

a) *Definition*: Incomplete endochondral ossification causes cartilage to remain, fissure in this cartilage creates a flap that may loosen causing a "joint mouse" [10]
b) *Cause*: Unknown but breed disposition (large breeds), genetic and dietary (overnutrition = rapid growth) factors contribute to condition, found in young dogs
c) *Clinical signs*: Forelimb lame (unilateral or bilateral), worse after exercise, improves with rest, pain on full shoulder extension
d) *Diagnosis*: Radiographs of shoulders, CT scan, US, arthroscopy (Figure 5.63).

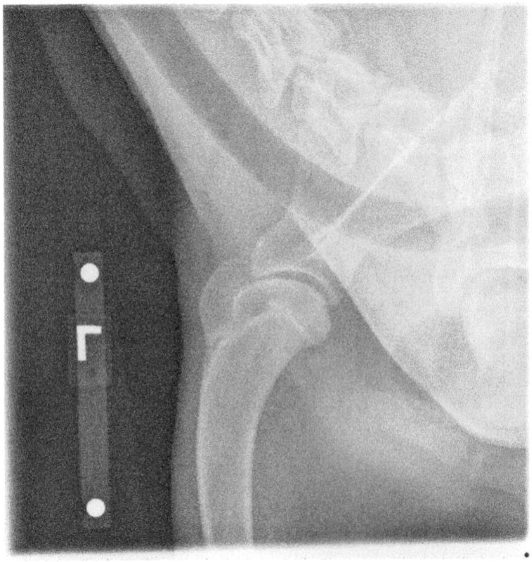

Figure 5.63 Pre-op radiograph – OCD visible. *Source:* Paul Manley, University of Wisconsin, Madison, WI. Reproduced with permission from Paul Manley.

Figure 5.64 Arthrotomy to elevate proximal humeral OCD. *Source:* Paul Manley, University of Wisconsin, Madison, WI. Reproduced with permission from Paul Manley.

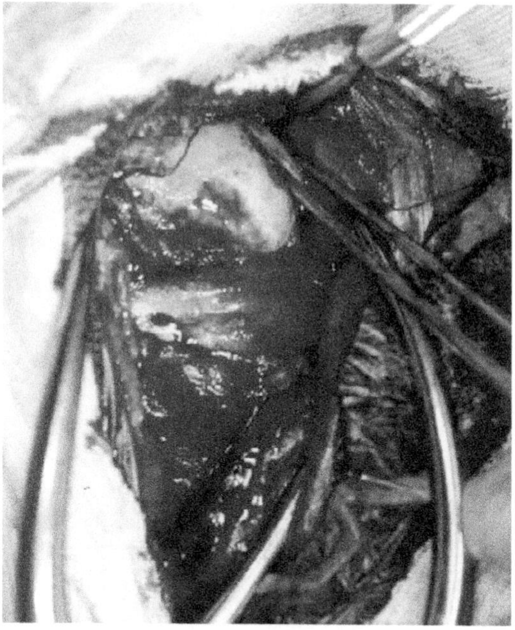

e) *Surgery*: Arthroscopic or open approach to remove cartilage flap (Figure 5.64).
f) *Positioning*: Lateral recumbency with surgical limb up
g) *Special instrumentation*:
   i) *Arthroscopy*: Arthroscope, arthroscopy instrumentation (cannulas, probes, graspers, shavers, shaver tips, camera, monitor, and tower)
   ii) *Open*: Ochsner forceps or other toothed forceps, bone curette, suction, electrosurgery, self-retaining retractor (Gelpi)
h) *Assistant's role*:
   i) *Arthroscopic*: Monitor fluid flow, manipulate limb, set up arthroscope
   ii) *Open*: Retraction of tissue, suction, cut sutures, occasionally screw hole drilling, securing plate on bone with bone forceps
i) *Postoperative care*: Cryotherapy, restricted activity, and physical rehabilitation

Elbow

Fragmented Coronoid Process (FCP)

a) *Definition*: Portion of medial coronoid process of ulna separates from parent bone
b) *Cause*: Unknown but several theories include OCD lesion disrupting endochondral ossification, developmental elbow incongruity, incongruence between radial head and radial notch, vascular abnormality of medial coronoid, tension from insertion of biceps brachii on ulna, secondary to low-grade trauma following a jump; breed disposition (large breeds), found in young dogs
c) *Clinical signs*: Forelimb lame, worse after exercise, stiff after rest, often bilateral, elbow pain with hyperextension and effusion
d) *Diagnosis*: Radiographs, CT of elbows, arthroscopy (Figure 5.65).
e) *Surgery*: Arthroscopy or open approach to remove fragment
f) *Positioning*: Dorsal recumbency to allow medial approach for both arthroscopic and open repair

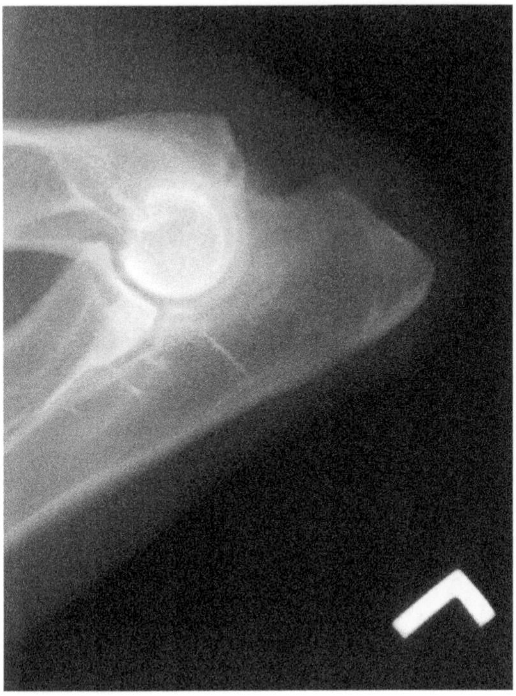

Figure 5.65 Radiograph of left-fragmented coronoid process after removal. *Source:* Paul Manley, University of Wisconsin, Madison, WI. Reproduced with permission from Paul Manley.

g) *Special instrumentation*:
   i) *Arthroscopic*: Arthroscope 30° 1.9 or 2.4 mm scope, blunt (preferred)/sharp trocar, cannula, camera, arthroscopic hand instruments, +/− motorized shaver, fluids, monitor, and tower
   ii) *Open*: Ochsner (or other toothed) forceps, osteotome and mallet OR oscillating bone saw, battery or nitrogen tank to power saw, suction, bulb syringe, electrosurgery
h) *Assistant's role*:
   i) *Arthroscopic*: Monitor fluid flow, manipulate limb for surgeon, set up arthroscope, set up motorized shaver if used.
   ii) *Open*: Assist with draping, set up suction/electrosurgery, retract tissue with hand-held retractors, lavage field, suction field, set up bone saw, cut sutures.
i) *Postoperative care*: Cryotherapy, restricted activity, and physical rehabilitation

Osteochondritis Dissecans (OCD) (Distal Humerus)

a) *Definition*: Incomplete endochondral ossification causes cartilage to remain, fissure in this cartilage creates a flap that may loosen causing a "joint mouse" (Figure 5.66).
b) *Cause*: Unknown but breed disposition (large breeds), genetic and dietary (overnutrition = rapid growth) factors contribute to condition, found in young dogs (five to seven months)
c) *Clinical signs*: Forelimb lame (unilateral or bilateral), worse after exercise, stiff after rest, pain and elbow effusion if osteoarthritis is present
d) *Diagnosis*: Radiographs of elbows, arthroscopy
e) *Surgery*: Arthroscopy or open approach to remove cartilage flap (Figures 5.67 and 5.68).
f) *Positioning*: Dorsal recumbency regardless of technique of repair

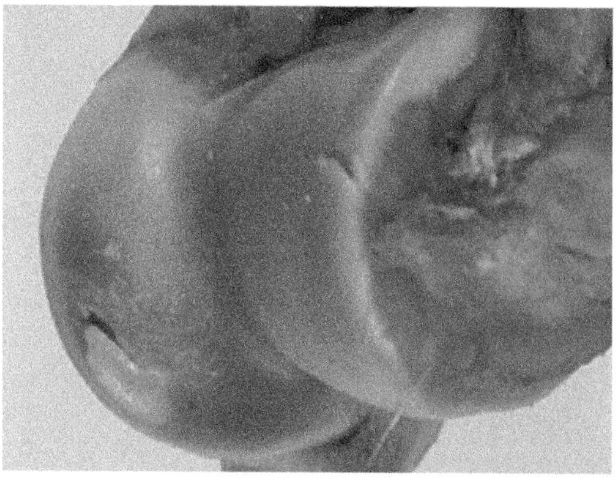

Figure 5.66 Distal humeral osteochondritis dissecans (OCD) flap. *Source:* Paul Manley, University of Wisconsin, Madison, WI. Reproduced with permission from Paul Manley.

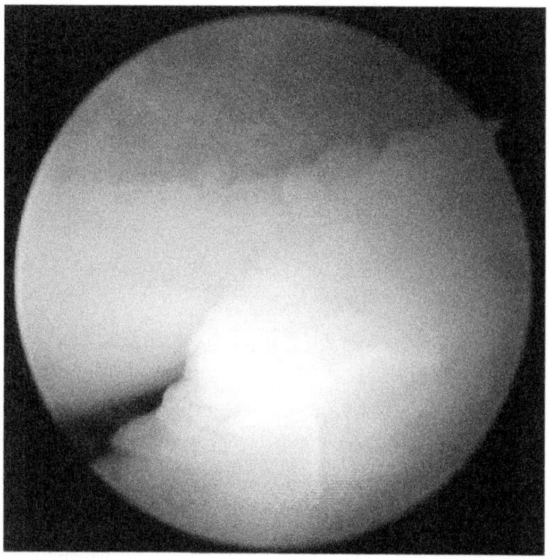

Figure 5.67 Arthroscopic view of distal humeral OCD flap. *Source:* Paul Manley, University of Wisconsin, Madison, WI. Reproduced with permission from Paul Manley.

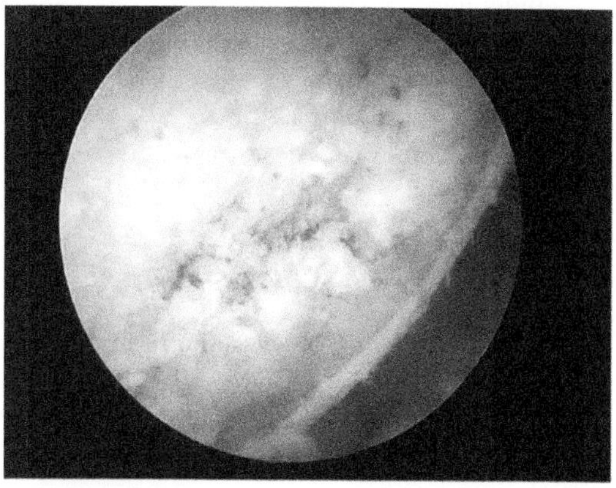

Figure 5.68 Arthroscopic view following removal of OCD. *Source:* Paul Manley, University of Wisconsin, Madison, WI. Reproduced with permission from Paul Manley.

g) *Special instrumentation*:
    i) *Arthroscopic*: Arthroscope 30° 1.9 or 2.4 mm scope, blunt (preferred)/sharp trocar, cannula, camera, arthroscopic hand instruments, +/− motorized shaver, fluids, monitor, and tower
    ii) *Open*: Ochsner (or other toothed) forceps, bone curette
h) *Assistant's role*:
    i) *Arthroscopic*: Monitor fluid flow, manipulate limb for surgeon, set up arthroscope, set up motorized shaver if used
    ii) *Open*: Assist with draping, set up suction/electrosurgery, retract tissue with hand-held retractors, lavage field, suction field, cut sutures
i) *Postoperative care*: No bandage or soft padded bandage, cryotherapy, restricted activity for up to eight weeks, physical rehabilitation

Ununited Anconeal Process

a) *Definition*: Anconeal process does not attach to proximal ulna
b) *Cause*: Center of ossification of the anconeus occurs separately from olecranon, disturbance of ossification of the juncture creates a fissure; large breed dogs, genetics, rapid growth, and trauma may contribute to condition; usual presentation at 6–12 months
c) *Clinical signs*: Intermittent forelimb lame (unilateral), worse after exercise, stiff after rest, pain and elbow effusion, decreased elbow range of motion, paw may rotate externally when dog is sitting or standing
d) *Diagnosis*: Radiographs (**after** five months of age) or CT scan of elbows (Figure 5.69).
e) *Surgery*: Open approach to elbow to remove anconeal process; dogs younger than one year with minimal joint damage may benefit from a combined ulnar osteotomy and lag screw placement procedure (Figure 5.70).
f) *Positioning*: For anconeal process removal only, lateral recumbency with affected limb up; For anconeal process removal, medical coronoid process excision and/or ulnar osteotomy – dorsal recumbency to allow medial approach
g) *Special instrumentation*: Gelpi self-retaining retractor, suction, electrosurgery, single-action ronguer, oscillating saw if doing ulnar osteotomy, bone screws, screw placement instrumentation, power drill for screw placement
h) *Assistant's role*: Assist with draping, suction during drilling, hydrate field during osteotomy, cut sutures, retract tissue if necessary, present screw placement equipment in proper order
i) *Postoperative care*: Bandage or soft padded bandage for up to one week, cryotherapy, restricted activity for four weeks, and physical rehabilitation

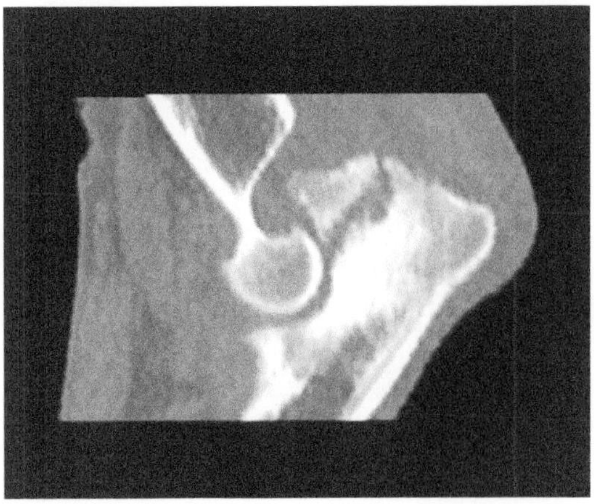

Figure 5.69 CT of united anconeal process (UAP).

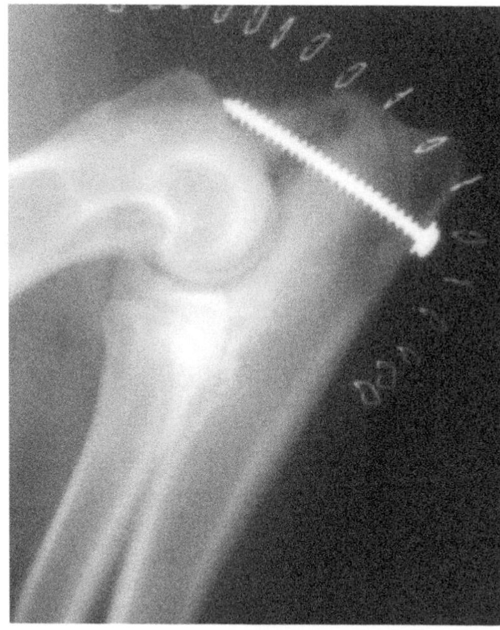

Figure 5.70 UAP repair with screw fixation. *Source:* Paul Manley, University of Wisconsin, Madison, WI. Reproduced with permission from Paul Manley.

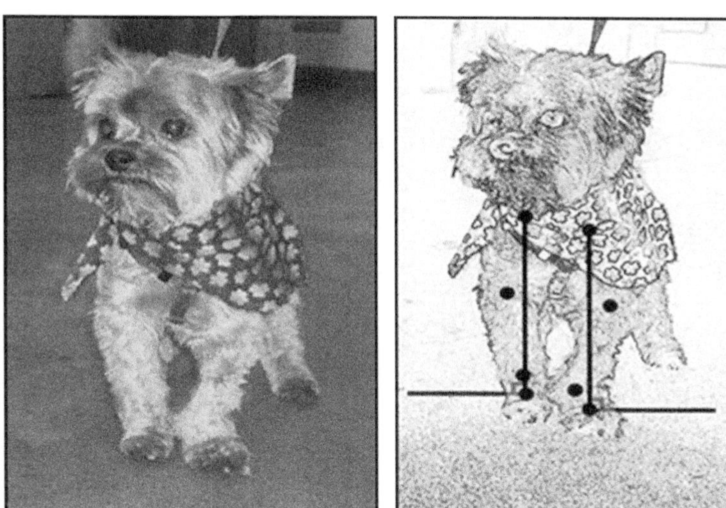

Figure 5.71 Valgus deformity of the distal portion of the radius. *Source:* Courtesy of Dr. Marcellin-Little.

Radius/Ulna

Valgus Deformity – Radial Valgus Deformity

a) *Definition*: The outward turning of the front limbs distal/proximal of antebrachium (Figure 5.71).
b) *Cause*: Genetic makeup that leads to the impairment growth of the appendicular skeleton and skull. Primarily seen in chondrodystrophic breeds including Dachshunds, Basset Hounds, Beagles, Corgis, and Bulldogs
c) *Clinical signs*: Limping consistently, pain from the outward turning of the limb, joint effusion, and OA in joints

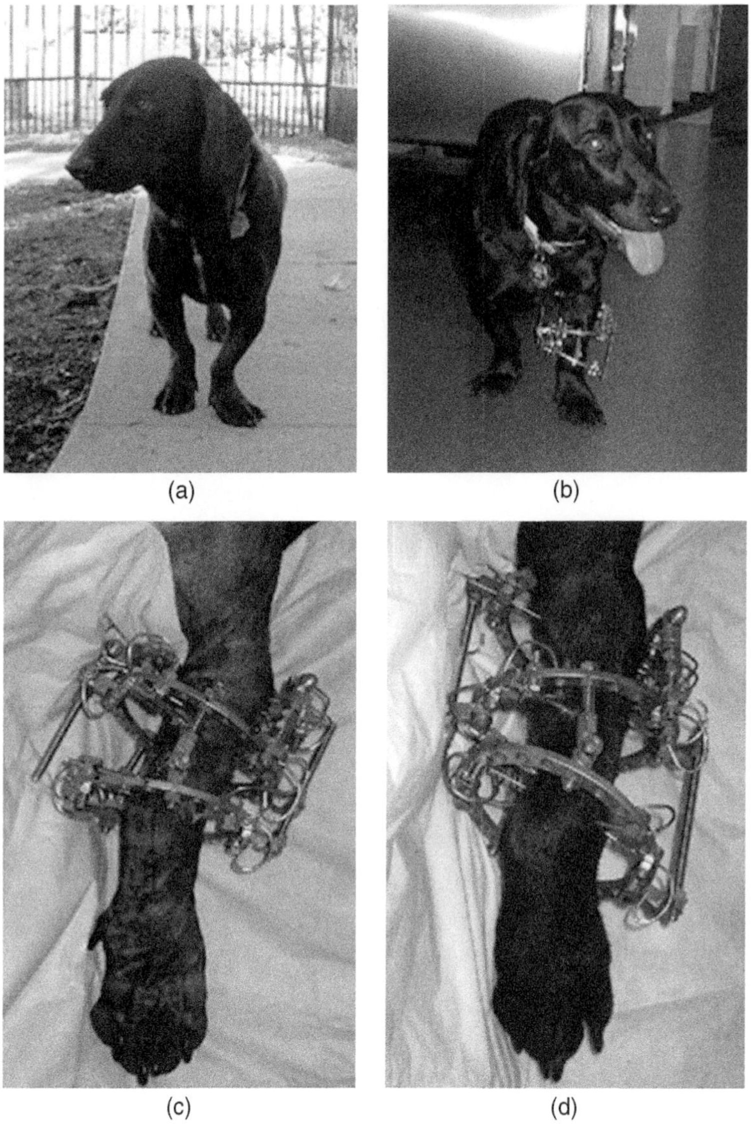

Figure 5.72 Semantic scholar correction of biapical radial deformities. (a) Pre-op, (b) four months post op, (c) post-op, (d) four months post op. *Source:* Courtesy of Dr. Marcellin-Little.

d) *Diagnosis*: X-ray, CT, and/or MRI of limbs
e) *Surgery*: Corrective osteotomy with the placement of a circular external skeletal fixation frame or special plate (Figure 5.72).
f) *Positioning*: Dorsal recumbency with the affected limb hanging from the ceiling with a lateral approach
g) *Special instruments*: Premade Ilizarov set (circular fixation frame), sterile leg hangers, small Hohmann retractors, small Gelpi self-retractors, cordless saw
h) *Assistant's role*: Assist with draping, hand instruments for screw placement in proper order (drill bit, drill guide, depth gauge, screw, screwdriver), keep drill bit clean between uses, hydrate field during osteotomy, cut sutures, retract tissue if necessary

i) *Postoperative care*: Wound care, maintaining limb range of motion in the carpus and elbow. Lengthening is accelerated after angular correction 15–30 days postoperative. Remove frame, when bone is healed, under sedation

Carpus

Arthrodesis of the Carpus

a) *Definition*: The fusion of two or more bones in a joint.
b) *Cause*: Ligaments and other support structures that stabilize the carpal and tarsal joints are torn or stretched, which could be from a hyperextension injury.
c) *Clinical signs*: Lameness, swelling, and pain with the carpus or tarsus dropping to the ground to a 180-degree hyperextension, palmigrade
d) *Diagnosis*: Palpation, X-ray, CT scan, MRI
e) *Surgery*: *Pancarpal arthrodesis*: Remove articular cartilage with burr, place bone graft, specific plate on dorsal aspect spanning from radius to metacarpal 3; *Partial carpal arthrodesis*: Similar approach – plate spans from radial carpal bone to metacarpal 3 (Figures 5.73 and 5.74).
f) *Special instruments*: Orthopedic pack, arthrodesis plates, screw sets, IM pin set, cordless drill, high-speed burr (Surgairtome), plate bender, fusion bone putty (bone graft), bone graft bowl, curettes (0, 00, 000), goniometer, small Gelpi self-retaining retractor.
g) *Positioning*: Lateral recumbency with the affected leg hanging; lateral approach
h) *Assistants role*: Assist with draping, support leg, hand instruments for screw placement in proper order (drill bit, drill guide, depth gauge [tap, tap sleeve if tapping needed], screw, screw-driver), keep drill bit/tap clean between uses, hydrate fields during screw placement, cut sutures, retract tissue if necessary.

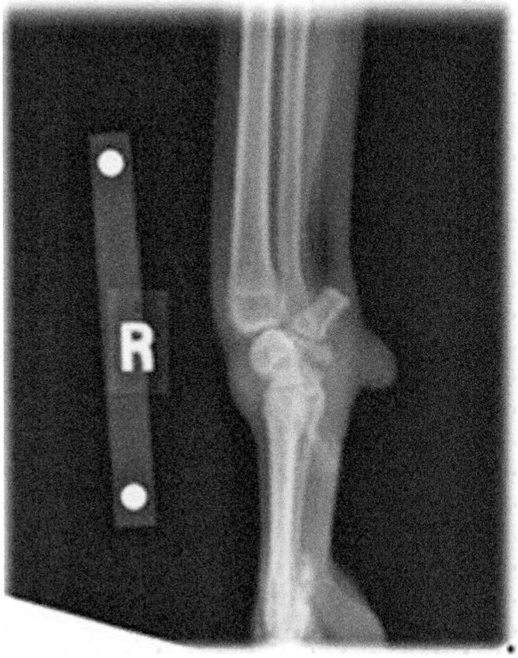

Figure 5.73 Pre-op lateral radiograph of carpal joint needing carpal arthrodesis. *Source:* Courtesy of Paul Manley University of Wisconsin retired.

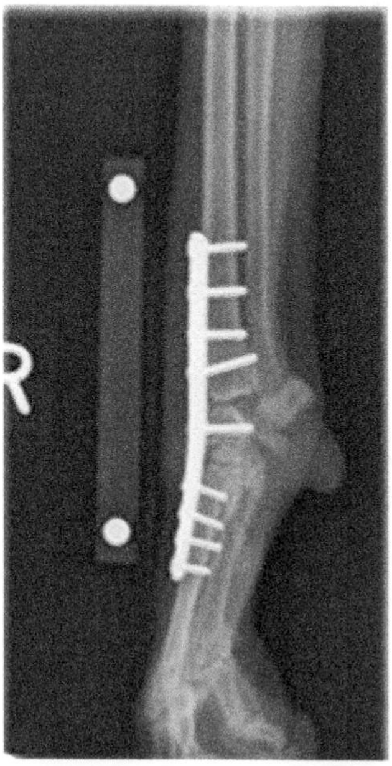

Figure 5.74 Post-op lateral radiograph following carpal arthrodesis. *Source:* Courtesy of Paul Manley University of Wisconsin retired.

i) *Postoperative care*: Place limb in a splint for six weeks postoperatively, or until there is radiographic evidence of union. Restrict activity until there is bony fusion of the joint, then start rehabilitation.

Digits

Onychectomy (Declaw) – Routine

Note: the editors and authors do NOT promote or condone onychectomy. They encourage non-surgical alternatives to declawing. Information is provided solely to aid veterinary technicians who must assist with this procedure.

a) *Definition*: Removal of the third phalanx of each digit, usually only performed on the front feet [11]
b) *Cause*: To prevent cats from scratching, usually reserved for extreme behavioral situations
c) *Clinical signs*: Normal kitten, fastest recovery when performed at early age
d) *Diagnosis*: Usually normal kitten, confirm number of toes as some cats may be polydactyl
e) *Surgery*: Third phalanx is flexed to facilitate dissection with a #12 or # 15 scalpel blade. All structures around third phalanx are transected including all tendons and ligaments (Figure 5.75).
f) *Positioning*: Lateral recumbency with surgical paw up
g) *Special instrumentation*: Tourniquet placed distal to elbow, #12/#15 scalpel blade, bandage material, tissue adhesive
h) *Assistant's role*: Apply tourniquet, stabilize/elevate limb
i) *Postoperative care*: Bandage feet for 12–24 hours, shredded paper litter or commercially available paper source litter for 2 weeks, monitor for hemorrhage as well as persistent lameness, pain management (Figures 5.76–5.81).

Onychectomy – Laser

a) *Definition*: Removal of the third phalanx of each digit, usually only performed on the front feet
b) *Cause*: To prevent cats from scratching
c) *Clinical signs*: Normal kitten, fastest recovery when performed at early age
d) *Diagnosis*: Usually normal kitten, confirm number of toes as some cats may be polydactyl

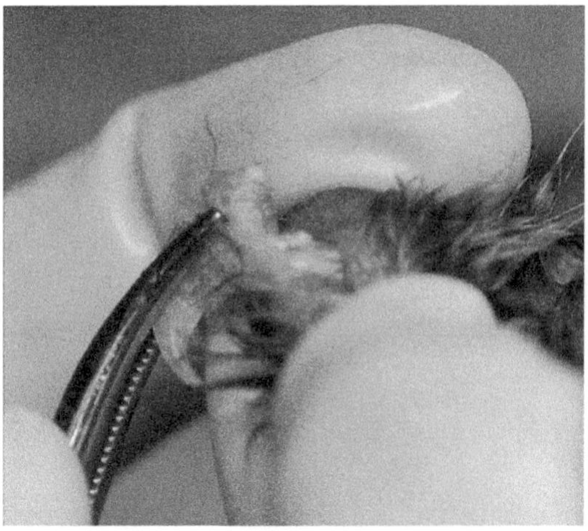

Figure 5.75 Dissection of claw and all surrounding tendons and ligaments. *Source:* Jonathan McAnulty, University of Wisconsin-Madison, Madison, WI. Reproduced with permission from Jonathan McAnulty.

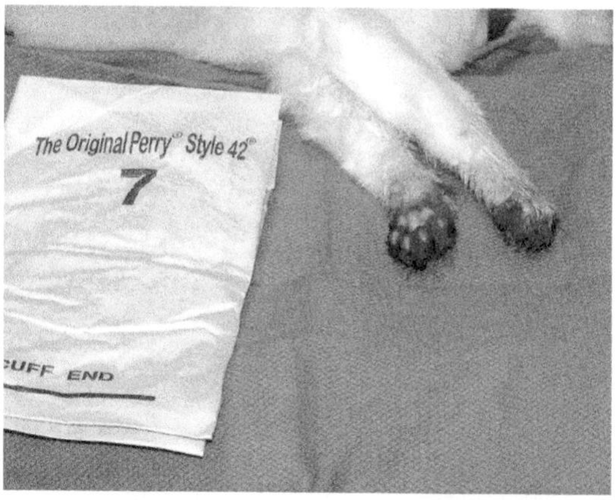

Figure 5.76 Declaw bandage step 1: After declaw procedure, open a package of size 7 sterile gloves.

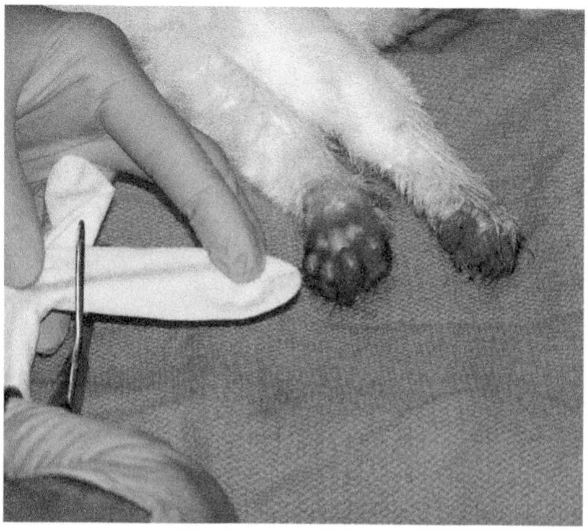

Figure 5.77 Declaw bandage step 2: Cut off middle finger of glove.

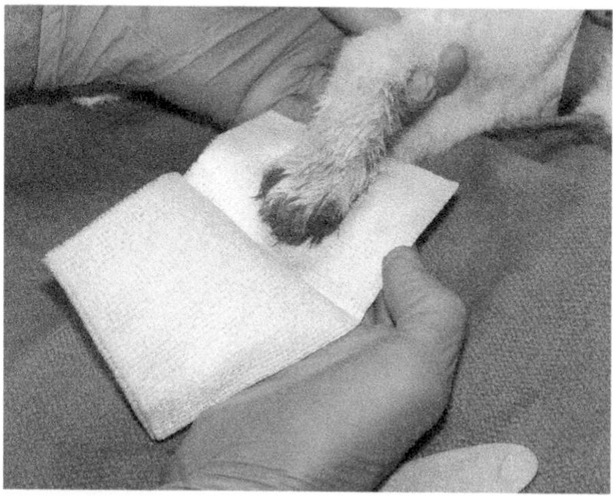

Figure 5.78 Declaw bandage step 3: Unfold two 3 × 3 gauze sponges, cover paw with gauze creating a tube shape.

e) *Surgery*: Third phalanx is flexed to facilitate dissection with the laser. Entire third phalanx is removed.
f) *Positioning*: Lateral recumbency with surgical paw up
g) *Special instrumentation*: CO_2 laser; **Note: NO ALCOHOL can be used in surgical prep of patient**, protective eyewear specific to laser wavelength should be worn by personnel and patient (Figure 5.82).

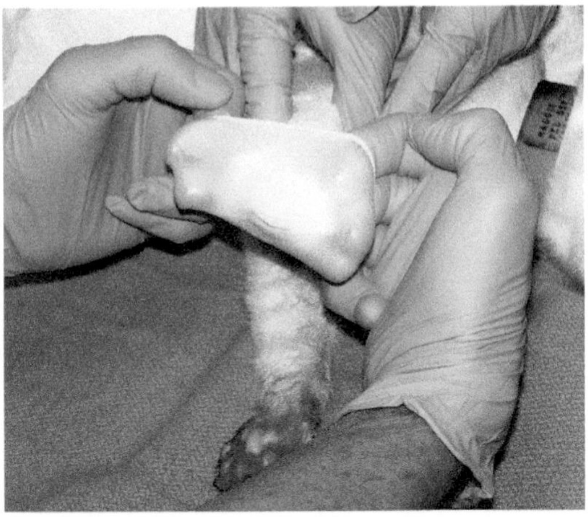

Figure 5.79 Declaw bandage step 4: Stretch glove finger over gauze to secure gauze in place.

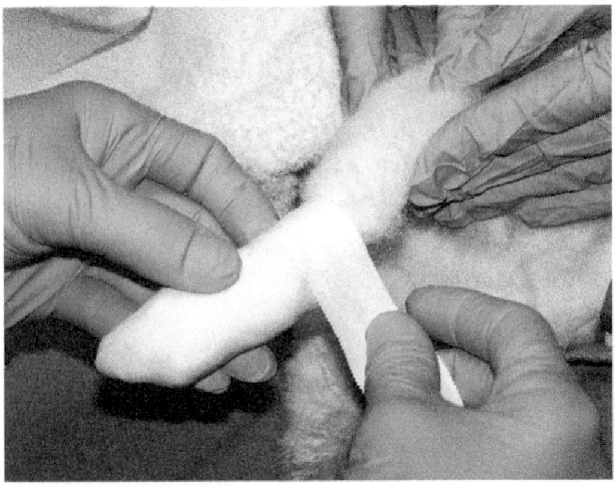

Figure 5.80 Declaw bandage step 5: Apply adhesive tape (1″) strip to edge of glove finger so one-half of the width of the tape is on the glove and the other half of the width is on the hair.

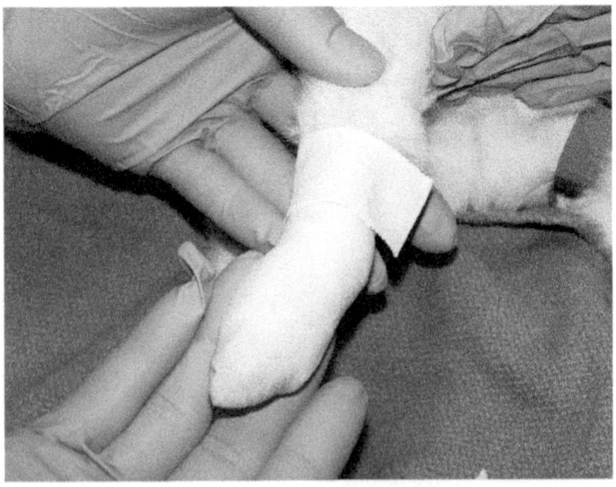

Figure 5.81 Declaw bandage step 6: Create "tab" on end of tape for ease removal. On the day after surgery, remove the bandages by gently detaching the tape strip and cutting the glove finger. Monitor the patient closely for bleeding.

h) *Assistant's role*: Suction smoke plume, monitor safety
i) *Postoperative care*: Bandage feet for 12–24 hours, shredded paper litter or commercially available paper source litter for two weeks, monitor for hemorrhage as well as persistent lameness, pain management

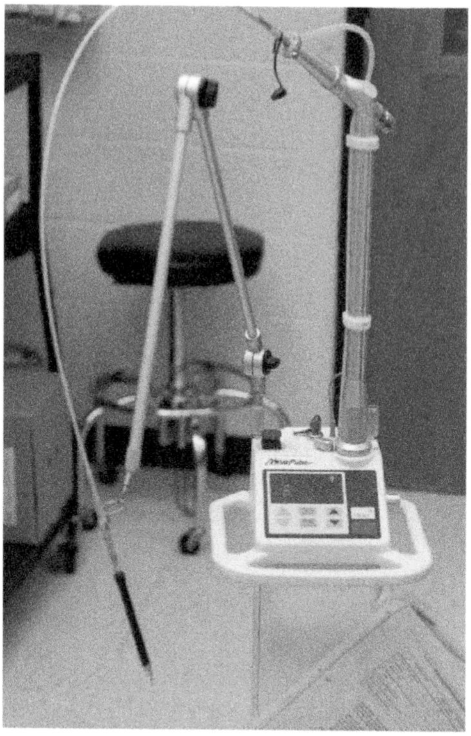

Figure 5.82 CO_2 laser.

Hindlimb

Pelvis

Hip Dysplasia

a) *Definition*: Malformation of the femoral head and acetabulum causing joint laxity, leading to degenerative joint disease, often bilateral
b) *Cause*: Genetic and environmental
c) *Clinical signs*: Reduced activity, difficulty rising, "bunny hopping" gait, muscle atrophy of rear limb(s)
d) *Diagnosis*: Radiographs, positive Ortolani sign (young, sedated patient), painful hip range of motion, crepitus in older patients (Figure 5.83).
e) *Surgery*: Conservative therapy consisting of exercise modification, medical and dietary management may be indicated pending the severity of the patient's clinical symptoms. The type of surgical procedure is dependent on the age of the patient, clinical severity, and the client's expectations. For example, a performance or working dog may have a better outcome and greater return to function with a total hip replacement than with a femoral head ostectomy.
   i) *Coxofemoral luxation*:
      a) *Definition*: Craniodorsal displacement of the femoral head.
      b) *Cause*: Trauma. Note: Assess for the presence of hip dysplasia – management will be different if dysplastic
      c) *Clinical signs*: Cannot bear weight on affected limb; limb may be externally rotated and adducted.
      d) *Diagnosis*: Examination of the length of the limbs, x-rays with two views (DV and lateral) – rule out dysplasia, fractures of femoral head, or acetabulum.

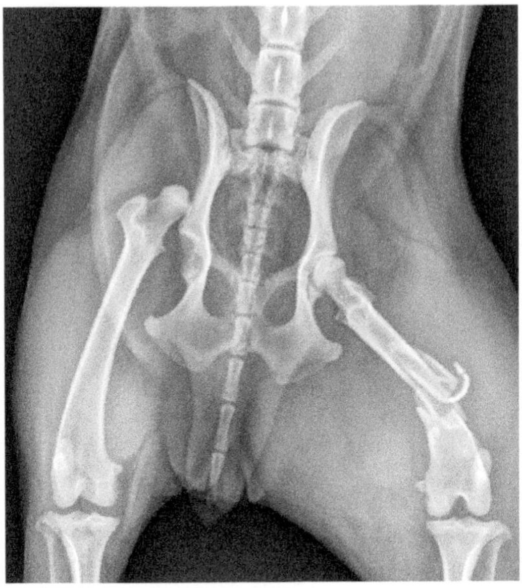

Figure 5.83 Pre-op VD coxofemoral luxation. *Source:* Courtesy of Paul Manley University of Wisconsin retired.

e) *Surgery*: Capsule repair, Toggle rod procedure – small toggle rod with suture threaded pushed through a hole drilled in medial wall of acetabulum, hole drilled from lateral femur to femoral head (using guide), suture pulled through hole and tied or crimped over button or rod on lateral femur (Figure 5.84).

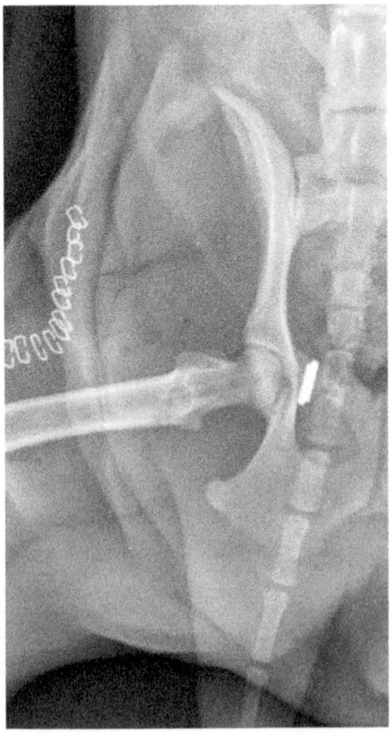

Figure 5.84 Post-op VD toggle placement. *Source:* Courtesy of Paul Manley University of Wisconsin retired.

f) *Position*: Lateral recumbency with a cranial lateral approach to the hip.
g) *Special instruments*: Suction, electrosurgery, standard orthopedic pack, Toggle Rod set (rod toggle, aiming device, insertion device, 3.2 mm drill bit, 2.0 mm drill bit, Nylon leader line, polypropylene button, small ASIF air drill).
h) *Assistant's role*: Assist with draping, support leg, hand instruments for screw placement in proper order (drill bit, drill guide, depth gauge, tap, tap sleeve [if tapping needed], screw, screwdriver), keep drill bit/tap clean between uses, hydrate fields, cut sutures, retract tissue if necessary.
i) *Postoperative care*: Restrict activity to short leash walking only for one month, then gradually increase activity

ii) *Femoral head and neck ostectomy (FHNO)* [12]: Removal of the head of the femur to create a fibrous false joint to relieve pain from bone-on-bone contact; surgery is a salvage procedure for end-stage degenerative joint disease (may also be performed following femoral head/neck fractures or acetabular fractures).

1) *Surgery*: A craniolateral approach to the hip is made to allow intentional luxation of the hip. The round ligament is incised (if still intact) and the femoral head is subluxated. The head and neck are then excised with an osteotome and mallet or bone saw (Figure 5.85).
2) *Positioning*: Lateral recumbency with affected limb up
3) *Special instrumentation*: Power saw, osteotome, mallet, ronguer, rasp, suction, electrosurgery, Gelpi self-retaining retractor, lavage fluid
4) *Assistant's role*: Lavage field, irrigate with saline as osteotomy is performed, cut sutures, rotate/stabilize limb, load saw blade on power saw
5) *Postoperative care*: Restricted activity for two weeks, then encourage limb use, physical rehabilitation to improve joint mobility, and increase muscle strength

iii) *Juvenile pubic symphysiodesis (JPS)* [13]: Pubic bone physis closure via stapling or electrocautery, causing improvement in the acetabular angle and thus more coverage of the femoral head by the acetabulum, degenerative joint disease (DJD) prevention, performed at 12–16 weeks of age. PennHIP radiographs determine a distraction index (DI) – if DI is greater than or equal to 0.70, surgery is not effective in preventing DJD [14] (Figure 5.86).

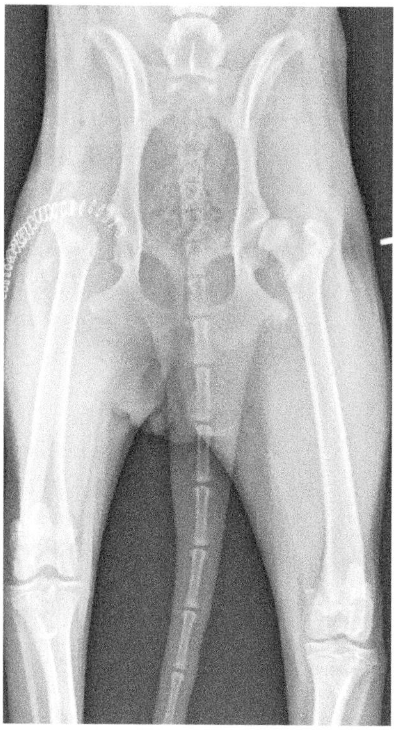

Figure 5.85 Post-op ventral–dorsal radiographic view of hips post-femoral head osteotomy (FHO). *Source:* Paul Manley, University of Wisconsin, Madison, WI. Reproduced with permission from Paul Manley.

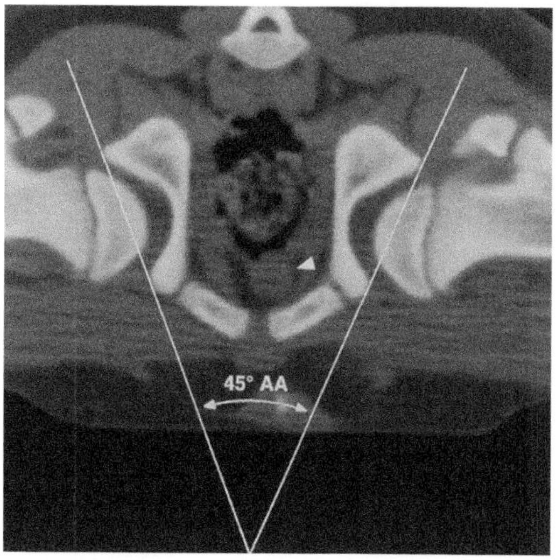

Figure 5.86 CT of pelvis indicating gap in pubic symphysis. *Source:* Courtesy of Paul Manley University of Wisconsin retired.

1) *Surgery*: A ventral midline incision over the pubis allows dissection/retraction of muscle to expose pubic symphysis. Electrosurgery unit is set at 40 W and ablation is performed every 2–3 mm along pubic symphysis (Figure 5.87).
2) *Positioning*: Dorsal recumbency
3) *Special instrumentation*: Small malleable retractor, suction, electrosurgery
4) *Assistant's role*: Retraction of muscle, suction, cut sutures
5) *Postoperative care*: Moderate exercise for two to three months

iv) *Total hip replacement/arthroplasty (THR/THA)* [15] – removal of the femoral head/neck and replacement with a stainless steel or titanium head/stem as well as reaming of the acetabulum and replacing it with a high-density polyethylene cup; surgery is a salvage procedure for end-stage degenerative joint disease (also may be performed for femoral head/neck fractures).

1) *Surgery*: A craniolateral approach is made to the hip. The hip is luxated and the round ligament is incised. The femoral head and neck are excised. The femoral canal is broached and prepped for implant placement. The acetabulum is reamed and prepped for acetabular placement. After implant placement, the hip is repositioned, range of motion is evaluated prior to closure.
2) *Positioning*: Lateral recumbency with surgical hip up, use THA positioner to ensure pelvic alignment (Figure 5.88).
3) *Special instrumentation*: Cemented/cementless femoral prosthesis, femoral head implant, acetabular implant, power saw/drill, total hip instrumentation set, Gelpi

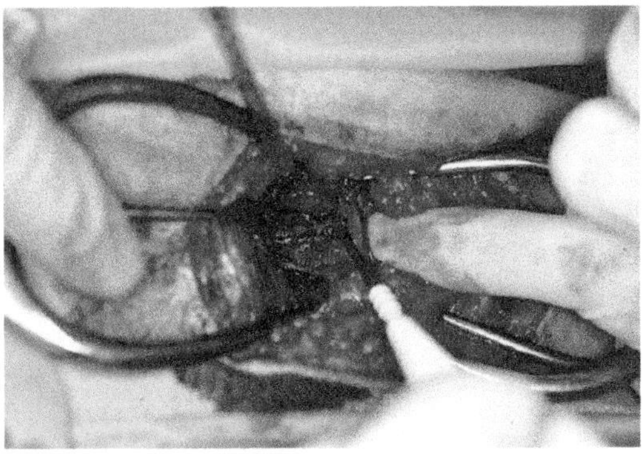

Figure 5.87 Blade cauterizing of pubic symphysis for JPS. *Source:* Courtesy of Paul Manley University of Wisconsin retired.

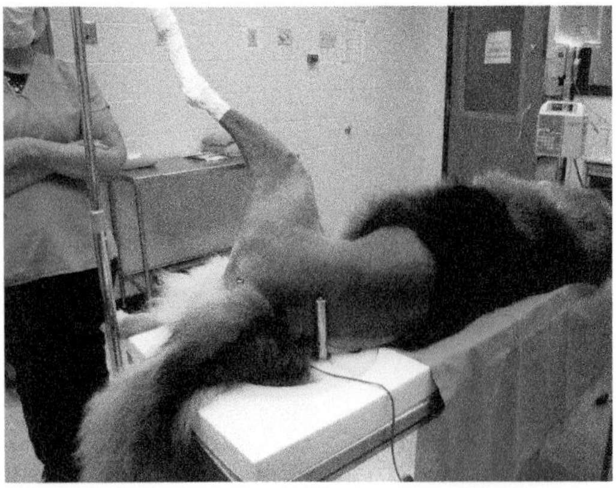

Figure 5.88 Patient positioner for THA. *Source:* Paul Manley, University of Wisconsin, Madison, WI. Reproduced with permission from Paul Manley.

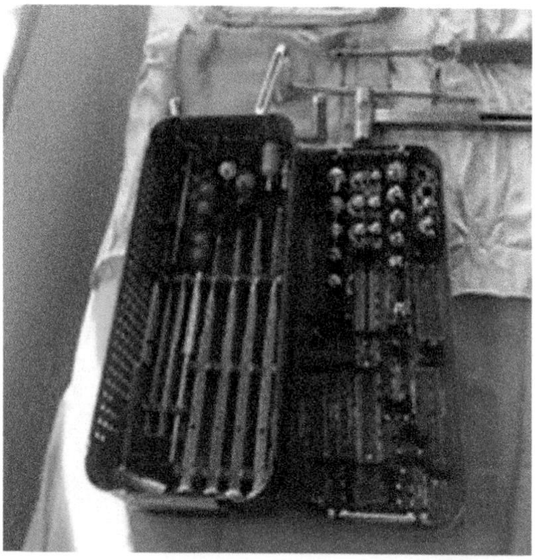

Figure 5.89 Total hip arthroplasty equipment.

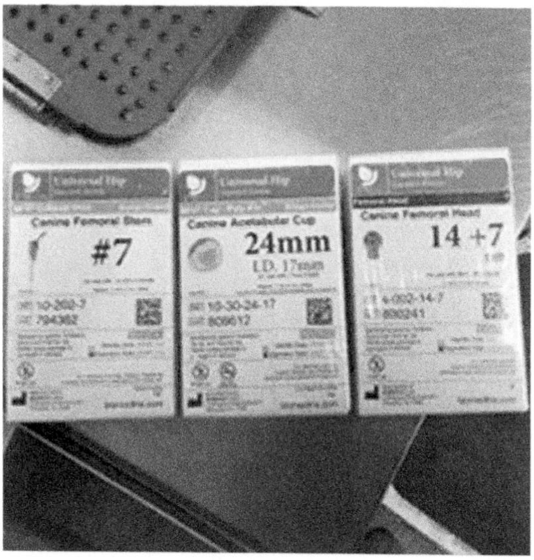

Figure 5.90 Total hip arthroplasty implants.

self-retaining retractor, deep muscle retractor (Myerding), Hohmann retractors, suction, electrosurgery, lavage fluid (Figures 5.89 and 5.90).

4) *Assistant's role*: Strict enforcement of asepsis, muscle retraction, stabilize limb, hand instruments during joint prep in correct order, keep instruments clean between use, cut sutures
5) *Postoperative care*: **VERY restricted** activity for four weeks, use of sling for walking at all times to avoid slipping and luxation of implants, rehabilitation starting two to four weeks postoperative, then slow increase in activity after four to eight weeks (Figure 5.91).

v) *Triple/double pelvic osteotomy (TPO/DPO)* [16]: Cuts made in the ilium and pubis (DPO) as well as ischium (TPO) to allow rotation of the acetabulum and provide more coverage of the femoral head, performed only in skeletally immature dogs (4–12 months) without degenerative changes, reduces degenerative joint disease from hip dysplasia (Figure 5.92).

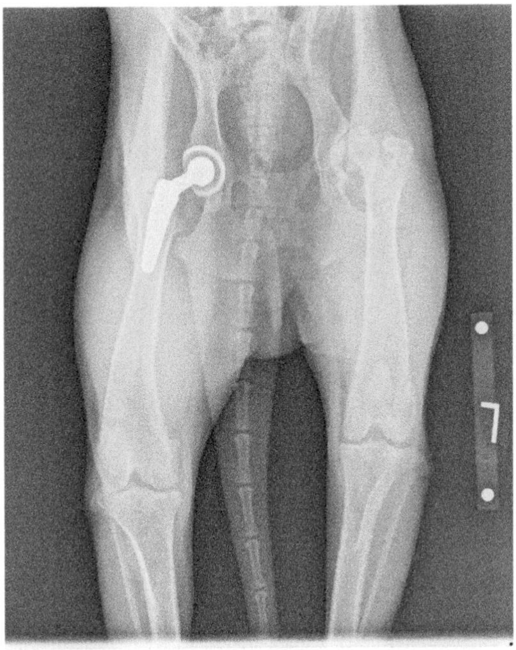

Figure 5.91 Post-op VD view of total hip arthroplasty (THA) implants. *Source:* Paul Manley, University of Wisconsin, Madison, WI. Reproduced with permission from Paul Manley.

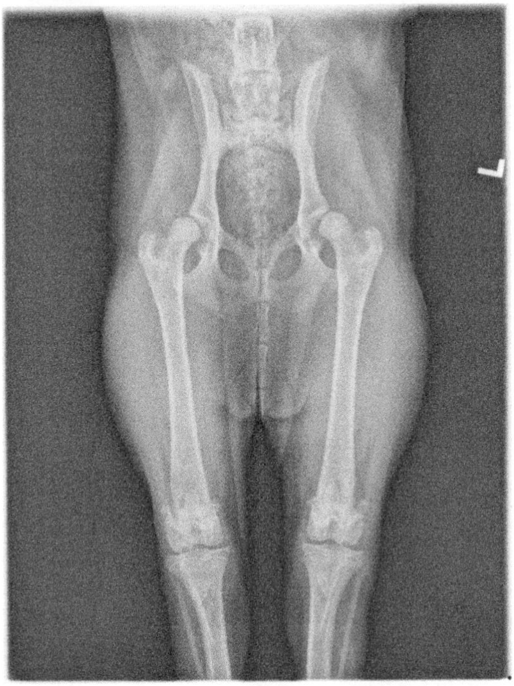

Figure 5.92 Pre-op VD radiograph of patient needing a triple pelvic osteotomy (TPO). *Source:* Paul Manley, University of Wisconsin, Madison, WI. Reproduced with permission from Paul Manley.

1) *Surgery*: An incision is made over the pectineus muscle to allow dissection and access to pubis. An osteotomy is performed on the medial wall of the acetabulum. The incision is closed. An ischial approach is made and the ischial osteotomy is performed. The ischial osteotomy is centered over the obturator foramen. Finally, the ilial approach and osteotomy are performed. The pelvis is re-aligned to permit application of a bone plate to stabilize the pelvis (Figure 5.93).

Figure 5.93 Post-op VD radiograph of patient having had a TPO performed. *Source:* Paul Manley, University of Wisconsin, Madison, WI. Reproduced with permission from Paul Manley.

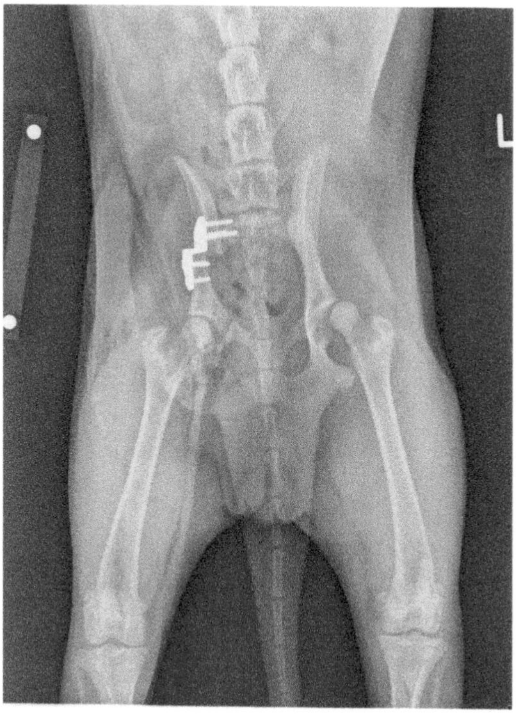

2) *Positioning*: Dorsal recumbency/lateral recumbency with affected hip up. *Note: Re-positioning of patient may be necessary to allow access to pelvic osteotomy sites*
3) *Special instrumentation*: Suction, electrosurgery, power bone saw, bone plates, bone screws, bone screw placement instrumentation, osteotome, mallet, bone-holding forceps, Gelpi self-retaining retractors, Hohmann retractors, periosteal elevator, second set of drapes, instruments (if re-positioning of patient is necessary to access pelvic osteotomy sites)
4) *Assistant's role*: Suction during osteotomies, lavage field as osteotomy performed, muscle retraction, handing of screw placement instruments in proper order when screws are being placed, cut sutures
5) *Postoperative care*: Exercise restriction for four to six weeks, physical rehabilitation, sling walk when on slippery surfaces

Stifle

Cranial Cruciate Ligament (CCL) Rupture

a) *Definition*: Partial or complete tearing of the CCL
b) *Cause*: Thought to be related to chronic inflammation of the CCL causing long-term deterioration and eventual tearing [17], most common in large breed dogs, may have a genetic component [18]
c) *Clinical signs*: Acute-to-chronic Grade 2–5/5 rear leg lameness, stifle effusion, painful during stifle manipulation, may sit to one side with affected leg in extension
d) *Diagnosis*: Positive cranial drawer test, positive tibial thrust test, radiographs to assess degree of inflammation, and degenerative joint disease

e) *Surgery*:
   i) *Extracapsular Repair, Lateral Fabellar Suture, "Fishing Line" Technique* [19, 20]: Stabilization of the stifle via suture technique outside the joint; suture material is monofilament nylon
      1) *Surgery*: Using heavy monofilament suture/leader line, a cruciate needle is passed around the fabella. Next, the suture is passed behind the patellar ligament. A hole is drilled through the tibial crest. With the stifle flexed, the sutures are passed through the hole and tied or crimped. Routine closure (Figure 5.94).
      2) *Positioning*: Lateral or dorsal recumbency
      3) *Special instrumentation*: Fishing or leader line, braided orthopedic suture, large monofilament non-absorbable suture, suction, electrosurgery, cruciate needle, metal crimper pieces, crimper tool
      4) *Assistant's role*: Stabilize the limb, suction field, provide hemostasis, cut sutures
      5) *Postoperative care*: Restricted activity for 8–10 weeks, physical rehabilitation to improve joint mobility and increase muscle strength
   ii) *Tightrope®*: Stabilization of the stifle via suture technique outside the joint; suture material is braided fiber wire
      1) *Surgery*: An ultra-high-strength, braided synthetic ligament is passed through bone tunnels created in the distal femur and proximal tibia. The "ligament" is pulled tight and secured with a femoral button, simulating the normal CCL.
      2) *Positioning*: Dorsal recumbency
      3) *Special instrumentation*: Power drill, drill bit, hand chuck, pin, ligament graft, femoral button, Gelpi retractor, suction, electrosurgery

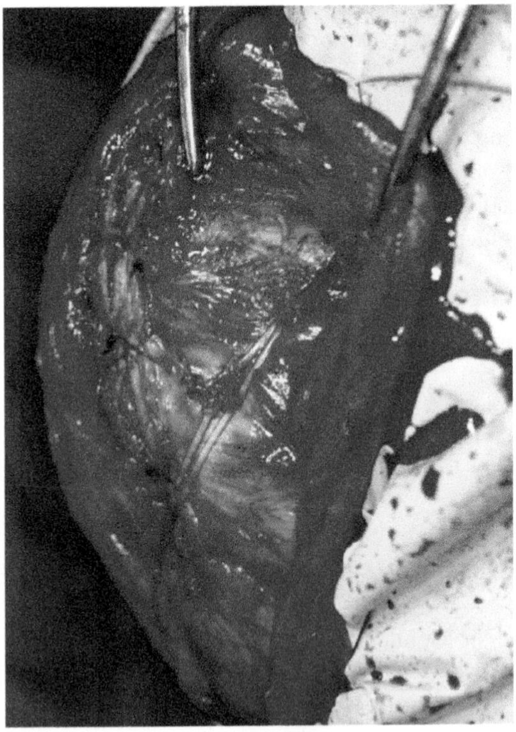

Figure 5.94 Leader line knotted for extracapsular repair. *Source:* Paul Manley, University of Wisconsin, Madison, WI. Reproduced with permission from Paul Manley.

4) *Assistant's role*: Stabilize limb while tunnels are created, suction, cut suture, stabilization of leg as graft is tightened
5) *Postoperative care*: Restricted activity for 8–10 weeks, physical rehabilitation to improve joint mobility and increase muscle strength

iii) *Tibial Plateau Leveling Osteotomy (TPLO)*: Mechanical stabilization of the stifle via a bone-cutting procedure to change the tibial plateau angle; TPLO limits the shear force created by compression of the stifle when weight-bearing and thus reducing tibial thrust [21]
1) *Surgery*: A medial approach to the joint provides visualization of the joint to allow for the bone saw to cut the tibia. As the osteotomy is completed, the tibial plateau slope decreases which allows for a more neutral or caudal cranial cruciate thrust. A TPLO bone plate is placed to stabilize the osteotomy site (Figure 5.95).
2) *Positioning*: Dorsal recumbency or dorsolateral oblique, tilted toward the affected limb, to allow the limb to lay flat on the surgery tabletop
3) *Special instrumentation*: Suction, electrosurgery, TPLO instrument set, TPLO bone plate, bone screw set (locking and regular), bone saw, power drill, Gelpi self-retaining retractor, Hohman retractor (meniscal probe/hook, stifle distractor for inspection of joint if arthroscopy not performed)
4) *Assistant's role*: Stabilize limb for sawing and/or drilling of screw holes, drill screw holes, place/remove K wires/pins, retraction of patellar tendon during osteotomy, suction, hydrate field during osteotomy and drilling, cut sutures (Figure 5.96).
5) *Postoperative care*: Restricted activity for 8–10 weeks until radiographs show bony healing, physical rehabilitation to improve joint mobility and increase muscle strength

iv) *Tibial Tuberosity Advancement (TTA)*: Mechanical stabilization of the stifle via a bone-cutting procedure to neutralize cranial tibiofemoral shear force [22]

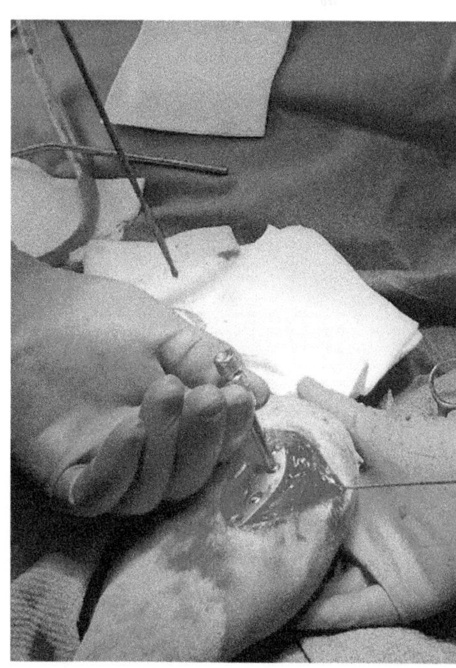

Figure 5.95 Locking axial drill guide with screw placement in TPLO plate.

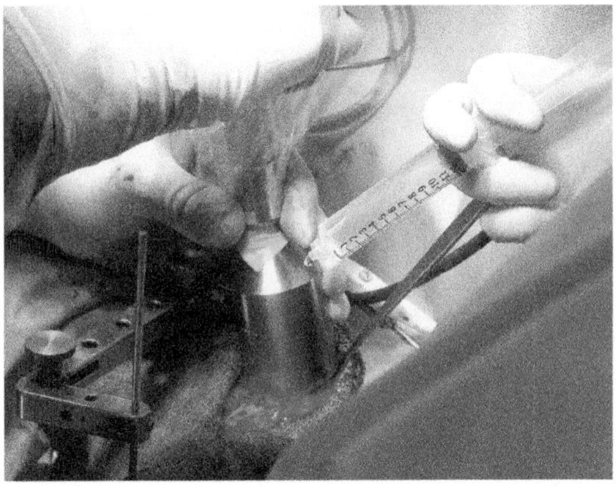

Figure 5.96 Using saw for tibial plateau leveling osteotomy (TPLO). Note: Assistant dripping fluid on bone to cool it while sawing.

1) *Surgery*: Using an open approach to the stifle joint, a partial tibial crest osteotomy is performed. A "cage" is secured with bone screws to keep the osteotomy site open. A TTA bone plate is used to stabilize the osteotomy site.
2) *Positioning*: Dorsal recumbency or dorsolateral oblique, tilted toward the affected limb, to allow the limb to lay flat on the surgery tabletop
3) *Special instrumentation*: TTA implant set, power saw, periosteal elevator, TTA instrumentation set, Gelpi self-retaining retractor (Figure 5.97).
4) *Assistant's role*: Stabilize limb, suction, cut sutures, hold plate while first screw holes are being drilled, irrigate during osteotomies or drilling
5) *Postoperative care*: Restricted activity for 8–10 weeks, physical rehabilitation to improve joint mobility and increase muscle strength (Figure 5.98).

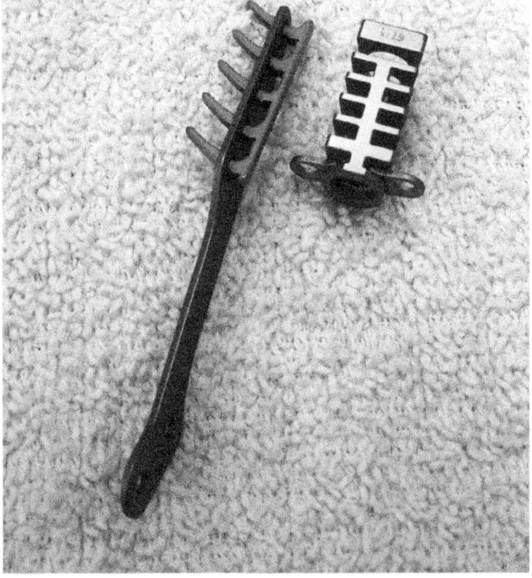

Figure 5.97 Tibial tuberosity advancement (TTA) cage, fork, and plate.

Patella Luxation

a) *Definition*: Displacement of the patella, either medially or laterally [23]
b) *Cause*: Congenital condition, medial luxation is most common, not only widespread in toy and miniature breeds but also occurs in large breeds and cats; bilateral complaint in 20–25% of patients
c) *Clinical signs*: Intermittent to continual non-weight-bearing lame on affected leg, divided into the following grades:
   1) Patella easily luxates, is easily reduced, spends most of the time in correct position (surgery generally not indicated)
   2) More frequent luxation than Grade 1; patella is easily reduced and most often in the correct position (may or may not require surgery)
   3) Patella always luxated, reducible with effort (requires surgical correction)
   4) Patella always luxated, not reducible (requires surgical correction)
d) *Diagnosis*: Stifle palpation, radiographs (Figure 5.99).
e) *Surgery*: A variety of surgeries correct this condition; they may be used singularly or in combination. The trochlear groove is deepened with a trochlear wedge, block recession, or trochlear resection procedure. Additional procedures may be done to maintain placement of the patella in the newly created groove: overlap of lateral or medial retinaculum, fascia lata overlap, patellar and tibial antirotational suture ligament, desmotomy and partial capsulectomy, quadriceps release, tibial tuberosity transposition (TTT) along with osteotomies if femoral deformities are present, semi-cylindrical recession tracheoplasty (SCRT) is an alternative to trochlear block or wedge recession
f) *Positioning*: Dorsal recumbency
g) *Special instrumentation*: Bone saw, #20 blade, suction, electrosurgery, hand/hobby saw, osteotome, mallet, ronguer, K wires, power drill, self-retaining retractor, is repetetive SCRT instrument set if that method performed
h) *Assistant's role*: Stabilize limb, suction site if bone saw used, lavage field, cut sutures
i) *Postoperative care*: Restricted activity for four weeks, physical rehabilitation to improve joint mobility and increase muscle strength, encourage weight bearing, sling support under abdomen to assist walking if bilateral procedure

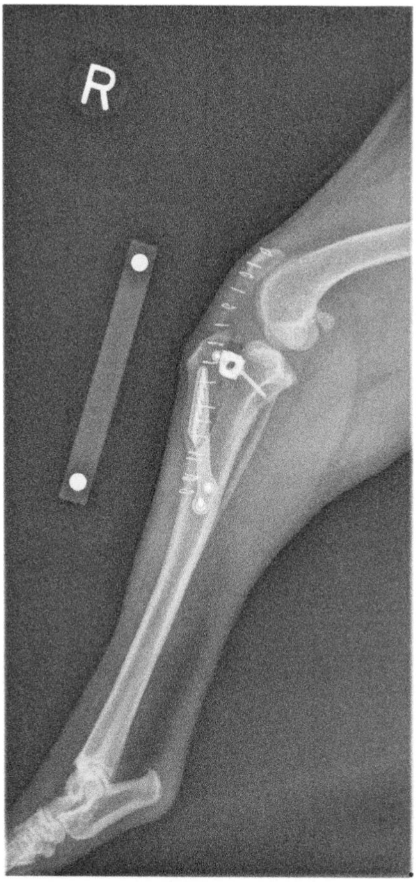

Figure 5.98 Post-op radiograph of TTA surgery. *Source:* Paul Manley, University of Wisconsin, Madison, WI. Reproduced with permission from Paul Manley.

Tarsus

Tarsus – Achilles Tendon Repair

a) *Definition*: Injury of the Achilles tendon.
b) *Cause*: Laceration, degeneration, tearing, or stretching of tendon. The cause may be chronic and degenerative, giving a gradual progression, or acute, with sudden collapse

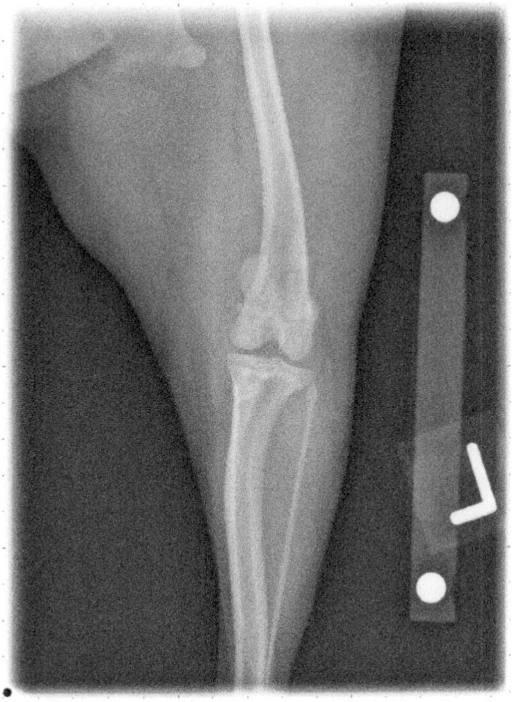

Figure 5.99 Cranial–caudal radiographic view of medial patellar luxation – pre-op. *Source:* Paul Manley, University of Wisconsin, Madison, WI. Reproduced with permission from Paul Manley.

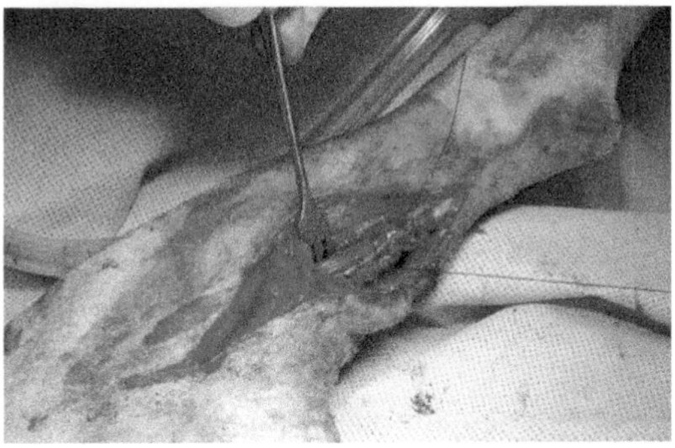

Figure 5.100 Repair of a lacerated calcaneal tendon using 0-prolene and a Kracow (locking loop) pattern. *Source:* Courtesy of Dr. Roe-NCSU-CVM.

c) *Clinical signs*: Lameness of the affected limb. An animal with a complete rupture will walk flat footed – plantigrade
d) *Diagnosis*: Exam, X-rays, US of the affected limb, CT scan, MRI.
e) *Surgery*: Attaching healthy ends of the tendon together with suture, mesh, or other types of graphs. Also, platelet-rich plasma (PRP) and stem cells may be used along with surgery. Depending on the severity of the injury, the affected limb may be treated with external support (cast, splint, and orthotics) (Figure 5.100).
f) Position: Lateral recumbency with a lateral approach.
g) *Special instruments*: Suction, electrosurgery, standard orthopedic pack, 0-prolene, blunt Senn retractors, baby Gelpi self-retaining retractor
h) *Assistant's role*: Assist with draping, support leg, hydrate fields, cut sutures, retract tissue if necessary.
i) *Postoperative care*: Very restrictive activity for 6–12 weeks while preventing flexion of the hock.

Arthrodesis

a) *Definition*: The fusion of two or more bones in a joint.
b) *Cause*: Ligaments and other support structures that stabilize the carpal and tarsal joints are torn or stretched, which could be from a hyperextension injury.
c) *Clinical signs*: Lameness, swelling, and pain. Tibiotarsal joint instability. Intertarsal joint – hyperflexion below the hock joint – toes often flexed. Achilles tendon tear – partial or complete collapse of hock – plantigrade
d) *Diagnosis*: Palpation, X-ray, CT scan, MRI
e) *Surgery*: *Pantarsal arthrodesis*: Remove articular cartilage – burr or saw, place bone graft, specific plate either on dorsal aspect (tibia to metatarsal) or medial aspect (medial malleolus removed); *Intertarsal arthrodesis*: Remove articular cartilage, plate on lateral aspect bridging calcaneus to metatarsals (Figures 5.101 and 5.102).
f) *Special instruments*: Orthopedic pack, arthrodesis plates and screw sets, IM pin set, cordless drill, high-speed burr (Surgairtome), plate bender, fusion bone putty (bone graft), bone graft bowl, curettes (0, 00, 000), goniometer, small Gelpi self-retaining retractor.
g) *Positioning*: Lateral recumbency with the affected leg hanging; lateral approach
h) *Assistants role*: Assist with draping, support leg, hand instruments for screw placement in proper order (drill bit, drill guide, depth gauge, [tap, tap sleeve if tapping needed], screw,

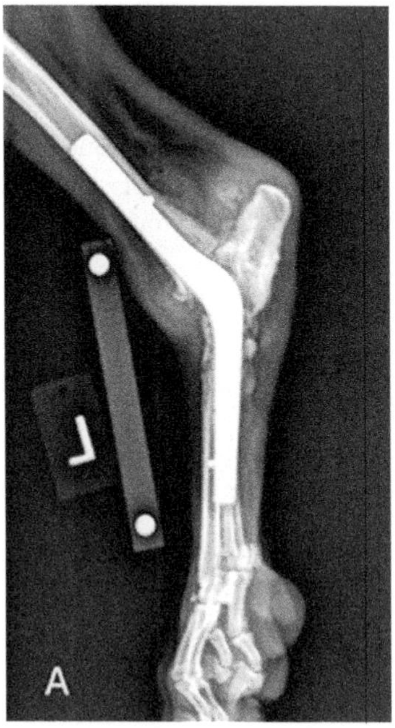

Figure 5.101 Pantarsal arthrodesis – lateral post-op radiograph. *Source:* Courtesy of Dr. Roe-NCSU-CVM.

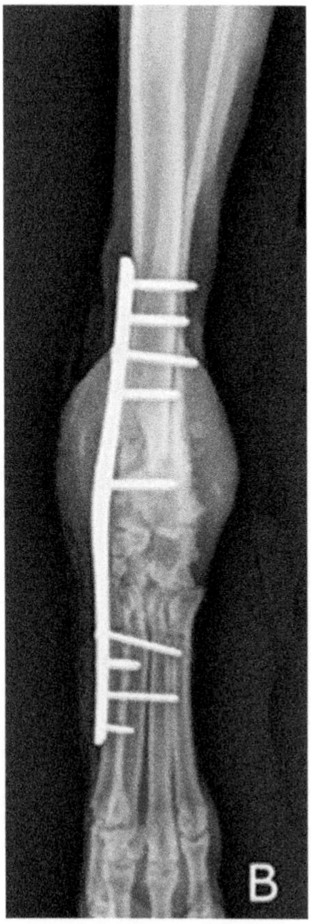

Figure 5.102 Pantarsal arthrodesis – CrCa post-op radiograph. *Source:* Courtesy of Dr. Roe-NCSU-CVM.

screwdriver), keep drill bit/tap clean between uses, hydrate fields during screw placement, cut sutures, retract tissue if necessary.

i) Place limb in a splint for six weeks postoperatively, or until there is radiographic evidence of union. Restrict activity until there is bony fusion of the joint, then start rehabilitation.

Thoracic

Cardiovascular

Thoracotomy / Patent Ductus Arteriosus (PDA)

a) *Definition*: Congenital conditions affecting the flow of blood through the heart and lungs (PDA/PRAA), tumors of various types, infection
b) *Cause*: PDA is a congenital condition; other reasons for thoracic surgery include trauma, neoplasia, lung torsion, infection, etc.
c) *Clinical signs*: Dependent on condition but generally decreased respiratory ability, increased lung sounds, low exercise tolerance, heart murmur, etc.
d) *Diagnosis*: Thoracic radiographs, chest auscultation, known trauma
e) *Surgery*: Thoracotomy [24] – surgical incision into the chest wall between two ribs or through the sternum. Surgical approach to the thoracic cavity can be accomplished with a ventral midline sternotomy or a lateral intercostal incision. Depending on the procedure, there may be vessel ligation, tissue resection, or organ resection. Closure depends on approach used (Figures 5.103–5.105).
f) *Positioning*: Dorsal recumbency or lateral recumbency, left or right lateral will be determined by procedure being performed
g) *Special instrumentation*: Finochietto retractor, lap pads, lavage fluid, chest tube, Heimlich valve, cardiovascular instruments, internal staplers, suction, electrosurgery, long instruments. If **sternotomy** is performed, bone saw, orthopedic wire, wire twister, wire cutter will be needed.
h) *Assistant's role*: Keep tissues moist, retract lungs, load internal staplers if used, suction, run suture, cut wires if sternotomy performed
i) *Postoperative care*: Close monitoring of respirations – if insufficient, radiograph for pneumothorax, evaluate blood gas for adequate ventilation, nasal oxygen or oxygen cage may be required, possible chest tube placement, provide pain control, critical care monitoring

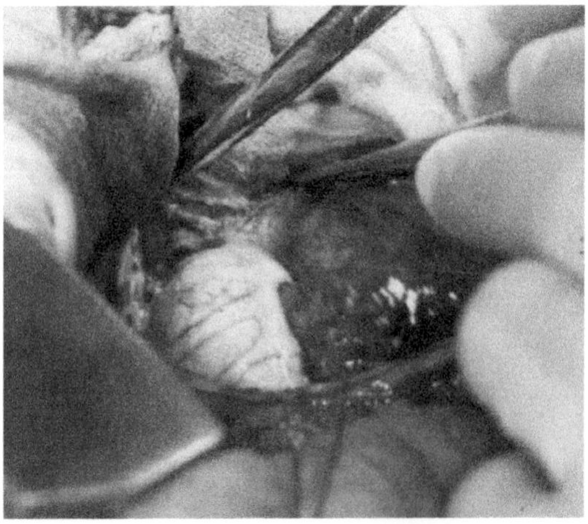

Figure 5.103 Patent ductus arteriosus (PDA) before ligation. *Source:* Dale Bjorling, University of Wisconsin, Madison, WI. Reproduced with permission of Dale Bjorling.

Figure 5.104 Patent ductus arteriosus (PDA) after ligation. *Source:* Dale Bjorling, University of Wisconsin, Madison, WI. Reproduced with permission of Dale Bjorling.

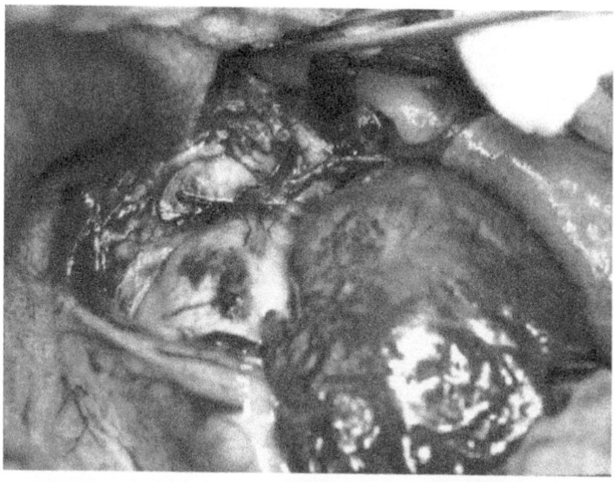

Figure 5.105 Patent ductus arteriosus (PDA) hemorrhaging. *Source:* Dale Bjorling, University of Wisconsin, Madison, WI. Reproduced with permission of Dale Bjorling.

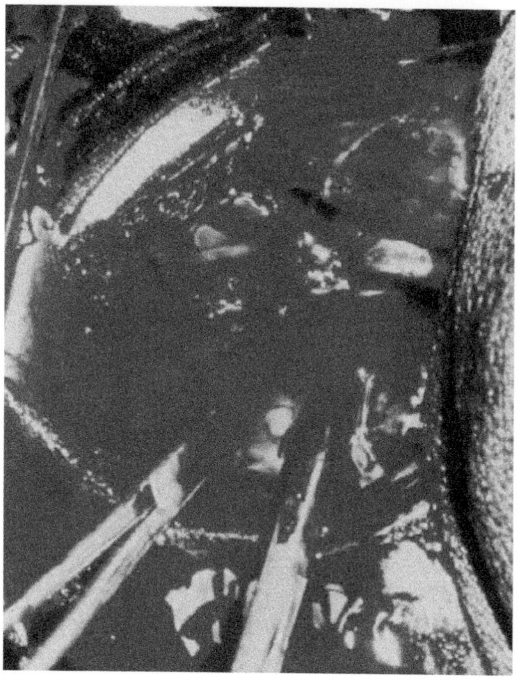

Persistent Right Aortic Arch (PRAA)

a) *Definition*: Persistent right aortic arch: the right aortic arch fails to regress normally, resulting in entrapment of the esophagus and trachea at the level of the heart base.
b) *Cause*: Genetics – vascular ring anomaly (Figure 5.106).
c) *Clinical signs*: Most common clinical sign is regurgitation (often noted at weaning), aspiration pneumonia
d) *Diagnosis*: CT, MRI, X-ray
e) *Surgery*: An incision is made on the left side of the chest and the fourth and fifth ribs are spread with a Finochietto rib spreader to expose the ligamentum arteriosum which is constricting the esophagus. The constricting band is isolated using a right-angle forceps and tied off with non-absorbable monofilament and cut (Figure 5.107). Monofilament sutures are used to close, and a chest tube is placed. An oral gastric tube is placed to ensure that there are no additional constrictions and then removed.

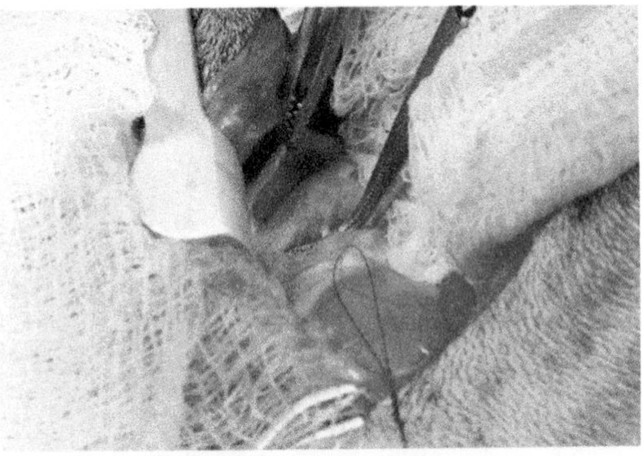

Figure 5.106 (Persistent right aortic arch (PRAA). *Source:* Courtesy of Dr. Mathews NCSU-CVM.

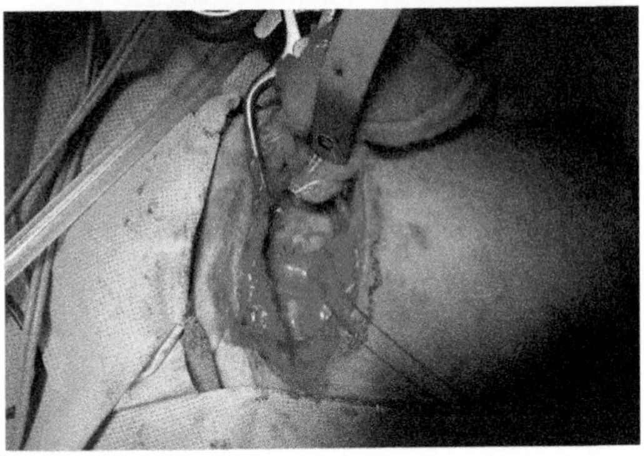

Figure 5.107 Occluded persistent right aortic arch (PRAA). *Source:* Courtesy of Dr. Mathews NCSU-CVM.

f) *Positioning*: Right lateral recumbency
g) *Special instruments*: Cardiothoracic pack, chest tube, Finochietto rib spreader, Gelpi self-retaining retractor, right-angle forceps, bipolar electrosurgery
h) *Assistants role*: Retract tissue, cut suture, cauterize vessels
i) *Postoperative care*: Pain management, IV fluids, removal of chest tube within 12–24 hours after surgery, soft food feeding increased for a month after surgery but can be discontinued when regurgitation stops, solid food can start when patient can swallow well and no regurgitation, exercise restriction for 3 weeks; complications include: incisional infection, aspiration pneumonia, never regain mobility of esophagus

Respiratory

Lung Lobectomy

a) *Definition*: Surgical resection of a lung lobe or part of the lung lobe
b) *Cause*: Metastatic (mammary adenocarcinoma, osteosarcoma, hemangiosarcoma, and oral melanoma) and malignant neoplasia (adenocarcinoma and alveolar carcinoma), abscess
c) *Clinical signs*: Chronic, non-productive cough; reduced exercise tolerance, tachypnea, dyspnea, wheezing
d) *Diagnosis*: CT, X-ray, US, MRI
e) *Surgery*: Depending on where the neoplasia is located, a lateral thoracotomy or a sternotomy will be performed. An incision is made on the chest with monopolar electrosurgery used to control bleeding. With a sternotomy, the ribs are cut with a saw. A Finochietto rib spreader or Gelpi is used to retract the ribs. If a lateral thoracotomy is made, incision will be made between

Figure 5.108 Finochietto retractor in chest.

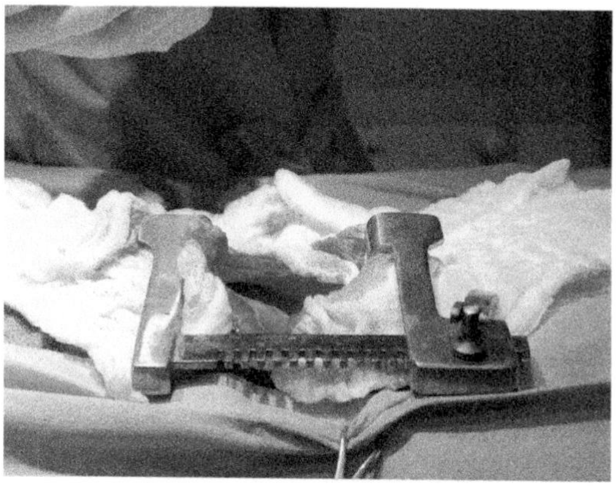

two ribs, depending on lung lobe affected (Figure 5.108). The affected lung is isolated, and a TA stapler or endo-GIA stapler is used to staple the lung and the neoplasia is cut away (Figures 5.109–5.111). If a sternotomy is performed, the ribs are brought together with wire, and monofilament sutures are used to close the layers of the skin. Regardless of approach used, the placement of a chest tube must occur (Figures 5.112 and 5.113).

f) *Positioning*: Lateral recumbency–lateral thoracotomy, dorsal recumbency–sternotomy
g) *Special instruments*: Cardiothoracic pack, Finochietto rib spreader, Gelpi self-retaining retractor, bipolar electrosurgery, chest tube, TA and endostapler and staples, hemoclips, surgical saw, Surgicel®
h) *Assistants role*: Retract tissue, cut suture, cauterize vessels, load hemoclips and staples, irrigate if bone saw used
i) *Postoperative care*: Pain management, removal of the chest tube 12–24 hours after surgery, exercise restricted for 10–15 days, some patients may need a light bandage, chemotherapy if neoplasia is malignant, chest X-ray twice a year to check for recurrence or spread of tumor

Tracheal Collapse

a) *Definition*: Trachea obstruction caused by cartilage flaccidity and flattening (Figure 5.114).
b) *Cause*: Cause is unknown, but most likely related to airflow dynamic changes genetically or trauma. Primarily seen in old, toy-breed dogs.

Figure 5.109 Caudal lung lobe abscess. *Source:* Dale Bjorling, University of Wisconsin, Madison, WI. Reproduced with permission of Dale Bjorling.

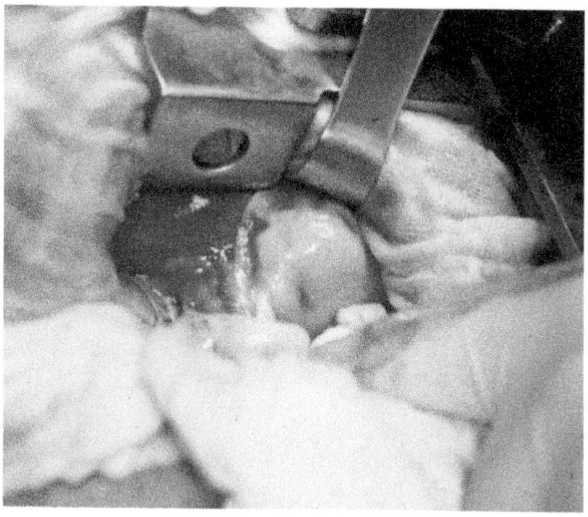

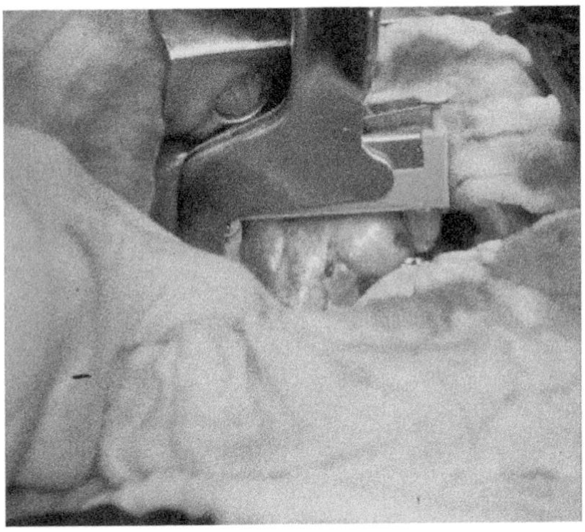

Figure 5.110 Internal stapler in position for lung lobectomy. *Source:* Dale Bjorling, University of Wisconsin, Madison, WI. Reproduced with permission of Dale Bjorling.

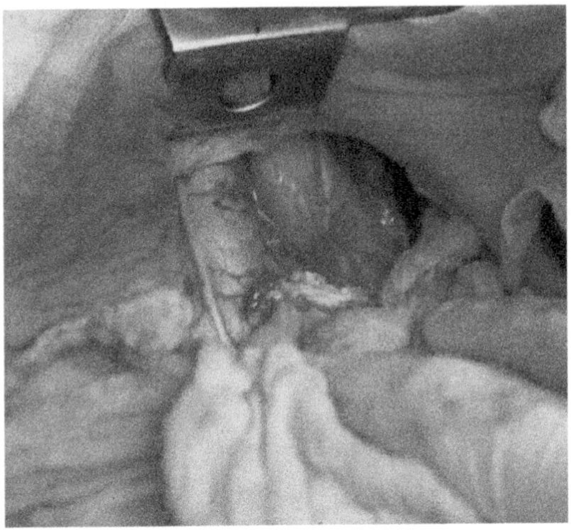

Figure 5.111 Post-lung lobectomy with internal stapler. *Source:* Dale Bjorling, University of Wisconsin, Madison, WI. Reproduced with permission of Dale Bjorling.

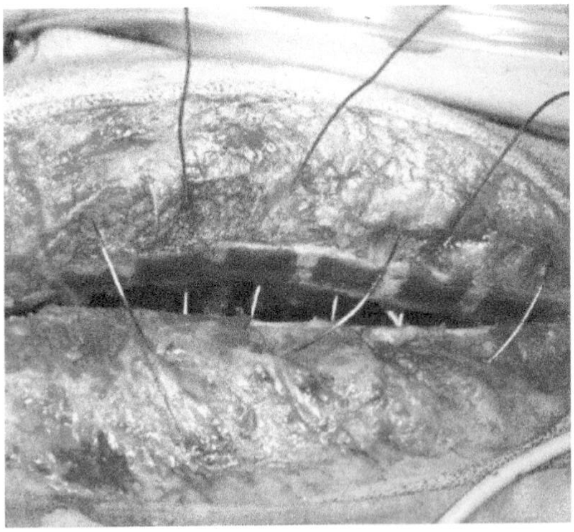

Figure 5.112 Orthopedic wire used to close the sternum.

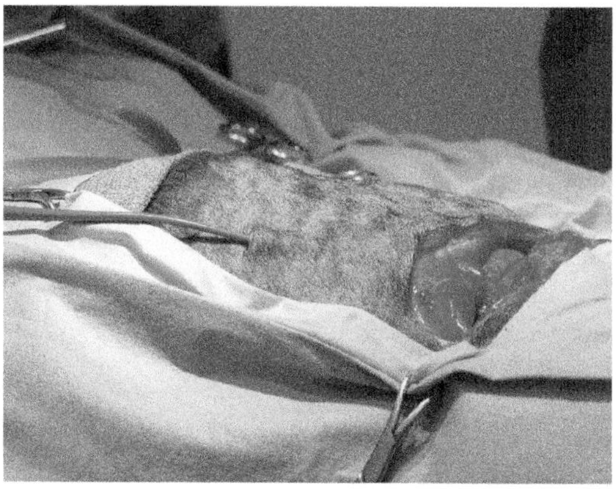

Figure 5.113 Chest tube exiting thoracic cavity.

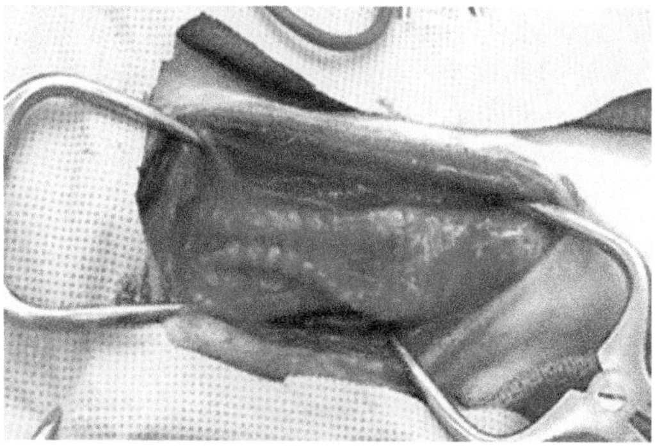

Figure 5.114 Tracheal collapse. *Source:* Courtesy of Dr. Mathews NCSU-CVM.

c) *Clinical signs*: Intermittent coughing is common. Fifty per cent of dogs have a characteristic "goose honk." Coughing may be exacerbated by stress, excitement, and mechanical stimulation of the trachea.
d) *Diagnosis*: Cervical and thoracic radiographs, fluoroscopy, laryngoscopy, tracheoscopy/bronchoscopy.
e) *Surgery*: The placement of a rigid support (extraluminal prosthesis) for the collapsed tracheal segment with non-absorbable suture (Figures 5.115 and 5.116).
f) *Positioning*: Dorsal recumbency with the front legs pulled back and a towel under the neck.

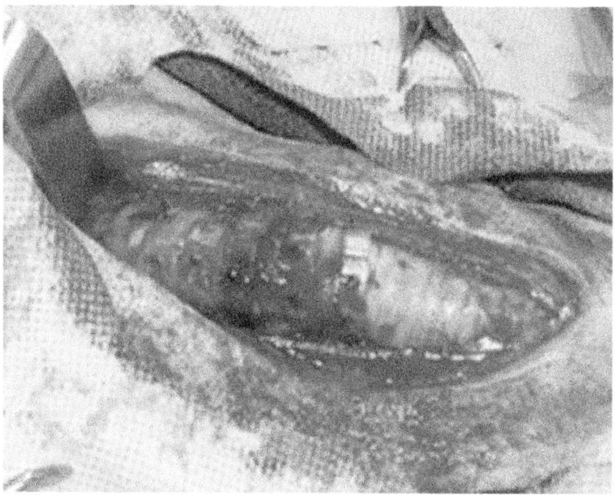

Figure 5.115 Tracheal rings. *Source:* Courtesy of Dr. Mathews NCSU-CVM.

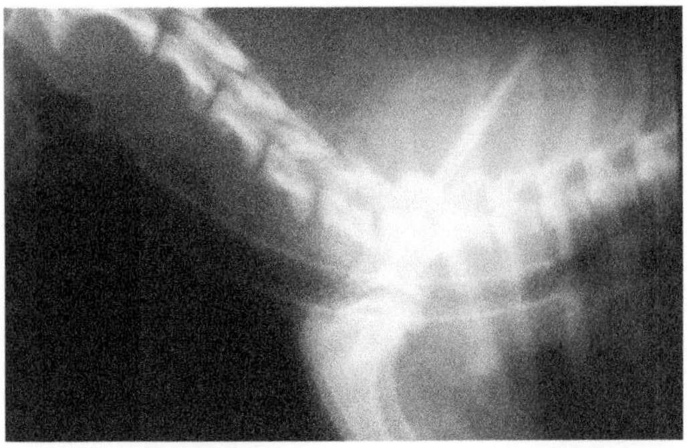

Figure 5.116 Tracheal stent. *Source:* Courtesy of Dr. Mathews NCSU-CVM.

g) *Special equipment*: Extraluminal stent, prosthetic tracheal rings or spirals made by cutting 3 ml polypropylene syringe cases, 4-0 polypropylene suture material with a tapered end, standard instrument pack, small Gelpi self-retaining retractors.
h) *Assistant role*: Lavage, tissue retraction, cut sutures.
i) *Post-op care*: Continuously monitor during recovery. Nasal insufflation of oxygen and a dose of corticosteroids may be helpful with animals that have edema and inflammation. Strict cage rest for three to seven days and then gradually increase exercise. A harness should be used for walks. Tracheoscopy one to two months after surgery and later if respiratory signs deteriorate.

   Grading Scheme for Tracheal Collapse
   Grade 1: Relatively normal tracheal cartilage; 25% decreased luminal diameter
   Grade 2: Mild-to-moderate flattening tracheal cartilage; 50% loss of luminal diameter
   Grade 3: Severe flattening of tracheal cartilage; 75% loss if luminal diameter
   Grade 4: Complete obstruction

Other Surgery

Anal Sacculectomy

a) *Definition*: The removal of the anal sacs
b) *Cause*: The treatment of chronically infected or impacted anal sacs that do not respond to medical treatment or for the removal of anal sacs tumors
c) *Clinical signs*: Inflammation within or around the anal sac or duct; enlargement and discomfort of the anal sacs
d) *Diagnosis*: Physical exam, rectum may have cellulitis or abscess, serum chemistry
e) *Surgery*: The procedure entails making an incision near the anus over the anal gland or glands. The gland is gently dissected from external and internal anal sphincters. Monofilament suture is used to close (Figure 5.117).
f) *Positioning*: Ventral recumbency in a Trendelenburg position (Figure 5.118).
g) *Special instruments*: General pack, Lonestar retractor, right-angle forceps, medium Gelpi retractor, Foley catheter, needle cautery tip, double skin hook, bipolar electrosurgery, hemoclips, small Frazier suction tip
h) *Assistant's role*: Placement of a purse string in anus, retract tissue, cut suture, and moisten tissue
i) *Postoperative care*: Place an E-Collar to prevent trauma; monitor for hemorrhage, infection, dehiscence, draining tracts, strictures, fecal incontinence, pain management

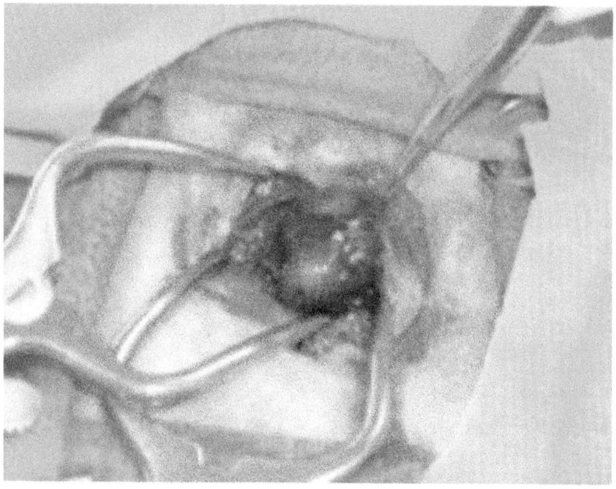

Figure 5.117 Anal sacculectomy.
Source: Courtesy of Dr. Mathews NCSU-CVM.

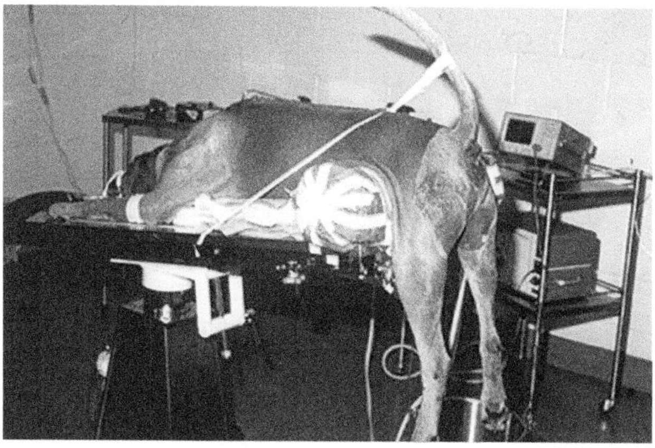

Figure 5.118 Perineal/perianal patient positioning. *Source:* Courtesy of Dr. Mathews NCSU-CVM.

Perineal Hernia

a) *Definition*: Herniation of the rectal wall
b) *Cause*: Muscular atrophy or stress from chronic straining can weaken the pelvic diaphragm, resulting in herniation of the rectal wall or abdominal organs (prostate, prostatic cysts, urinary bladder, and intestines) into the perineal region (Figure 5.119).
c) *Clinical signs*: Tenesmus, dysphasia, perineal swelling
d) *Diagnosis*: Rectal examination, serum chemistry, urinalysis evaluation for metabolic abnormalities, CT, US, X-ray
e) *Surgery*: Unilateral and/or bilateral repair of the rectal wall (Figure 5.120).
f) *Positioning*: Ventral recumbency in Trendelenburg position
g) *Special instruments*: General pack, monopolar and bipolar electrosurgery, Lonestar retractor, mini-vessel loops, fine Metzenbaum scissors, right-angle forceps, polypropylene mesh
h) *Assistant's role*: Retract tissue, cut suture, and moisten tissue; anal purse-string suture placement
i) *Postoperative care*: Rectal exam to confirm that the hernia is repaired, low-residue diet and stool softener is prescribed to reduce straining, Elizabethan for 1 week to prevent self-trauma

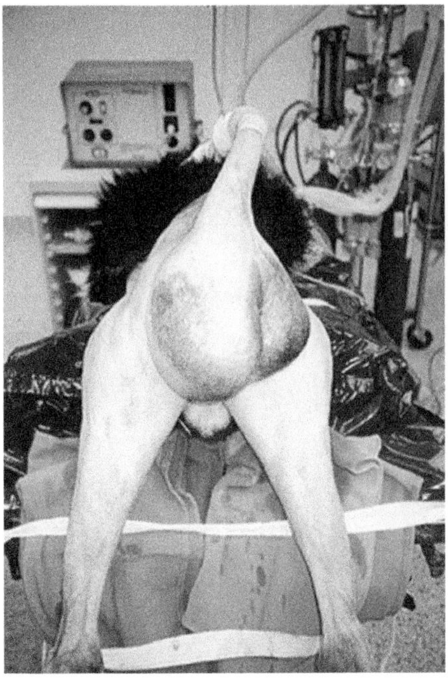

Figure 5.119 Perineal hernia.
Source: Courtesy of Dr. Mathews NCSU-CVM.

Mastectomy

a) *Definition*: The surgical removal of mammary tissue, most often for neoplasia
b) *Cause*: Non-inflammatory mammary neoplasia or inflammatory carcinomas incidence: For dogs, 0.5% and 8% spayed before the first and second estrus; 26% spayed and left intact; for cats, much less common.
c) *Clinical signs*: Non-inflammatory neoplasia: non-painful incident finding on exam; inflammatory carcinomas: anorexia, weight loss, weakness, rapid tumor growth, swelling, redness, pain, and diffuse involvement of multiple glands
d) *Diagnosis*: Thoracic radiographs to check for metastases, abdominal US, cytology of the mass, lymph node cytology, serum chemistry to check for disseminated intravascular coagulation (DIC)
e) *Surgery*: Non-inflammatory: mass removal; inflammatory carcinomas: bilateral or unilateral radical mastectomy which is based on lymphatic drainage (Figures 5.121 and 5.122).
f) *Positioning*: Dorsal recumbency
g) *Special instruments*: General pack, Metzenbaum scissors, Debakey forceps, monopolar electrosurgery,

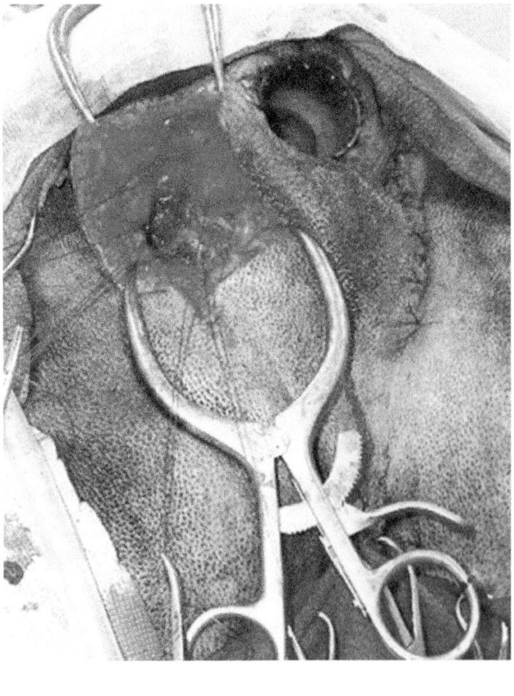

Figure 5.120 Intra-operative perineal hernia.
Source: Courtesy of Dr. Mathews NCSU-CVM.

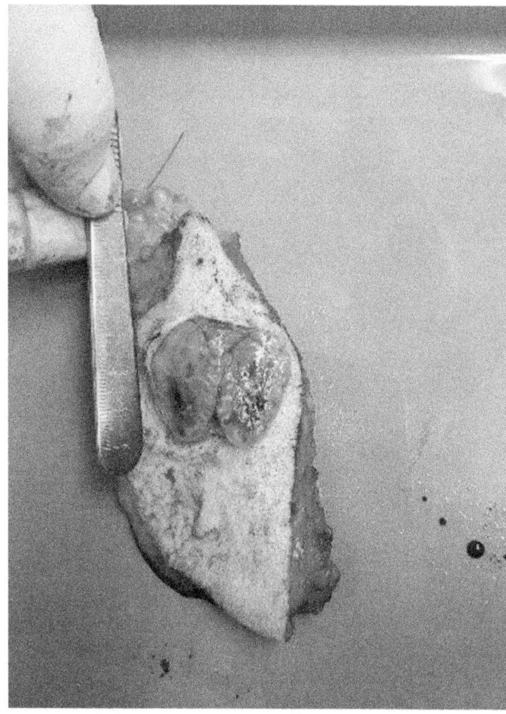

Figure 5.121 Mammary tumor removed. *Source:* Courtesy of Mindi James NCSU-CVM.

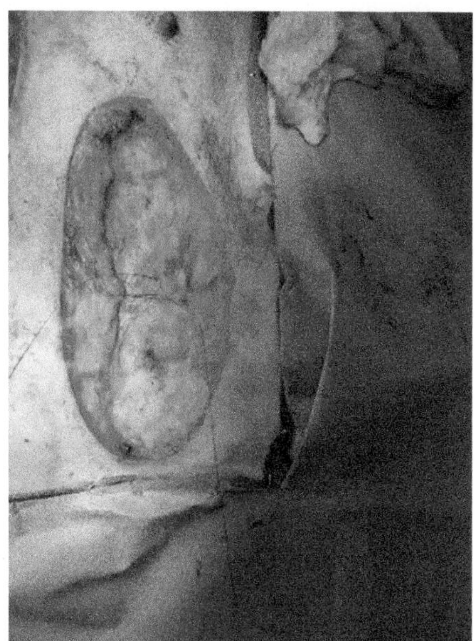

Figure 5.122 Mastectomy closure site. *Source:* Courtesy of Mindi James NCSU-CVM.

ENSEAL™/harmonic vessel sealing device, Jackson Pratt drainage tube, formalin for tissue submission, microscope slides for impression smears

h) *Assistant's role*: Retract tissue, hemostasis, cut suture, and moisten tissue
i) *Postoperative care*: Submission for histologic evaluation of neoplasia, bandage of the incision, E-Collar, exercise restriction, removal of drains 24–48 hours after surgery, pain management

References

1 Hedlund, C.S. & Fossum, T.W. (2007) Surgery of the digestive system. In: Fossum, T.W. (ed), *Small Animal Surgery*, 3rd edn. Mosby Elsevier, St. Louis, MO, pp. 425–433 and 462–467.

2 Fossum, T.W. (2007) *Small Animal Surgery*, 3rd edn. Mosby Elsevier, St. Louis, MO, pp. 317–322.

3 Fossum, T.W. (2007) *Small Animal Surgery*, 3rd edn. Mosby Elsevier, St. Louis, MO, pp. 539–553.

4 http://en.wikipedia.org/wiki/Portosystemic_shunt.

5 Hedlund, C.S. (2007) Surgery of the reproductive and genital systems. In: Fossum, T.W. (ed), *Small Animal Surgery*, 3rd edn. Mosby Elsevier, St. Louis, MO, pp. 702–720.

6 Fossum, T.W. (2007) *Small Animal Surgery*, 3rd edn. Mosby Elsevier, St. Louis, MO, pp. 624–629.

7 Fossum, T.W. (2007) *Small Animal Surgery*, 3rd edn. Mosby Elsevier, St. Louis, MO, pp. 698–701.

8 Hedlund, C.S. (2007) Surgery of the upper respiratory system. In: Fossum, T.W. (ed), *Small Animal Surgery*, 3rd edn. Mosby Elsevier, St. Louis, MO, pp. 817–838, 842–846.

9 Shores, A. (1985) Intervertebral disk disease. In: Newton, C.D. & Nunamaker, D.M. (eds), *Textbook of Small Animal Orthopaedics*. Lippincott, Williams & Wilkins, Philadelphia, PA.

10 Schulz, K.S. (2007) Diseases of the joints. In: Fossum, T.W. (ed), *Small Animal Surgery*, 3rd edn. Mosby Elsevier, St. Louis, MO, pp. 1176–1197.

11 Hedlund, C.S. (2007) Surgery of the integumentary systems. In: Fossum, T.W. (ed), *Small Animal Surgery*, 3rd edn. Mosby Elsevier, St. Louis, MO, pp. 251–253.

12 Piermattei, D.L., Flo, G. & DeCamp, C.E. (eds) (2006) *Handbook of Small Animal Orthopedics and Fracture Repair*, 4th edn. WB Saunders Co., Philadelphia, PA, pp. 501–506.

13 Piermattei, D.L., Flo, G. & DeCamp, C.E. (eds) (2006) *Handbook of Small Animal Orthopedics and Fracture Repair*, 4th edn. WB Saunders Co., Philadelphia, PA, p. 491.

14 Dueland, R.T., Adams, W.M., Patricelli, A.J. *et al.* (2010, 2010) Canine hip dysplasia treated by juvenile pubic symphysiodesis. Part I: two year results of computed tomography and distraction index. *Veterinary and Comparative Orthopaedics and Traumatology*, 23(6), 472.

15 Piermattei, D.L., Flo, G. & DeCamp, C.E. (eds) (2006) *Handbook of Small Animal Orthopedics and Fracture Repair*, 4th edn. WB Saunders Co., Philadelphia, PA, pp. 495–501.

16 Piermattei, D.L., Flo, G. & DeCamp, C.E. (eds) (2006) *Handbook of Small Animal Orthopedics and Fracture Repair*, 4th edn. WB Saunders Co., Philadelphia, PA, pp. 483–489.

17 Muir, P. (2010) Role of synovial immune responses in stifle synovitis. In: Muir, P. (ed), *Advances in the Canine Cranial Cruciate Ligament*. American College of Veterinary Surgeons and Wiley-Blackwell, Ames, IA, pp. 87–91.

18 Wilke, V. (2010) Genetics of cranial cruciate ligament rupture. In: Muir, P. (ed), *Advances in the Canine Cranial Cruciate Ligament*. American College of Veterinary Surgeons and Wiley-Blackwell, Ames, IA, pp. 53–58.

19 Schulz, K.S. (2007) Diseases of the joints. In: Fossum, T.W. (ed), *Small Animal Surgery*, 3rd edn. Mosby Elsevier, St. Louis, MO, pp. 1255–1276.

20 Cook, J.L. (2010) Extracapsular Stabilization. In: Muir, P. (ed), *Advances in the Canine Cranial Cruciate Ligament*. American College of Veterinary Surgeons and Wiley-Blackwell, Ames, IA, pp. 163–168.

21 Milovancev, M. & Schaefer, S.L. (2010) Tibial plateau leveling osteotomy. In: Muir, P. (ed), *Advances in the Canine Cranial Cruciate Ligament*. American College of Veterinary Surgeons and Wiley-Blackwell, Ames, IA, pp. 169–175.

22 Boudrieau, R.J. (2010) Tibial tuberosity advancement. In: Muir, P. (ed), *Advances in the Canine Cranial Cruciate Ligament*. American College of Veterinary Surgeons and Wiley-Blackwell, Ames, IA, pp. 177–187.

23 Piermattei, D.L., Flo, G. & DeCamp, C.E. (eds) (2006) *Handbook of Small Animal Orthopedics and Fracture Repair*, 4th edn. WB Saunders Co., Philadelphia, PA, pp. 562–582.

24 Fossum, T.W. (2007) *Small Animal Surgery*, 3rd edn. Mosby Elsevier, St. Louis, MO, pp. 867–879.

Additional Resources

References

1 Marcellin-Little, D. (2017) Canine angular limb deformities. In: Bojrab, M.J. & Monnet, E. (eds), *Mechanisms of Disease in Small Animal Surgery*, 3rd edn. Teton NewMedia, Jackson, WY.

2 Kwan, T.W., Marcellin-Little, D. & Harrysson, O. (2014) Correction of biapical radial deformities by use of bi-level hinged circular external fixation and distraction osteogenesis in 13 dogs. *Veterinary Surgery*, 43, 316–329.

3 Birchard, S.J. & Sherding, R.G. (1994) *Saunders Manual of Small Animal Practice*. W.B. Saunders Company, Philadelphia, PA, pp. 1004–1005; 1055–1056.

4 Birchard, S.J. & Sherding, R.G. (1994) *Saunders Manual of Small Animal Practice*. W.B. Saunders Company, Philadelphia, PA, pp. 1014–1021.

5 Birchard, S.J. & Sherding, R.G. (1994) *Saunders Manual of Small Animal Practice*. W.B. Saunders Company, Philadelphia, PA, pp. 380–386.

6 Fossum, T.W. (2013) *Small Animal Surgery*, 4th edn. Mosby Elsevier, St. Louis, MO, pp. 325–344.

7 Birchard, S.J. & Sherding, R.G. (1994) *Saunders Manual of Small Animal Practice*. W.B. Saunders Company, Philadelphia, PA, pp. 389–395.

8 Fossum, T.W. (2013) *Small Animal Surgery*, 4th edn. Mosby Elsevier, St. Louis, MO, pp. 325–344.

9 Birchard, S.J. & Sherding, R.G. (1994) *Saunders Manual of Small Animal Practice*. W.B. Saunders Company, Philadelphia, PA, pp. 1185–1188.

10 Fossum, T.W. (2013) *Small Animal Surgery*, 4th edn. Mosby Elsevier, St. Louis, MO, pp. 307–311.

11 Birchard, S.J. & Sherding, R.G. (1994) *Saunders Manual of Small Animal Practice*. W.B. Saunders Company, Philadelphia, PA, pp. 1185–1188.

12 Birchard, S.J. & Sherding, R.G. (1994) *Saunders Manual of Small Animal Practice*. W.B. Saunders Company, Philadelphia, PA, pp. 389–395.

13 Fossum, T.W. (2013) *Small Animal Surgery*, 4th edn. Mosby Elsevier, St. Louis, MO, pp. 320–324.

14 Fossum, T.W. (2013) *Small Animal Surgery*, 4th edn. Mosby Elsevier, St. Louis, MO, pp. 300–303.

15 Birchard, S.J. & Sherding, R.G. (1994) *Saunders Manual of Small Animal Practice*. W.B. Saunders Company, Philadelphia, PA, pp. 548–550; 556–558.

16 Fossum, T.W. (2013) *Small Animal Surgery*, 4th edn. Mosby Elsevier, St. Louis, MO, pp. 937–943.

17 Birchard, S.J. & Sherding, R.G. (1994) *Saunders Manual of Small Animal Practice*. W.B. Saunders Company, Philadelphia, PA.

18 Fossum, T.W. (2013) *Small Animal Surgery*, 4th edn. Mosby Elsevier, St. Louis, MO, pp. 628–630.

19 Tams, T.R. & Rawlins, C.A. (2011) *Small Animal Endoscopy*. Elsevier Mosby, St. Louis, MO, pp. 397–477.

20 Tams, T.R. & Rawlins, C.A. (2011) *Small Animal Endoscopy*. Elsevier Mosby, St. Louis, MO, pp. 479–506.

21 Tobis, K.M. (2010) *Manual of Small Animal Soft Tissue Surgery*. Wiley-Blackwell, Ames, IA, pp. 331–337.

22 Tobis, K.M. (2010) *Manual of Small Animal Soft Tissue Surgery*. Wiley-Blackwell, Ames, IA, pp. 57–66.

23 Tobis, K.M. (2010) *Manual of Small Animal Soft Tissue Surgery*. Wiley-Blackwell, Ames, IA, pp. 339–346.

24 Tobis, K.M. (2010) *Manual of Small Animal Soft Tissue Surgery*. Wiley-Blackwell, Ames, IA, pp. 433–440.

25 Fossum, T.W. (2013) *Small Animal Surgery*, 4th edn. Elsevier Mosby, St. Louis, MO, pp. 735–755.

26 Fossum, T.W. (2013) *Small Animal Surgery*, 4th edn. Elsevier Mosby, St. Louis, MO, pp. 705–719.

27 Fossum, T.W. (2013) *Small animal surgery*, 4th edn. Elsevier Mosby, St. Louis, MO, pp. 798–799, 806–807.

28 Tobis, K.M. (2010) *Manual of Small Animal Soft Tissue Surgery*. Wiley-Blackwell, Ames, IA, pp. 125–133.

29 Fossum, T.W. (2013) *Small Animal Surgery*, 4th edn. Elsevier Mosby, St. Louis, MO.

Webliography

1 https://www.vetsurgeryonline.com/subcutaneous-ureteral-bypass-sub [accessed on 20 February 2023].

2 https://www.vscvets.com/surgery/surgery-procedures/subcutaneous-ureteral-bypass-sub [accessed on 26 February 2023].

3 https://www.merckvetmanual.com/respiratory-system/respiratory-diseases-of-small-animals/neoplasia-of-the-respiratory-system-in-dogs-and-cats?query=lung%20lobectomy [accessed on 15 February 2023].

4 https://www.merckvetmanual.com/circulatory-system/congenital-and-inherited-anomalies-of-the-cardiovascular-system/persistent-right-aortic-arch-in-animals [accessed on 28 January 2023].

5 https://www.animalsurgicalcenter.com/persistent-right-aortic-arch [accessed on 19 January 2023].

6 https://todaysveterinarypractice.com/ophthalmology/eyelid-tumors-dogs-cats) [accessed on 30 January 2023].

7 https://www.acvs.org/small-animal/achilles-tendon-injuries [accessed on 20 December 2023].

8 Conzemius, M. https://www.youtube.com/watch?v=lELMsHHN1Lc [accessed on 14 December 2023].

6

Wound Management

Gerianne Holzman[1] and JoAnne Mead[2]

[1] *University of Wisconsin, School of Veterinary Medicine, Emerita, Madison, WI, USA*
[2] *College of Veterinary Medicine, North Carolina State University, Raleigh, NC, USA*

Patients come to the veterinary hospital with a huge variety of wounds. They range from simple scrapes to burns to huge gaping contaminated injuries. While basic wound management starts the same for any injury, the extent of care varies greatly. A Labrador Retriever with a pad laceration from stepping on a piece of glass needs far different care than a Chihuahua attacked by a Mastiff causing bite wounds and internal abdominal damage or a cat caught in a house fire. Postoperatively and sometime preoperatively, patients require wound and surgical incision care that may include drains, bandages, and external coaptation. The veterinary technician is an integral part of the team in daily (or more frequent) assessment of patients' wounds. A wound is damaging to the skin and to the underlying structures [1]. There are many types of injuries.

Types of Wounds

1) *Abrasion*: Although painful, abrasions are less than full skin thickness deep, have a minimal amount of bleeding, and heal quickly with little intervention
2) *Puncture*: Fully penetrating injury, punctures go deep into the tissues through a small opening, resulting in contamination and destruction – examples include stick penetration, bites, and gunshot wounds
3) *Laceration*: Sharp skin edges characterize lacerations although the edges may be ragged, and they may be deep or superficial and include surgical incisions
4) *Degloving*: Much skin and underlying tissue is lost or torn away, thus severing the blood supply, most often found on distal limbs
5) *Burn*: Resulting from a heat, or cold, source near or directly on the skin; burns vary in severity: superficial partial (epithelial), deep partial (epithelial and partial dermal), and full thickness; and burns may worsen in severity over time due to delayed microvascular damage
6) *Decubital ulcer*: A compression injury, decubital ulcers form when skin and soft tissues are compacted between a bony prominence (e.g. elbow, hock, and hip) and a hard surface (e.g. deficiently padded bed), and tissue damage can be extensive and is most common in recumbent patients

Surgical Patient Care for Veterinary Technicians and Nurses, Second Edition.
Edited by Gerianne Holzman and Teri Raffel Kleist.

Companion website: www.wiley.com/go/holzman/patient

Phases of Wound Healing

Wounds follow a specific pattern of healing (Table 6.1).

The steps and signs of healing are defined as:

1) *Inflammation*: When a wound occurs, inflammation begins [2]. Endothelin protein is produced along with other mediators; it initially causes vasoconstriction. The coagulation cascade begins to create hemostasis. Thrombin and growth factors attract cells to the site to begin wound healing. Neutrophils and macrophages travel to the wound within 24–48 hours to remove bacteria. These cells die as they ingest material and produce fluid. This is the purulent material seen in wounds (Figure 6.1). Soon after, prostaglandins, histamine, and other factors initiate vasodilation and increase blood flow to the area. This creates the characteristic inflammatory signs of redness, heat, and swelling (Figure 6.2).
2) *Proliferation*: This constructive phase begins after wound debridement from about day 4 through day 12 following injury. It is delayed when foreign material, infection, necrotic debris, and a hematoma are present. The scope of the wound, its location, and patient's condition influences the duration of this period (Figure 6.3). Capillaries grow into the wound from surrounding vasculature, collagen is produced and the wound contracts, and eventually closes. A network of small blood vessels within the wound provides oxygen and nutrients and eventually develops into granulation tissue, which is very resistant to infection (Figure 6.4).

Table 6.1 Wound healing chronology.

Time	Wound
1–3 days	Cellular debridement and inflammation in minimally traumatized (ideal) wound
3–5 days	Granulation bed forming and visible
7 days	Collagen deposition increases with minimal increase in wound strength
7–14 days	Rapid increase in wound strength
14 days	Wound begins to strengthen
6 weeks	Full contracture of properly managed wound
Months to years	Scar maturation and gradual strengthening

Source: Courtesy of Jonathan McAnulty, DVM, PhD.

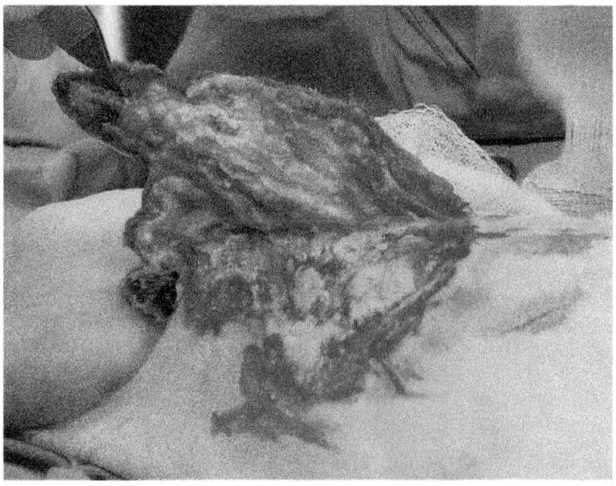

Figure 6.1 Phase 1 of wound healing is characterized by purulent material accumulating within the wound from cell death.
Source: Courtesy of Robert J. Hardie.

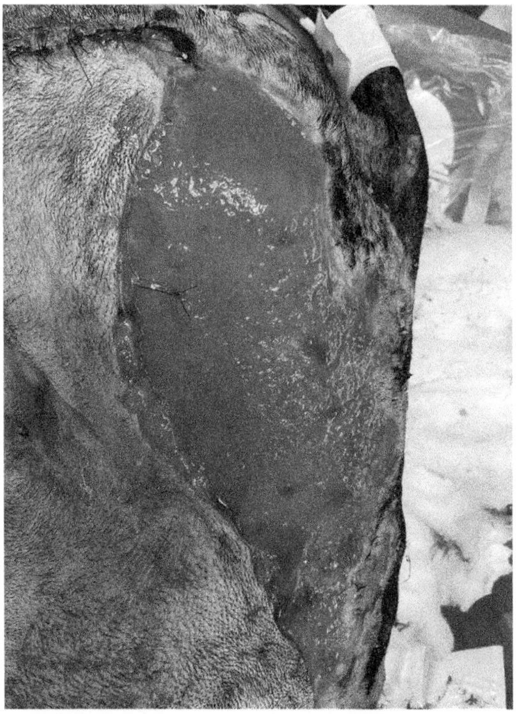

Figure 6.2 Phase 1 of wound healing is characterized by **inflammation** within the wound. *Source:* Courtesy of Kenneth Carroll.

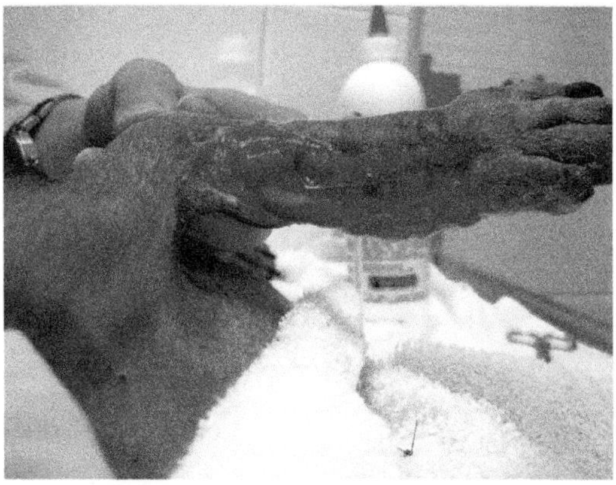

Figure 6.3 Phase 2 of wound healing includes **proliferation** of tissue and granulation bed formation. *Source:* Courtesy of Robert J. Hardie.

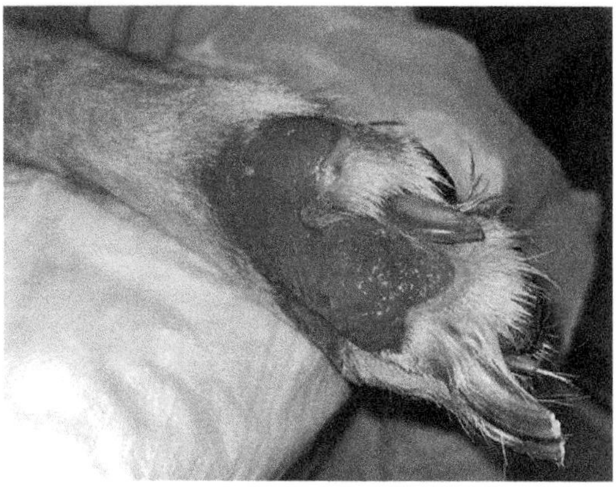

Figure 6.4 Phase 2 of wound healing showing extensive granulation bed. *Source:* Courtesy of Kenneth Carroll.

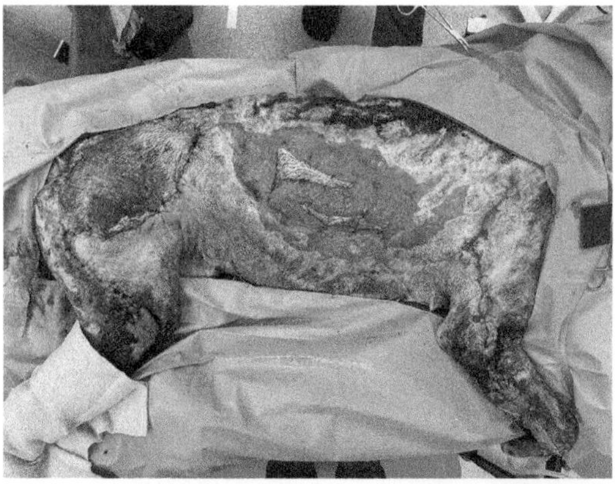

Figure 6.5 Phase 3 of wound healing is the **maturation** of the cells as collagen forms and strengthens while the wound continues to shrink in size. *Source:* Courtesy of Kenneth Carroll.

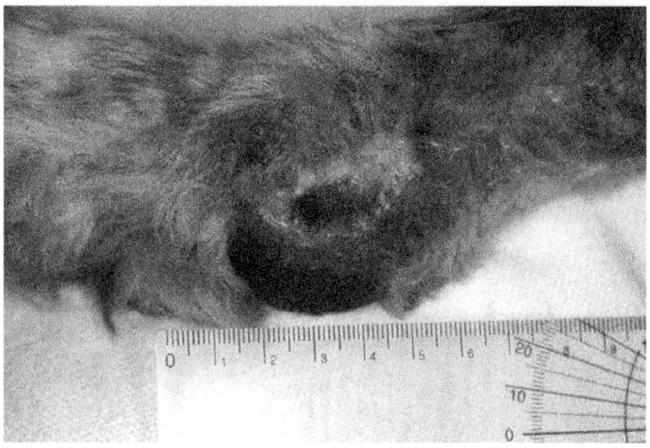

Figure 6.6 Phase 3 of wound healing near a joint. *Source:* Courtesy of Robert J. Hardie.

3) Maturation: The remodeling and strengthening phase is the longest, primarily it begins in 5–9 days and lasts 4–5 weeks but can extend to 18 months. During this time, the initial type of collagen changes and becomes stiffer, stronger, and thicker collagen (Figure 6.5). If continual bending occurs at the wound site, such as over a joint, this phase of healing is prolonged. The first collagen continues production and abnormal healing occurs by contracture causing decreased function of the joint (Figure 6.6).

Delays in Wound Healing

In addition to contamination with foreign material, infection, and necrotic tissue, other factors can affect wound healing. Patients' general conditions can delay healing. Systemic disorders such as diabetes, Cushing's disease, chronic steroid use, renal and liver disease, cancer, starvation, and chemotherapy all affect a patient's ability to heal. Wounds must be well perfused to provide oxygen critical to healing. Systemic antibiotics cannot reach the injury without sufficient blood flow. Shock and hypotension as well as arterial and venous impairment limit hemoglobin (oxygen) delivery to the wound. Hematomas and seromas impair healing by physical disruption, increased pressure on the wound bed, increasing dead space, and providing an ideal environment for bacterial growth. Large wounds heal slower due to the greater affected surface area than smaller wounds. Partial wound closure, where appropriate, reduces this factor.

Good surgical techniques can **DECREASE** delays in healing. These include minimizing tissue trauma, minimizing debris, maintaining moist tissues, minimizing surgical time, avoiding tension on the wound (incision), and providing drainage as needed. Factors that can **INCREASE surgical wound infection** are many.

1) Bacterial contamination: Surgeries are classified according to their likelihood of infection [3] and higher classifications have a much increased chance of postoperative complications. Wounds are classified as:
   I) *Clean*: No trauma, infection, or inflammation and respiratory, and gastrointestinal, genitourinary, and oropharyngeal cavities are NOT entered – infection rate: 2–4.8%
   II) *Clean-contaminated*: Respiratory, gastrointestinal, genitourinary, and oropharyngeal cavities are entered under controlled conditions – infection rate: 3.5–5%
   III) *Contaminated*: Open, fresh, accidental wounds, operations with major breaks in sterile technique, or gross spillage from gastrointestinal tract – infection rate: 4.6–12%
   IV) *Dirty and infected*: Old traumatic wounds with devitalized tissue, existing clinical infection, foreign bodies, perforated colon, and infective organisms present prior to surgical procedure – infection rate: 6.7–18.1% [4]
2) *Propofol use* [5]: Lipid-based emulsions may support microbial growth. Prompt use of prepared syringes of propofol and avoiding the use of the same syringe on multiple patients decreases this source of infection.
3) *Operating room personnel*: Inadequate aseptic technique and increased number of personnel in the surgical suite increases the source of contamination.
4) *Patient's sex*: Intact males produce androgenic hormones leading to immunomodulation. [6]

Despite best surgical practices, surgical wound infection remains a concern in small animal hospitals. The Centers for Disease Control created guidelines defining surgical site infection (SSI) (Table 6.2).

Table 6.2 Centers for disease control criteria for defining a surgical site infection (SSI).

Type of infection	Timing	Infected tissue	Signs – at least one present
Superficial incisional SSI	Within 30 d of surgery	Skin or subcutaneous	1) Superficial purulent discharge 2) Positive culture 3) Pain, tenderness, swelling, redness, or heat
Deep incisional SSI	Within 30 d of surgery or 1 yr if implant is in place, and infection is related to procedure	Deep soft tissue of incision: fascia or muscle	4) Deep purulent discharge 5) Incision spontaneously dehisces 6) Abscess present in deep tissue
Organ/space SSI	Within 30 d of surgery or 1 yr if implant is in place, and infection related to procedure	Any part of anatomy opened or manipulated during surgery, excluding incision	7) Purulent drainage from drain placed into organ or space 8) Positive culture 9) Abscess present in organ/space

Source: Adapted from Centers for Disease Control Guideline For Prevention Of Surgical Site Infection, 1999 Alicia J. Mangram, MD; Teresa C. Horan, MPH, CIC; Michele L. Pearson, MD; Leah Christine Silver, BS; William R. Jarvis, MD.

General Wound Care

Upon admittance, along with evaluating the entire patient, an assessment is made of the patients' wounds for degree and duration of injury. Patient's life-threatening injuries are always addressed first, including the ABCs – airway, breathing, and circulation. Despite the initial reaction to want to manage huge gaping wounds, even these do not generally require immediate attention unless the patient is hemorrhaging.

The facilitation of healing without infection is the goal of wound management. Contamination is the presence of bacteria on the surface of a wound. If unattended, this leads to colonization where the microbes are increasing. If still not addressed, colonization becomes infections where the bacteria and other organisms invade the tissues. Class 1 wounds are less than 6 hours old with minimum contamination and trauma. These first 6 hours are the *golden period* where there are an insufficient number of microbes to cause infection. Class 2 wounds, 6 to 12 hours old, show organism replication but they may not have reached the critical level (10^5 colony-forming units [CFU] per gram of tissue) to create infection. Class 3 wounds of greater than 12 hours show great bacterial and other organism growth and develop infection.

First-intention healing occurs when the surgeon **primarily closes** a wound within hours of its occurrence. Most Class 1 injuries and surgical incisions are secured by this method. Class 2 wounds may be amendable to primary closure if there is minimal wound contamination and trauma. Surgical debridement occurs prior to closure and includes the removal of devitalized tissue, bacteria, and foreign matter. In the face of mild contamination and trauma, Class 2 wounds benefit from **delayed primary closure** happening within three to five days of injury.

Second-intention healing occurs when a wound is left to heal without primary closure. This occurs, over time, by **granulation and contraction**. While many wounds can heal this way, it is a long, often inefficient process and may create an unfavorable result. Excessive granulation tissue may form keeping the skin edges from completely constricting. Likewise, abnormal wound contracture may cause scarring and decreased function of the injured area. Wounds most suited for open wound management (second-intention healing) are dirty and contaminated. They often require extensive and prolonged cleaning and debridement. With time, these wounds may progress enough for secondary closure.

Third-intention healing occurs when a wound is repaired by **secondary closure** – more than three to five days after injury. These wounds have undergone extensive cleansing to remove severe contamination. The tissue is healthier and granulation tissue is present protecting the wound from infection. The surgeon closes the wound over the granulation bed.

Open wound management allows for lavage and debridement to remove debris and microbial contamination (Figure 6.7).

Isotonic saline in large volumes or under high pressure aids in cleaning wounds. The use of an administration set attached to a fluid bag produces copious amounts of irrigation at low pressure. An 18-gauge needle attached to a 35 ml saline-filled syringe creates high pressure of 7–8 psi. Commercial jet pressure (70 psi) units quickly remove contaminants but may force more bacteria into underlying tissues and cause edema. The addition of antiseptics to the irrigation solution is usually unnecessary and can have cytotoxic effects [7] (see Table 6.3).

The goal of open wound management is to convert a contaminated, traumatized wound into one that is clean and healthy. This creates an injury that can be closed with great confidence of healing successfully with minimal complications.

Debridement of a wound removes any remaining foreign material and necrotic tissue. The clinician may surgically remove damaged skin and fascia to clean up the wound. Assorted topical treatments also provide wound debridement and care (Table 6.4).

Figure 6.7 Irrigating a wound with saline removes debris, contaminants, and purulent material.

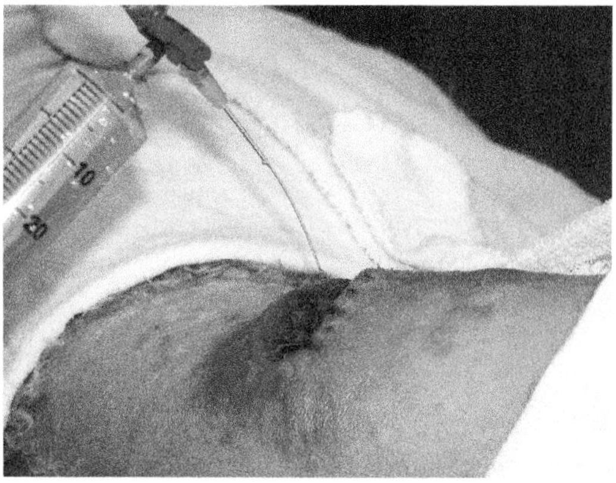

Table 6.3 Wound cleaners.

Product	Advantages	Disadvantages
Balanced electrolyte solution: • Lactated Ringer's solution (LRS) • Normosol®	• Isotonic • Least cytotoxic	• Not antimicrobial
Chlorhexidine 0.05%	• Wide antimicrobial spectrum • Good residual activity • Not inactivated by organic matter	• More than 0.05% of concentrated solutions are cytotoxic • Corneal toxicity
Chlorhexidine 0.05% with Tris-EDTA	• Increases antimicrobial effectiveness 1000-fold over plain diluted chlorhexidine	• More than 0.05% of concentrated solutions are cytotoxic • Corneal toxicity • Precipitates in electrolyte solution
Commercial cleaners • Allclenz® • Sur-Clenz® • Cara-Klenz® • Ultra-Klenz®	• Breaks bonds between foreign bodies and wound • Convenient	• Toxic to cells • Delays wound Healing • Expensive
Normal saline solution (0.9%)	• Isotonic	• Slightly more acidic than LRS • Not antimicrobial
Povidone–iodine 0.1%	• Wide antimicrobial spectrum	• Inactivated by organic material • Limited residual activity • Cytotoxic at concentrations greater than 1% • Contact hypersensitivity • May cause thyroid disorders if absorbed
Tap water	• Readily available	• Cytotoxic trace elements • Hypotonic • Not antimicrobial

Source: Adapted from Fossum [8].

Table 6.4 Topical treatments.

Material	Indication	Example
Alginate	Absorbs excessive exudate and promotes granulation while keeping wound moist	Calcium alginate dressings
Enzymatic agents	Debridement	Trypsin and collagenase
Gauze – wet to dry	Debridement[a]	Sterile gauze moistened with sterile saline
Honey	Antibacterial, reduces inflammation and edema, and augments granulation and epithelialization	Medical grade honey
Hydrocolloid	Absorbs moderate exudate and promotes granulation while keeping wound moist	Hydrocolloid dressings
Hydrogel	Minimal exudate and keeps wounds moist	Hydrogel dressings
Hypertonic saline dressing	20% saline and antimicrobial	Commercially available hypertonic saline gauze
Maggots	Digestive enzymes dissolve necrotic tissue	Medicinal maggots
Polyelectrolyte matrix	Absorbs wound fluid, contours to wound, and maintains a moist microenvironment	Microlyte vet
Silver	Infected wounds	Silver sulfadiazine or silver-impregnated dressing
Sugar	Hyperosmotic effect	Sugar from store shelf
Topical antibiotic ointment	Lessens surface bacteria	Triple antibiotic

Source: Adapted from Hosgood [1].

[a] The use of wet–dry gauze bandage is controversial. Based on the author's consultation with veterinary surgeons, this continues to be a viable wound management technique.

Based on the extent of the injury, debridement may be a one-time occurrence or continue for several days, or even be performed more than once per day. Infected sites benefit from extended treatment to minimize microorganism growth prior to wound closure. This may be achieved with the use of a tie-over bandage that is changed as needed (Figures 6.8–6.12). This may include a combination of lavage and debridement to remove purulent and necrotic tissue.

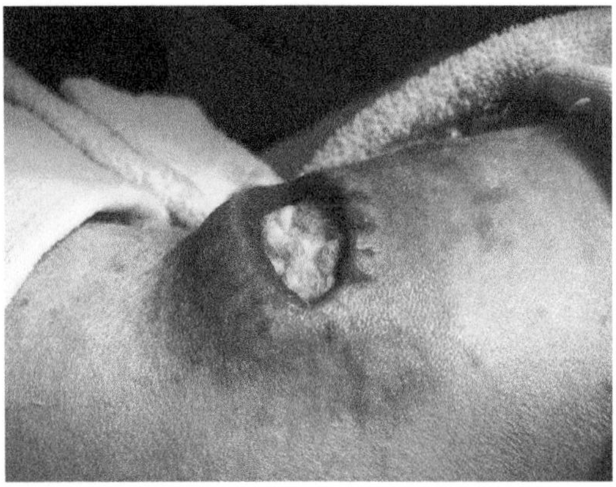

Figure 6.8 Wet gauze applied to a wound is a traditional method of removing accumulating discharge. This is the first step to a tie-over bandage.

Figure 6.9 Loose sutures are placed as step 2 of a-tie-over bandage.

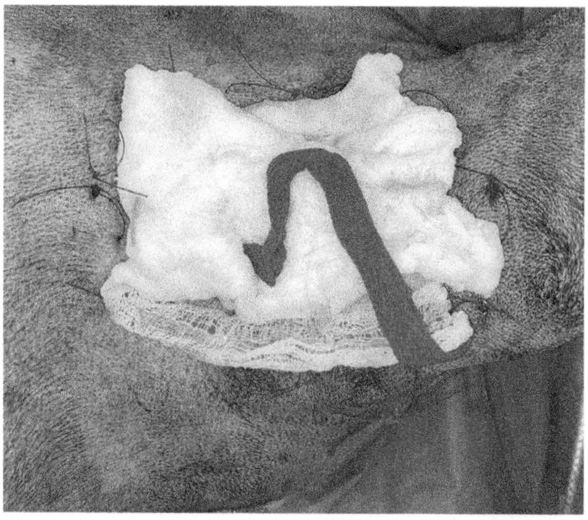

Figure 6.10 The dry part of a wet–dry bandage (and step 3 of a tie-over) absorbs drainage while maintaining moisture within the "wet" layer.

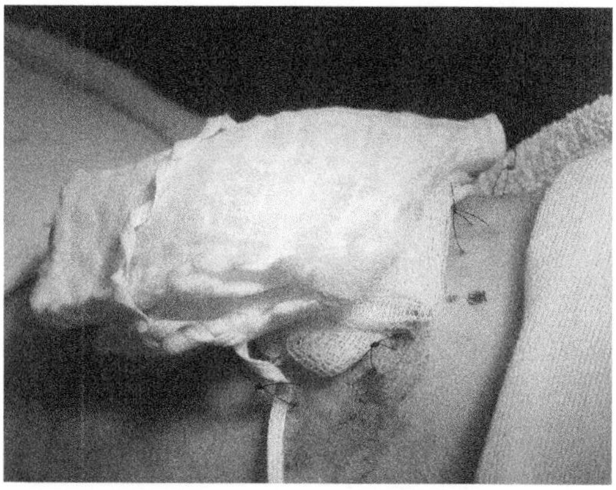

Figure 6.11 A tie-over bandage is secured in place with loose sutures acting as loops for lacing umbilical tape in step 4.

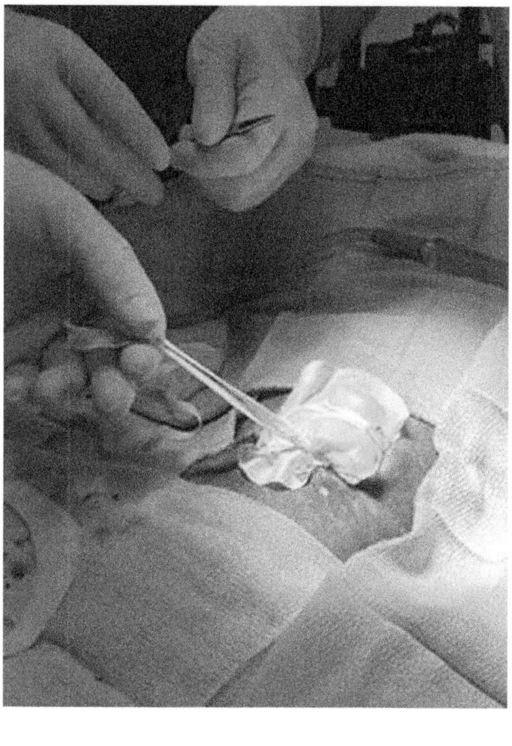

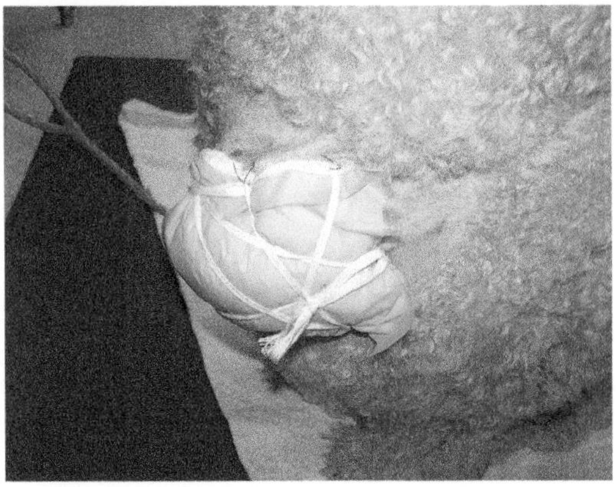

Figure 6.12 A tie-over bandage in place on an open wound over the hip. This difficult location to bandage is served well with this type of wrap. Chux padding covers the underlying gauze to protect it from contamination.

Topical broad-spectrum antimicrobial ointments, gels, and creams applied to a wound aid in controlling contamination and decreasing microbe population. **Collection of a wound culture and sensitivity PRIOR to applying antimicrobials provides important information for choosing a systemic antibiotic.** Narrowing the spectrum of coverage of a systemic antibiotic based on culture-sensitivity results reduces the incidence of developing resistant microorganisms. [1]

Honey is used for cleaning and accelerating the healing of wounds (Figure 6.13). The biological effects of honey in wounds include: decrease of inflammatory edema, stimulation of macrophage migration, increase of sloughing of dead skin, production of protective layer of proteins, development of healthy granulation bed, and an antibacterial effect. [8, 9] Because of its naturally occurring hydrogen peroxide content, it helps stimulate angiogenesis within the wound. Honey is effective against a wide variety of gram-positive and gram-negative bacteria.

Contaminated or infected wounds are lavaged after surgical debridement. A surgical gauze is soaked with sterile regular honey or manuka honey and then placed on or in the wound. (Manuka honey is harvested from bees that harvest pollen only from *Leptospermum scoparium* trees, native to Australia and New Zealand.) Absorbent dressing is applied on the wound and should be changed one to three times per day depending on the amount of strikethrough. Caution is exercised when using honey on large wounds because of its hydrophilic properties of drawing fluid from the wound. Monitoring the patient's hydration, electrolytes, and protein levels are essential.

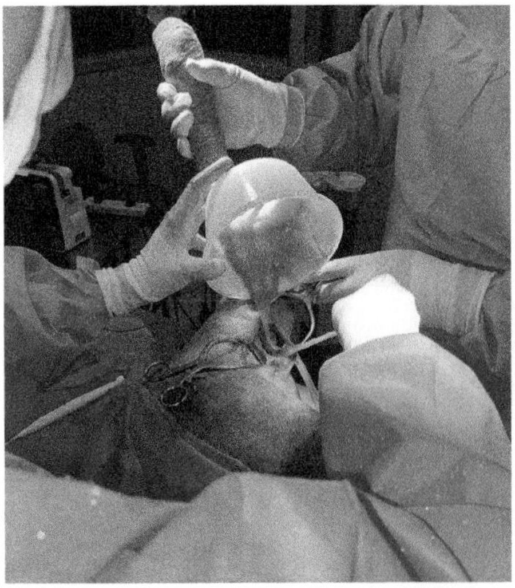

Figure 6.13 Sterilized Manuka honey provides antimicrobial treatment to a wound. *Source:* Courtesy of Kenneth Carroll.

Sugar has the same biological effects as honey. After wounds are cleaned and lavaged, at least 1 cm of sugar is poured into the wound and an adsorbent bandage is placed. The bandage should be changed when strikethrough occurs or at least twice per day to maintain the osmolality of the wound. Once healthy granulation is present with no sign of infection, discontinue the use of sugar. Hyperglycemia does not occur in patients treated with sugar because the sugar molecule is not absorbed from the wound. Care should be exercised with sugar just like honey.

Topical antimicrobials are of little use after a healthy granulation bed has formed. The topical treatment may impede healing and a sound granulation bed is resistant to infection.

Application of a dressing following lavage, debridement, and topical treatment shields the wound from further contamination. The bandage also absorbs exudate and protects newly forming granulation tissue from trauma. Traditionally, the first layer of a protective bandage is a non-adherent dressing, which comes in many types, sizes, and shapes. Telfa® pads, while non-adherent, do not allow exudate to migrate away from the wound. Sterile oil-emulsion gauze sponges do not stick to the skin and allow fluid to move away from the wound into surrounding padding. This type of bandage is commercially available or readily created in the clinic (Figure 6.14).

Silver-coated antimicrobial barrier dressing may be used for wounds that have a heavy exudate and that are very hard to heal (Figure 6.15). Silver-impregnated products provide a sustained release of positively charged silver ions at the wound surface, which can promote wound healing and decrease infection by killing bacteria. There are multiple varieties of silver-coated sheets. They may be left in place for three to seven days depending on the product.

Some silver-coated dressings contain a high silver level which may lead to cellular toxicity that can slow healing. [10] Studies show that a reduced rate of silver provides the same benefit without the risks. Another form of silver dressing, Microlyte Vet®,[1] conforms to wounds with a "shrink fit," providing direct contact while providing a lower level of silver than traditional dressings. The

Figure 6.14 Oil-emulsion gauze is easily made in a clinic following the recipe. *Source:* Recipe is courtesy of the UW Veterinary Care Surgical Suite Technicians.

Oil Impregnated Gauze

- Stainless steel container with cover, e.g., cold sterilization tray
- 4 × 4 or 4 × 8 gauze sponges
- Petrolatum (Vaseline®)

Put gauze in container and cover with petrolatum. Autoclave until petrolatum melts. This does not sterilize the gauze but the process melts the petrolatum to permeate the gauze sponges. Sponges are removed individually with a sterile forceps. The entire tray is autoclaved weekly to prevent bacteria growth.

1 https://www.theveterinarynurse.com/opinion/article/introducing-microlyte-vet-a-new-generation-of-wound-technology-for-optimal-wound-healing.

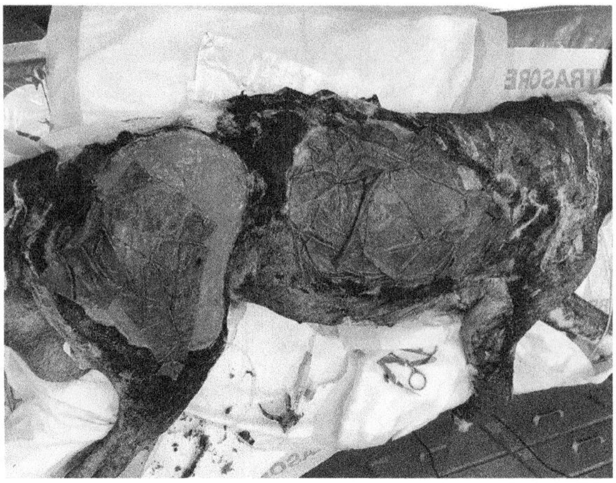

Figure 6.15 Silver-coated antimicrobial dressing applied to burn injuries. *Source:* Courtesy of Kenneth Carroll.

intimate contact avoids any dead space where microbes may grow. The material is not changed for four days, thus not disturbing the healing wound bed. The wound is covered with a traditional dressing as follows.

The primary layer of protection is applied, e.g. oil-impregnated gauze, silver-coated dressing, etc. All areas of the wound bed are covered to provide protection and maintain moisture. (Petrolatum applied to the normal skin surrounding the wound protects it from irritation and scald from any exudate.) The next bandage layer is absorbent to soak up wound fluid and pull it away from the wound surface. Roll cotton and cast padding are great products for this purpose. The thickness of the layer depends on the amount of exudate expected and the amount of additional support needed, e.g. wounds on limbs may also need support for bone or tendon injuries. Following the padding layer, stretch gauze is applied to hold the cotton in place. Depending on the amount of padding applied as well as the area to be bandaged and the needs of the bandage, the stretch gauze may be applied tightly to provide compression. (Never apply a bandage tight enough to restrict breathing or inhibit blood flow – unless needed to stop hemorrhage.) The final bandage layer is impermeable. Its primary purpose is to keep the underlying layers clean and avoid environmental contaminants. The layer is made of self-adhering flexible bandage tape (e.g. Vetrap™ – 3M™), adhesive elastic bandage tape (e.g. Elastikon™ – Johnson & Johnson), or white adhesive tape. Care is taken to avoid over-tightening the bandage from tapes with elastic properties. (See Chapter 7, Postoperative Care, for detailed instructions on bandage application.)

Negative Pressure Wound Therapy

Negative pressure wound therapy (NPWT) or vacuum-assisted closure (VAC) is a treatment for patients requiring skin grafts as well as those suffering from infected wounds and burns among other conditions. This treatment is now commonly used in human as well as veterinary medicine. A study performed at Michigan State University experimentally compared healing by traditional open wound management methods and with negative pressure wound therapy. [11] Identical wounds were created on both forelimbs of 10 dogs to resemble a minor shear injury. One side was treated as a control using traditional open wound care of absorbent dressing and padding until a granulation bed formed. Upon granulation, a non-adherent dressing and padding covered the wound until the close of the study at 21 days postinjury. The bandages were changed at appropriate intervals following standard wound care. The dogs' opposite limbs received negative pressure wound therapy (NPWT). Foam or gauze covered the wounds followed by an impermeable adhesive drape incised with an evacuation tube leading to the vacuum apparatus. The NPWT was continued throughout the study and the bandages changed at the same intervals as the control limb. Wound measurements, granulation tissue assessment, biopsies, and cultures were obtained throughout the study. The study found advantages and disadvantages of NPWT over traditional open wound therapy. If initialized, negative pressure wound therapy should continue for no more than 10 days to lessen its effects on contraction and epithelialization.

- Advantages
  - earlier granulation tissue
  - superior smoother granulation tissue
  - less exuberant granulation tissue
  - earlier acute inflammatory stage
  - potential for longer time interval between dressing changes
  - decreased need for patient sedation for traditional bandage changes
- Disadvantages
  - initially more retraction of wound edges
  - decreased wound contraction and epithelialization
  - higher bacterial load but no clinical infection was noted in the study
  - erythema in the tissue surrounding the wound
  - vacuum system requires monitoring to maintain negative pressure
  - commercial system to deliver constant vacuum required

Figure 6.16 shows a Greyhound that had undergone a right rear leg amputation. The surgical wound dehisced. Due to the location of the wound and the thinness of the patient's pelvis, traditional bandaging and wound care were unsuccessful. The patient underwent NPWT. The suction tubing attached to the wound is connected to a VAC unit (Figure 6.17). The unit contains a cassette that collects the wound exudate (Figure 6.18). This cassette is changed as it fills with material.

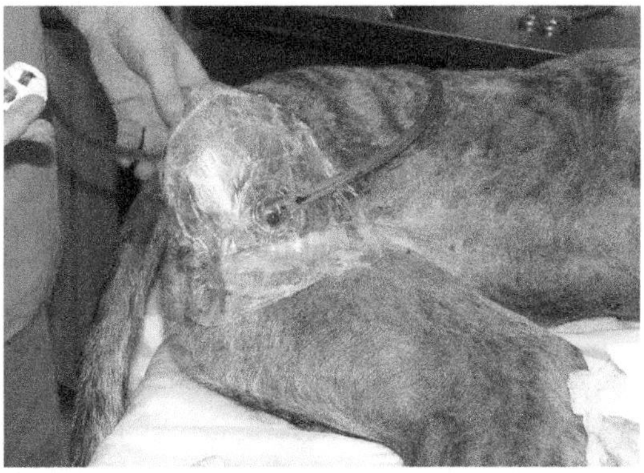

Figure 6.16 Negative pressure wound therapy (NPWT) is applied to a non-healing wound, postamputation, in a Greyhound dog.

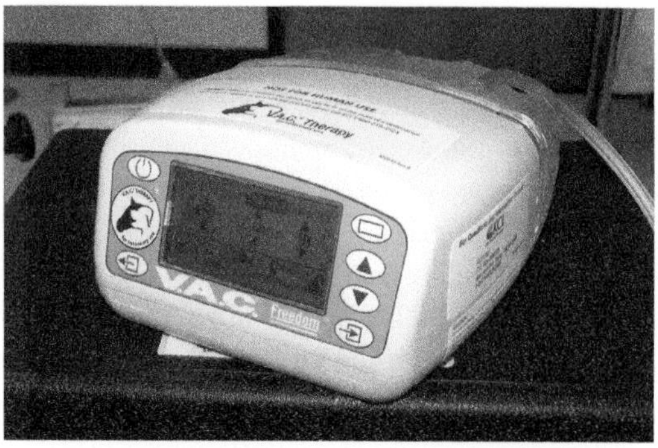

Figure 6.17 Vacuum-assisted closure (VAC) units provide constant negative pressure for negative pressure wound therapy.

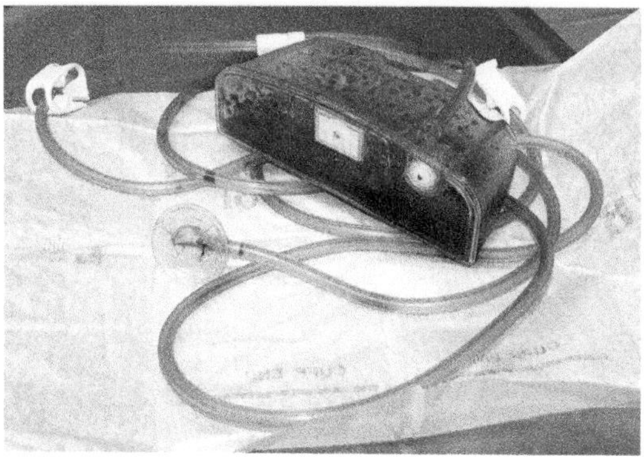

Figure 6.18 Cassette within the VAC system collects fluid removed via NPWT.

Burns

Severe burns are one of the most difficult injuries to treat in human and veterinary medicine. They range greatly in severity – burns that are more extensive carry a graver prognosis. Burns are classified according to the source of injury, depth of wound, and percentage of patient that is injured. The source of the burn divides into three main types of injury. Burns are ***thermal*** from either extreme heat or extreme cold (frostbite). Most often, however, thermal burns are considered to come from a heat source. This may be fire, liquids (scalds), hot objects, superheated air in a house fire, or radiation. ***Chemical*** burns occur when a chemical interacts with the skin and/or produces a hyperthermic or hypothermic reaction. Animals chewing on electric cords can suffer from ***electric*** burns.

Thermal Burns

Thermal burns are graded according to the degree of injury based on the depth of tissue affected [12] (Figure 6.19 and Table 6.5).

This section concentrates on thermal injuries due to hyperthermia. (Hypothermic burns [frostbite] are described in a separate section.) Burn injuries occur rapidly. A skin temperature of 104–111 °F can begin cell death. Partial thickness burns can happen in 1 second if the skin temperature reaches 140 °F, and full thickness in less than a second if temperature exceeds 158 °F. Depending on the source of the flame, house fires can exceed 1000 °F.

Another, perhaps more accurate classification for assessing burn injury is based on percentage of body surface area affected. The "Resuscitation or Veterinary Burn Card" is based on the size (8.5 × 5.3 cm or 45 cm^2) of an ordinary credit card (Figure 6.20a, b). The burn is compared to the size of the card (or multiple cards) to determine the square centimeters of body surface injured compared to the patient's entire body surface area. The patient's body surface area is taken from standard body weight to surface area chart. The number of cards is multiplied by 0.45 and divided by body surface area in square meters (m^2) to reach a percentage of total body surface area (TBSA) affected.

Burned tissue is divided into three areas:

1) *Zone of coagulation (or necrosis or destruction)*: Center of the wound, area of greatest injury, and no viable tissue
2) *Zone of stasis*: Next farthest out from zone of coagulation, less blood perfuses this area, and tissue may remain viable if no further damage occurs
3) *Zone of hyperemia*: Furthest away from center of wound, tissue is viable, and inflammation occurs to aid in healing

Burn wounds heal slower than other wounds due to the lack of normal wound-healing cytokines and other growth factors.

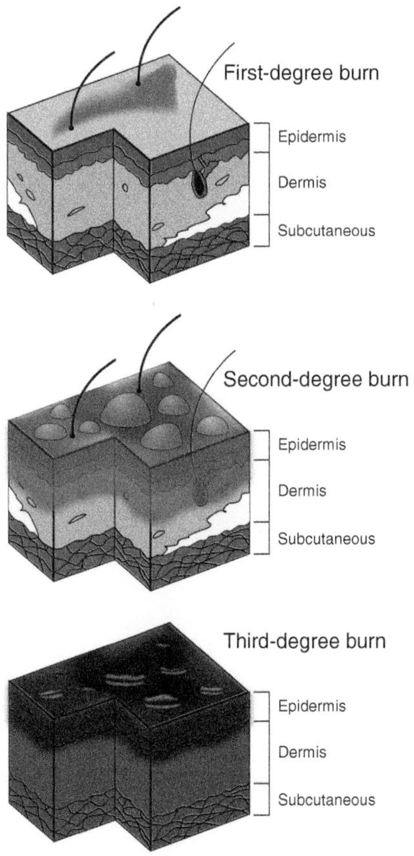

Figure 6.19 Burn diagram demonstrating the depth of injury in the three degrees of thermal burns. *Source:* Diagram courtesy of Wikimedia commons, GNU Free Documentation License.

Thermal Burn Treatment

Patients caught in building fires commonly suffer smoke inhalation in addition to thermal injuries. Home materials produce toxic substances, and carbon monoxide from the smoke inhibits the lungs and other systems from absorbing and producing oxygen. As with all emergencies, airway, breathing, and circulation are addressed prior to treating other injuries.

Table 6.5 Degree of classification of thermal burns.

Degree	Symptoms	Depth	Treatment
First	Erythema, premature skin sloughing, and mild discomfort	Partial skin thickness – epidermis	First aid
Second – superficial	Fluid exudate, blistering, and sensitive to light touch	Partial skin thickness – epidermis and superficial dermis	First aid and pain control
Second – deep	Skin white and poorly vascularized, and less sensitive	Partial thickness – epidermis and most of dermis	May require wound excision +/− grafting
Third	Skin dry and leathery without blisters	Full thickness – epidermis, dermis, and into subcutaneous	Wound excision and grafting
Fourth	Skin leathery or missing	Full thickness – extends to muscle and/or bone	Extreme measures to preserve area of injury

Source: Adapted from http://www.medstudentlc.com/page.php?id=84.

Veterinary Burn Card

To calculate the burn percentage of the total body surface area (%TBSA):

1. Measure the burn with this card. How many cards are needed to cover the burn?
2. Weigh the patient. Convert the weight to surface area in m^2 using the conversion table on the back.
3. Apply numbers to the following:
   Number of cards × $0.45/m^2$ = %TBSA burn

Example: 21 kg dog, burn size 15.5 burn cards

(a)

Dogs — Weight to surface area — Cats

Kg	m²	Kg	m²	Kg	m²	Kg	m²
1	0.1	20	0.74	48	1.32	1.0	0.100
2	0.15	21	0.76	50	1.36	1.5	0.131
3	0.2	22	0.78	52	1.41	2.0	0.159
4	0.25	23	0.81	54	1.44	2.5	0.184
5	0.29	24	0.83	56	1.48	3.0	0.208
6	0.33	25	0.85	58	1.51	3.5	0.231
7	0.36	26	0.88	60	1.55	4.0	0.252
8	0.40	27	0.90	62	1.58	4.5	0.273
9	0.43	28	0.92	64	1.62	5.0	0.292
10	0.46	29	0.94	66	1.65	5.5	0.311
11	0.49	30	0.96	68	1.68	6.0	0.330
12	0.52	32	1.01	70	1.72	6.5	0.348
13	0.55	34	1.05	72	1.75	7.0	0.366
14	0.58	36	1.09	74	1.78	7.5	0.383
15	0.60	38	1.13	76	1.81	8.0	0.400
16	0.63	40	1.17	78	1.84	8.5	0.416
17	0.66	42	1.21	80	1.88	9.0	0.432
18	0.69	44	1.25			9.5	0.449
19	0.71	46	1.28			10	0.464

(b)

Figure 6.20 (a,b) Veterinary Burn Card (same size as a credit card) used to measure the area of the body that is burned. *Source:* Adapted from Bohling [12].

Many body systems are affected by burns. After establishing a patent airway and providing ventilation support, other metabolic areas are treated in addition to the burn itself. Among the many systems affected by burns are the following.

1) *Cardiovascular*: The vascular system's leakage of plasma and evaporation cause hypovolemia, the heart has decreased contractility in very severe burns, and carbon monoxide causes decreased cardiac output
2) *Gastrointestinal*: Gastrointestinal barrier is compromised allowing translocation of bacteria, endotoxins, and cytokines, leading to septic shock and decreased gut motility
3) *Renal*: High burn percentages, of total body surface area, are linked to acute renal failure, decreased cardiac output provides less blood flow to the kidneys
4) *Neurologic*: Severe pain is present in all burns. It occurs initially, while being treated, and during healing.

Burn patients are treated using diligent aseptic techniques to minimize contamination. Initially, first aid is applied to wounds, and then aggressive fluid therapy is initiated, as well as treating inhalation damage and pain, and providing nutritional support. Finally, the burn wound itself is addressed.

Initial care of a burn is application of cold running water (35–60 °F). This provides analgesia and improves healing as it stops the burning. Treatment with ice **is not indicated** and it does not provide benefit to the patient. Many ointments, creams, herbs, and plants have been used as burn remedies. None of these has been scientifically proven as superior to plain, cold running water. After initial cooling, the wound is covered with a sterile non-adherent dressing. Small partial-thickness wounds often mend well from second intention healing with minimal scars. Patients are provided with analgesia and the injury is protected from further damage including infection. A topical antibiotic is applied to the wound followed by a moist layer. Padding and bandaging follow as with any open wound.

Deep partial-thickness and full-thickness wounds require surgical intervention. The wound is debrided to remove all non-viable and necrotic tissue. Over time, more tissue may lose its viability and require excision. Small wounds may be primarily closed at this time and large wounds may require grafting.

Patients with extensive wounds covering large portions of the body also benefit from NPWT. The patient shown in Figures 6.21–6.24 underwent treatment for second- and third-degree burns. Silver-impregnated dressing was used in combination with negative pressure wound therapy and bandaging.

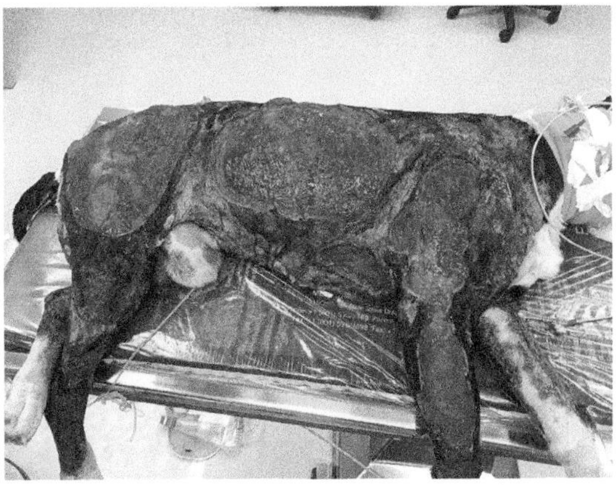

Figure 6.21 Debridement of second- and third-degree burns. *Source:* Courtesy of Kenneth Carroll.

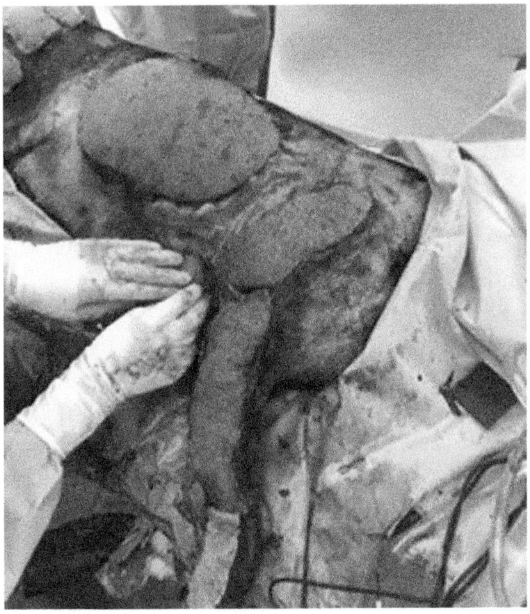

Figure 6.22 Insertion of silver-coated dressing into a deep wound. *Source:* Courtesy of Kenneth Carroll.

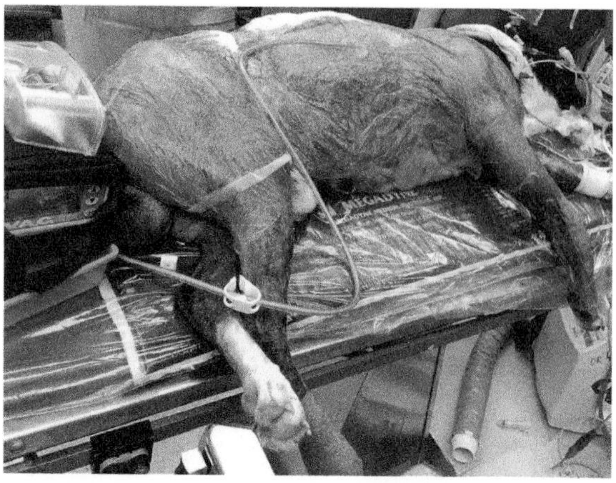

Figure 6.23 Application of NPWT to the burn wounds. *Source:* Courtesy of Kenneth Carroll.

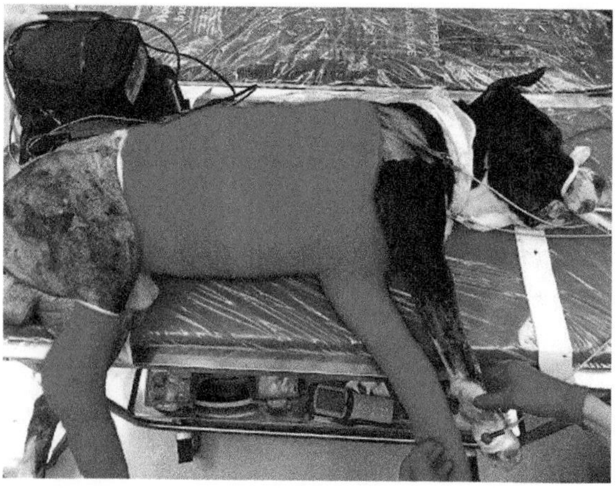

Figure 6.24 The burn patient is bandaged and attached to the VAC unit. *Source:* Courtesy of Kenneth Carroll.

Frostbite

Lengthy exposure to cold can cause hypothermic burns or frostbite. Areas most often affected are extremities and pinnae. Thin skin of the flank folds may also be injured. Iatrogenic damage may occur from misuse of a cryotherapy unit. Frostbite causes:

1) *Tissue freezing*: Ice crystals create intracellular and extracellular damage through disruption of the cell membrane and cell lysis.
2) *Hypoxia*: Cold causes vasoconstriction which decreases blood flow.
3) *Release of inflammatory mediators*: Activation of the inflammatory cascade causes clotting and intravascular thrombosis.

Frostbite Treatment

Initial first aid includes rapid but gentle re-warming of the affected area. Lukewarm water (104–108 °F) immersion is the most effective treatment. This is not initiated until there is no chance of re-freezing as a "freeze–thaw–freeze" cycle creates more damage. Along with thawing, fluid therapy is initiated to improve circulation, and anti-inflammatory medications are provided.

Final treatment of frostbite begins after the extent of injury is recognized. Debridement and open wound management are as described under thermal burns.

Chemical Burns

Chemicals cause burns via a variety of actions. Acids (toilet and drain cleaners) are oxidizers that disrupt the cellular protein structure. Alkaline or base chemicals (bleach and ammonia) are reducers causing a denaturing of proteins and other reactions that can lead to a thermal burn. Vesicants are blistering agents generally used in chemical terrorism. The chemotherapeutic drug doxorubicin may cause tissue toxicity and blistering.

Chemical Burn Treatment

Neutralization of the agent is of primary importance. Until this happens, the burning continues. The chemical is neutralized via tissue components, another chemical, copious washing/ and or dilution. Warning labels attached to household cleaning products provide information for treatment of chemicals. Poison control hotlines are also excellent sources of information. Doxorubicin blistering treatment includes surgical removal, local treatment with hyaluronidase for dilution, and infiltration of the site with dimethyl sulfoxide.

Following initial first aid, chemical burns are treated as thermal burns dependent upon their degree and severity.

Electrical Burns

Puppies and kittens suffer oral burns from chewing on cords. Other patients may receive electrical burns from improperly grounded electrocautery units in surgery. Joule's law states that tissues with a higher electrical resistance (e.g. bone) will sustain greater damage than tissues with lower resistance (skin). Electrical wounds may appear superficial on the skin while underlying muscle, bone, and adjoining structures are severely injured as the electric energy is met with resistance while traveling through the site. Surgical debridement of electrical wounds is required.

References

1 Hosgood, G. (2012) Open wounds. In: Tobias, K.M. & Johnston, S.A. (eds), *Veterinary Surgery – Small Animal*. Volume II. Elsevier, St. Louis, MO, pp. 1210–1220.
2 Cornell, K. (2012) Open wounds. In: Tobias, K.M. & Johnston, S.A. (eds), *Veterinary Surgery – Small Animal*. Volume 1. Elsevier, St. Louis, MO, pp. 125–129.
3 Mangram, A.J., Horan, T.C. & Pearson, M.L. (1999). Guideline for prevention of surgical site infection. Centers for Disease Control and Prevention. The Hospital Infection Control Practices Advisory Committee. US Department of Health and Human Services.
4 National Research Council Wound Classification System Range of reported surgical infection rates in dogs and cats. In: Tobias, K.M. & Johnston, S.A. (eds), *Veterinary Surgery – Small Animal*. Volume 1. Elsevier, St. Louis, MO, pp. 135–139.
5 Brown, C.B. (2012) Wound infections and antimicrobial use. In: Tobias, K.M. & Johnston, S.A. (eds), *Veterinary Surgery – Small Animal*. Volume 1. Elsevier, St. Louis, MO, pp. 628–646.

6 Brown, C.B. (2012) Wound infections and antimicrobial use. In: Tobias, K.M. & Johnston, S.A. (eds), *Veterinary Surgery – Small Animal*. Volume 1. Elsevier, St. Louis, MO, pp. 135–139.
7 McAnulty, J. (2013) *Proceedings Presented During Junior Surgery Lectures*. University of Wisconsin School of Veterinary Medicine. Madison, WI.
8 Fossum, T.W. (2013) *Small Animal Surgery*, 4th edn. Mosby Elsevier, St. Louis, MO, p. 196.
9 Swaim, S.F. (2006) *Veterinary Clinics of North America- Small Animal Practice*. Volume 36. W.B. Saunders Co, Philadelphia, PA, pp. 748–749.
10 Herron, M., Agarwal, A., Kierski, P. *et al.* (2014) Reduction in wound bioburden using a silver-loaded dissolvable microfilm construct. *Advanced healthcare materials.*, 3. doi:10.1002/adhm.201300537.
11 Demaria, M., Bryden, J.S., Hauptman, J.G. *et al.* (2011) Effects of negative pressure wound therapy on healing of open wounds in dogs. *Veterinary Surgery*, 40(6), 658–669.
12 Bohling, M.W. (2012) Burns. In: Tobias, K.M. & Johnston, S.A. (eds), *Veterinary Surgery – Small Animal*. Volume II. Elsevier, St. Louis, MO, pp. 1291–1301.

7

Postoperative Care

Gerianne Holzman[1] and Sandra Engelmeyer[2]

[1] *University of Wisconsin, School of Veterinary Medicine, Emerita, Madison, WI, USA*
[2] *Blue Pearl Veterinary Partners, Golden Valley, MN, USA*

All patients deserve quality care while hospitalized. Patients recovering from surgery have special needs to maintain their comfort. This includes both the immediate postoperative period of anesthesia recovery and any further hospitalization required until discharged. Postoperative pain control is essential to healing and patient well-being. (Note: Pain control is covered in Chapter 2 *Preoperative Planning*.)

Anesthesia Recovery

Patients must be directly monitored while recovering from anesthesia. After stopping the flow of anesthetic gas, patients are maintained at an appropriate rate of oxygen flow until they are breathing well on their own. They are never left alone while an endotracheal tube is in place. Once a patient shows signs of consciousness, it is appropriate to deflate the endotracheal tube cuff and extubate the patient. Brachycephalic breeds require extended respiratory monitoring and are not extubated until fully awake or chewing at the endotracheal tube [1]. Some patients may become very restless and begin thrashing during this time. It is important to assess the patient's pain level to determine if pain is causing the behavior. If pain is noted, appropriate pain medications are provided to maintain analgesia. If pain does not appear to be causing the patient distress, it is possible for the patient to be negatively reacting to anesthetic or analgesic medications. Many of these drugs can cause dysphoria. A tranquilizer may be indicated for these patients to calm them down while the drugs are dissipating from the body.

Even after the endotracheal tube is removed, patients recovering from surgery must be closely watched. (This is also a great time to trim toenails. Clients appreciate this extra benefit.) The patient's body temperature is monitored for changes. Hypothermia is very common, especially during long surgical procedures. The intraoperative and postoperative use of circulating hot water blankets, hot-air warming units, blankets, towels, and so on lessens the incidence of hypothermia. Patients are warmed to a body temperature of 99 °F before removing supplemental heating sources. Some patients, particularly cats, may develop hyperthermia after surgery. This appears to be an

Surgical Patient Care for Veterinary Technicians and Nurses, Second Edition.
Edited by Gerianne Holzman and Teri Raffel Kleist.

Companion website: www.wiley.com/go/holzman/patient

abnormal reaction to certain narcotic medications [2, 3]. These patients are cooled by housing in a stainless steel cage with no bedding, applying cool, wet towels over their back or groin area, and using fans. The patient is continuously monitored until a normal temperature is achieved.

While recovering from anesthesia, patients may not have complete control of their bladder or bowels. Keeping the patient and cage clean are imperative to avoid contamination of the surgery site and to maintain patient comfort.

Once a patient is fully awake and able to stand (assuming it is expected to stand after surgery), it is safe to return the patient to its normal hospital cage. Dogs are walked, prior to returning to their cage or run, to urinate and defecate. Orthopedic and neurologic patients may need the assistance of a sling, towel, or blanket to aid their ambulation. Patients must not be allowed to slip and fall after any procedure. (See Chapter 8 *Aftercare and Home Care* for more information on postoperative supportive devices.)

Self-Trauma

The surgical incision is at risk of self-trauma from licking, chewing, and scratching. The most common method of prevention is the use of an Elizabethan collar or E-Collar (Figure 7.1). E-Collars come in various sizes and materials. Cats often do very well with flexible E-Collars while determined dogs require rigid ones. Inflatable collars can prevent access to thoracic or abdominal incisions, but some patients can still get to extremities. T-shirts, socks, and custom-made body suits can be used as well [4].

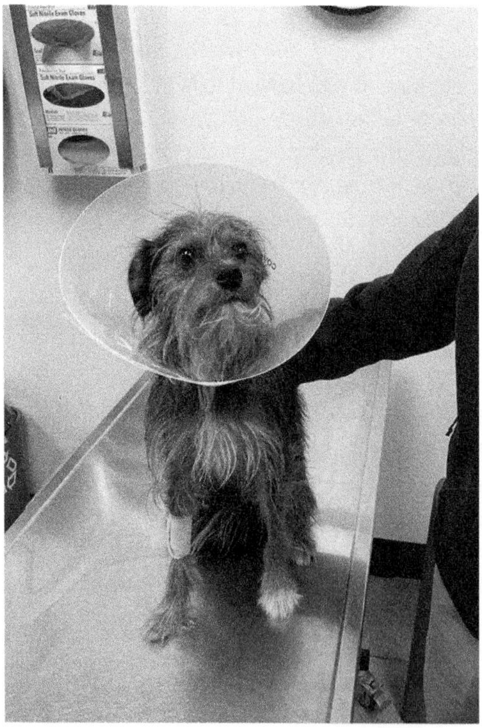

Figure 7.1 Rigid Elizabethan Collars (E-Collar) prevent self-trauma.

Housing

Patients become stressed when not in their home environment and surrounded by their families. They are exposed to new smells, sounds, and handlers. Providing them with a comfortable and safe area, away from noise and hospital traffic, calms their fears and aids in healing.

Bedding

Many forms of bedding and housing are available to maximize patient care and comfort. Blankets and towels provide warmth and padding from cage and run floors. They must always be laundered and sanitized between patients. Monitor bedding frequently for patient soiling and change bedding as needed. Patients must never be allowed to reside in their urine, feces, or other body fluids. When soiled bedding is found, it is imperative to also check and clean the patient. Urine and feces left on the hair and skin may cause scalding and wound contamination. ***Treat patients as one would want one's own pet taken care of.***

Pads

Foam rubber pads provide extra comfort for recumbent patients as well as those recovering from surgery (Figure 7.2). To avoid cross-contamination between patients, the foam rubber is enclosed in an impermeable material. These pads can be custom-made in sizes that partially or completely cover the floors of cages and runs. They are also made in a variety of thicknesses depending upon the depth of foam rubber interior. The pads are covered with waterproof material and should be cleaned and disinfected between patients. They are monitored for patient chewing or damage. If damaged, prompt repair is important to prevent patient ingestion from chewing the internal foam rubber as well as contamination and wetting of the foam.

Perforated Mats

Rubber and plastic mats come in a variety of sizes and configurations. Commercially available mats are made in sizes specifically made for different brands of cages and runs or available by the roll and cut, in clinic, to custom sizes. They come ribbed or with circular holes to allow drainage (Figure 7.3). While they aid in keeping a patient out of urine, some urine may still be trapped

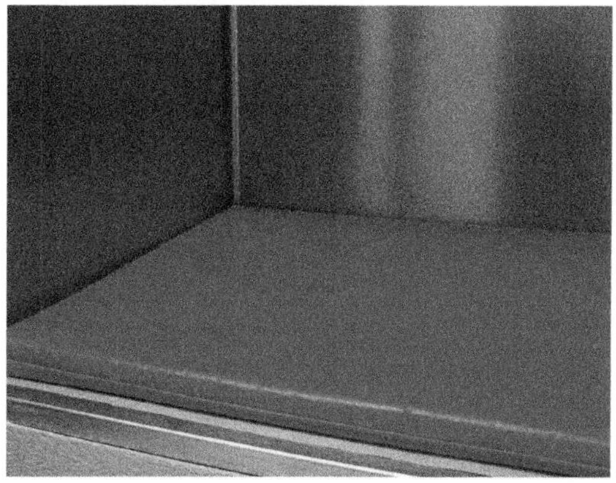

Figure 7.2 Cage pads provide comfortable conditions for patients. They must be impermeable and easy to disinfect.

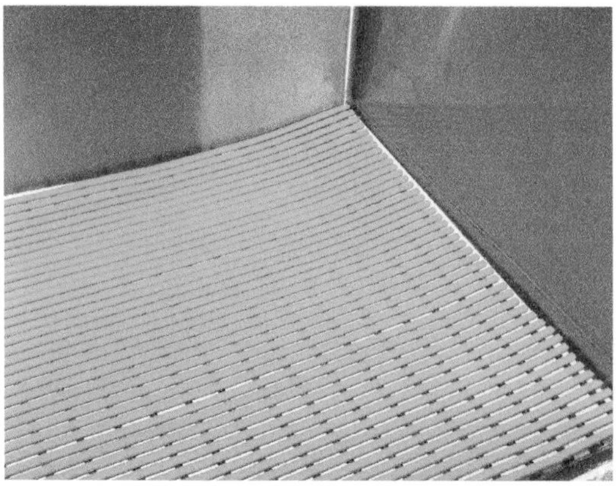

Figure 7.3 Perforated cage mats allow urine and other fluids to pass away from the patient, however, they are not soft and provide minimal padding.

between the mat and the patient. Close patient monitoring reduces this problem. These mats also provide traction for patients needing extra footing. However, they are generally hard plastic or rubber and provide minimal padding.

Other Mats

Yoga and other commercially available mats are generally thin, providing minimal padding. However, they are great for providing extra traction for patients in cages. They, also, are beneficial for performing patient exams – both for patient and technician/veterinarian comfort. Thin mats provide stability for standing exams. They provide padding for personnel standing, kneeling, or sitting while examining or restraining a patient.

Other Bedding

A wide variety of beds is commercially available for added patient comfort. These include covered corrugated foam rubber which help to prevent pressure sores. Four-legged "hammock" type beds made of plastic mesh aid in keeping recumbent patients comfortable, allow urine flow, and provide cooling and air circulation (Figure 7.4).

Air and water mattresses are especially beneficial for preventing skin ulcerations. However, they are susceptible to leakage caused by patients' nails and teeth. They also do not allow urine to flow away from the patient. These mattresses provide the best patient comfort when covered with a

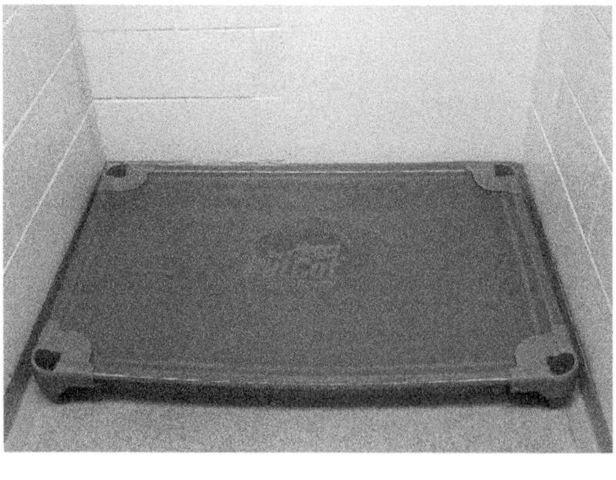

Figure 7.4 Hammock beds allow fluids to pass away from the patient, are soft, and help to cool a patient with air circulating beneath the bed.

blanket or towel. If any of these types of beds are not available, rotating a patient frequently helps to alleviate pressuresores in recumbent patients.

Cage Lining

Cages can be lined with absorbent pads to provide patient traction and absorb urine and spilled water. They also provide cold protection from the metal, plastic, or fiberglass cage floor. Commercially available cage paper can be ordered to custom-fit cages.

Boxes/Hiding Spots

Plastic litter pans and covers, boxes, and crates provide stressed patients with comfort and help to keep small patients warm. Cats, especially, are anxious when hospitalized. Arranging a place for them to hide may help to calm them. Extra blankets or towels allow for burrowing. The top of a covered litter pan placed on a blanket is a great place for a cat to hide (Figure 7.5). It can easily be lifted up to allow patient access. Simply covering the front of the cage with a towel can give a kitty a feeling of safety by lessening visual stimulation.

Blanket-lined boxes and large litter pans, either upright or on their side, give cats and small dogs a compact, warm-resting area. The sides of the box/pan must be low enough to allow the patient to move in and out. Caution is taken to monitor the patient for box chewing to avoid gastrointestinal obstruction.

Crates of assorted sizes and configurations provide a safe, warm, and closed environment for small dogs and cats. They also provide ease of transporting the patient around the hospital. If a patient arrives at the clinic with a crate, housing the patient in its own crate while in a cage is helpful. This is especially useful for calming stressed patients by providing them with the "smell of home." Placed in the patient's cage, the crate's door is left open for patient access. Crates are inspected and cleaned as needed to avoid post-op contamination and soiling.

Cage Height

Housing cats in upper cages helps to relieve their stress. However, this is not practical with fractious patients – cats or dogs. These patients should always be housed in lower or mid-height cages to allow easier patient access and to protect personnel from injury. Patients in middle-height cages

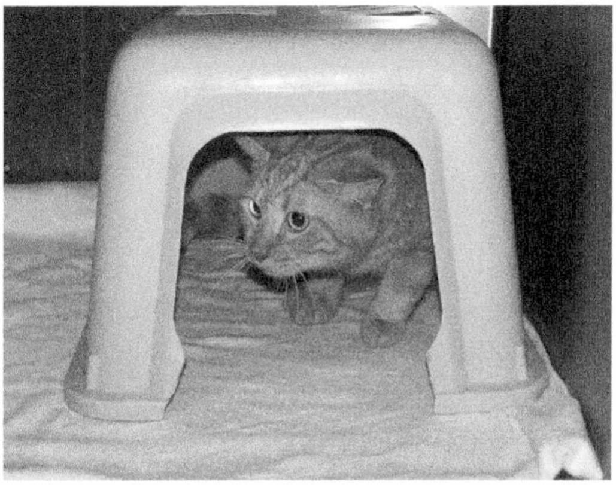

Figure 7.5 Boxes, crates, and litter pan covers provide a great secure "hiding place" for feline patients.

can be coaxed onto a gurney at the same height level. Fractious and fearful patients are easiest to manage in low cages and runs. Patients will often walk out of an open cage or run door if they do not feel threatened. Minimal personnel in the area help the patient to feel less intimidated. When leaving an lower cage or run door open, the surrounding kennel doors must be secured to avoid patient escape. When drastic removal measures are needed, e.g. rabies pole, the only safe area for accessing a patient is a lower cage or a run.

Pheromones

Feline facial pheromones sprayed on blankets or as atomizers in rooms help to soothe cat patients. It calms and relaxes them during hospitalization and during venous catheterization [5]. Canine pheromones as sprays or atomizers in kennels may calm anxious dogs.

Nutritional Support

Patients are continually monitored for eating behavior both before and after surgery. Maintaining them on their home diet helps to encourage eating and reduces dietary upset from a change in the type of food. Trauma, surgery, pain, and the stress of hospitalization may lead to anorexia, as does the use of narcotics and anti-inflammatory medications. The body has a higher metabolic demand as it is recovering from surgery, infections, burns, and tumors [6]. Long-term hospitalization accompanied by anorexia leads to malnutrition. The use of feeding tubes is advisable in these patients. Clients can be taught how to maintain the tube at home and provide parenteral nutrition.

Stress-related diarrhea may occur in surgical patients. Providing them with a bland but nutritional diet may aid in reducing diarrhea. Homemade diets of boiled hamburger or chicken and rice are bland and often enticing to the patient. Many commercially available diets provide excellent nutrition to fit a variety of metabolic conditions.

Urinary Bladder Care

Following surgery, especially involving the spinal cord, patients may develop the inability to urinate. Many techniques are available for emptying a bladder. While in the hospital, a patient may have an indwelling catheter or repeated catheterization episodes. Care is taken to maintain sterile technique and minimize the risk of introducing bacterial cystitis. Catheterization of a male dog is much easier than a female dog, and dogs are easier than cats. Using a catheter of the appropriate size for the patient provides the best results while limiting urethral trauma. Highly pliable red rubber and Foley catheters decrease the chance of bladder and urethral perforation when compared to stiff polypropylene catheters. Indwelling catheters are sutured in place. Attached to an administration set and empty intravenous fluid bag or urine collection bag creates a closed system for urine collection. Patients are monitored closely to keep from chewing the catheter and often need an Elizabethan collar.

Bladder expression is tailored to individual patients. Cats and small dogs have easily palpable bladders that can be held in one hand. Grasping the bladder in one hand and providing gentle but firm compression may achieve the desired results. ***Never attempt to express the bladder of a patient with a potential urethral stricture***. *Struggling to express the bladder in these patients may result in a bladder rupture.* For larger patients, a two-handed technique is required. The patient may be laying in lateral recumbency or standing with support. Using the flat surfaces of the hand, not the tips of the fingers, palpate the bladder. While isolating the urinary bladder, the hands are pushed together, while also pushing toward the patient's back. This traps the bladder between the hands and the back, thus allowing only one path for the urine – out of the urethra.

Patients with bladder control are difficult if not impossible to express due to their sphincter control. Animals recovering from different types of intervertebral disc disease may have a neurogenic bladder thus lacking bladder control. This includes under or over activity of the detrusor muscle and the urinary sphincter depending on the site of the protruding disc.

Lower motor neuron (LMN) signs originate from lesions in the sacral spinal cord. LMN bladders are distended and easily expressed. Over discharge of the sympathetic nerves to the urethral sphincter causes failure of urethral relaxation in LMN patients.

Upper motor neuron (UMN) signs come from lesions to the thoracolumbar spine as well as the brain and brain stem. UMN bladders are distended but difficult to express. An accurate diagnosis by the attending veterinarian provides appropriate medical management of these conditions to aid in bladder expression.

Patients with overly distended bladders may leak urine leading to a misdiagnosis of their ability or inability to urinate. Unless a full voluntary stream of urine is observed, the presumption is that the patient is experiencing overflow urination. Palpating the bladder's size, and/or imaging the bladder, confirms this assumption. Patients with "overflow" have a distended bladder. This must be addressed immediately to avoid permanent damage to the bladder musculature.

Bandages

External Coaptation Concepts

External coaptation devices include external skeletal fixators (ESF), bandages, casts, splints, and slings [7]. Most of these apparatuses serve a specific purpose in orthopedic patient care. However, soft tissue patients require bandages for wound protection, active, and passive drainage control and for support. For example, a non-healing full-thickness wound of the hock may heal better with a splint support that decreases bending and stretching of the wound while allowing wound healing. Figures 7.6 and 7.7 show an example of an Irish wolfhound with a non-healing pressure sore treated with a custom-made orthotic splint. Multiple primary closure attempts were performed on this patient. However, due to the location of the wound, several incidences of dehiscence occurred.

The wound eventually closed by second intention after protection and support of the orthotic splint and topical therapy.

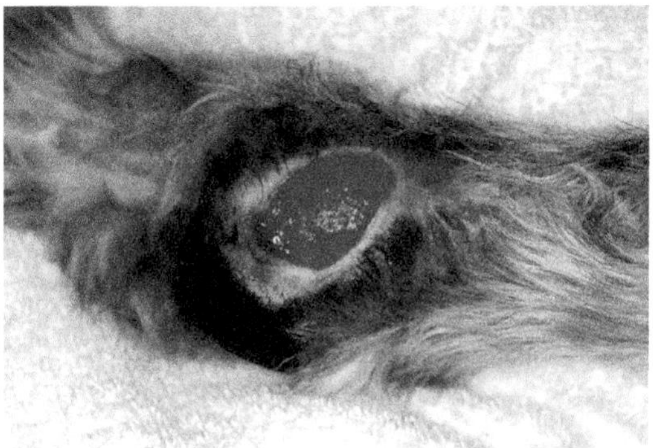

Figure 7.6 Wolfhound is shown with a non-healing granulating wound on the lateral side of the hock. The patient laying on the wound and motion within the hock decreased the ability to heal the wound. *Source:* Courtesy of Robert J. Hardie.

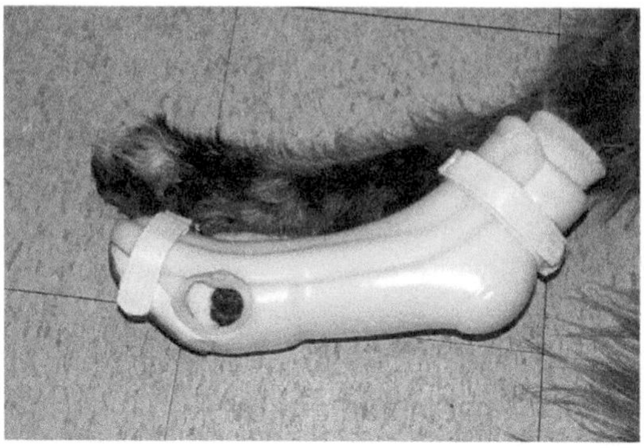

Figure 7.7 The same patient as seen in Figure 7.6 with an orthotic device to allow wound care, stop motion at the wound site, and protect the open lesion from lying on the ground. *Source:* Courtesy of Robert J. Hardie.

External coaptation serves the following functions:

1) *Immobilizes* a body part with external support: fractures, luxations, tendon ruptures, and wound protection all benefit from short-term or long-term protection. This may be temporary stabilization of a fracture prior to internal fixation or permanent support until healed such as a comminuted tibia fracture repaired with an external fixation device.
2) *Provides* control of fracture bending and some control of torsion but does not control compression or distraction. Fracture ends are still able to compress and distract within a cast or splint perhaps causing grinding and rounding of the fracture edges. ESF may provide control of all forces placed on a fracture.

To be effective in stabilizing a fracture, the entire bone must be supported. To do this requires the joint proximal and distal to the fracture to be immobilized. This is easily accomplished with injuries to the tibia/fibula by supporting the hock and the stifle. Correspondingly, fractures of the radius/ulna require immobilization of the carpus and elbow. Humerus and femur fractures require a spica splint for temporary stabilization. A spica bandage involves applying the bandage completely up the leg and incorporating the trunk. Splint material, extended from toes to body midline, is added to the bandage to keep the shoulder/hip from moving. If this type of bandage is not possible to apply, it is best to leave femur and humerus fractures with no protection. Coaptation that does not include the joint "above and below" the fracture may terminate at a fracture site, thus creating a fulcrum and putting more pressure on the injury [8].

Types of Support

Temporary Support

Bandages, splints, and casts provide *temporary support*. Applied to a fracture, prior to internal fixation, they control pain by limiting the movement of fractured bones. Further soft tissue damage is decreased from any sharp fracture ends that may cut or puncture muscles, veins, arteries, and skin. Stabilization with a bandage or splint may keep a closed fracture from becoming open with the bones' edges protruding through the skin. Provided as first aid; bandages, splints, and casts limit further trauma while allowing for safe transportation of a patient to a treatment facility.

Supplemental Support

External coaptation delivers *supplemental support* when applied after internal fixation for fracture or tendon repair.External skeletal fixators add stability, and control rotational forces of intramedullary pin fracture repair. Acute tendon tear and laceration repair require additional reinforcement to prevent bending and stretching as the tendon heals. Following many soft tissue and orthopedic procedures, postoperative bandages, applied for 24–48 hours, may control pain and swelling while keeping the incision clean and absorbing postoperative drainage. Recent studies show no reduction in swelling by bandaging patients after tibial plateau leveling osteotomy (TPLO) surgery [9].

Primary Support

Casts, splints, and external skeletal fixation devices offer *primary support* for certain fractures and chronic tendon strains. A young animal with a non-displaced fracture of the radius and an intact ulna may heal very well with a splint or cast. Greenstick or incomplete fractures also require less support than more serious injuries. However, petite dogs with a forelimb fracture often **do not** heal with only external coaptation [10]. Patients with chronic strains of the calcaneal (Achilles) tendon or tendon repair benefit from long-term support via a bandage/splint combination or a custom-made orthotic splint or brace (Figure 7.8). The orthotic can be made with a hinge to allow the ability to increase its range of motion over time.

Considerations

Not all orthopedic patients require external coaptation. Internal fixation of a fracture or ligament tear provides strong stabilization. They, most often, do not require any additional support other than a soft-padded bandage for 24 hours to control postoperative swelling. The veterinarian's decision to apply long-term external coaptation has several considerations.

1) *Tolerance*: Will a patient tolerate a bandage or an external fixator? Despite the use of an Elizabethan collar, dogs and cats may still aggressively try to pull a bandage apart or lick the pins of a fixator.

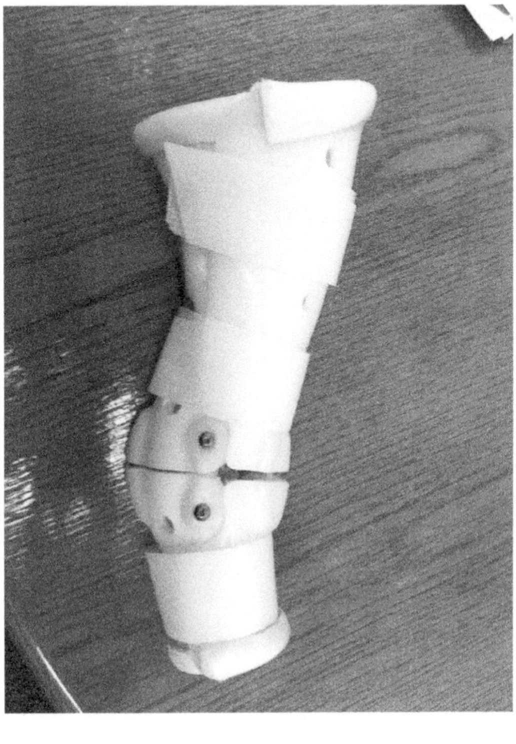

Figure 7.8 A custom-created orthotic with a hinge for treating a patient with a calcaneal tendon strain. The range of motion of the hinge is increased over time to allow more freedom of movement as the patient heals. *Source:* Courtesy of James T. Lewellen.

2) *Wound care*: The presence of open wounds often requires daily or more frequent treatment. Applying a Robert Jones bandage that requires much staff time, materials, and potentially patient sedation may not be the best option for these patients. However, the use of an easily replaced bi-valved cast will provide support for a fracture while allowing multiple quick bandage changes to attend to a wound. Very long-term wound care may benefit from a custom-designed splint for support, ease of removal, and minimization of bandage sores.
3) *Environment*: The patient's home living condition is a factor when determining the appropriateness of extended use of an external coaptation device. For example, dogs housed in outdoor pens and cats living on farms quickly soil bandages. Bandages that become wet and damaged provide no support and swiftly cause skin irritation. External skeletal fixation devices may become hooked on protruding home objects. This apparatus must also be kept clean from soil, water, and other contaminants. Other pets in the home may also be attracted to the patient's bandage, splint, etc. and must be monitored.
4) *Client compliance*: Veterinarians and veterinary technicians can provide the best care and support for the patient; however, it is imperative for the client to follow home care instructions. They must be educated in monitoring the external coaptation for problems. Clients need to provide the proper environmental conditions and monitor their pet's tolerance of the external coaptation device. (See more information on *Home Care* in Chapter 8.) If a client cannot or will not attend to the patient's needs, external coaptation may not be appropriate.

Anatomy of a Bandage

All bandages require the same "ingredients." As discussed with open wound management, these include the primary wound cover, a padding layer, a compressive layer, and a protective layer (Figure 7.9).

Additional components are added depending on the patient's condition and the bandage's purpose. Splint or cast material is added for support and tape stirrups aid in decreasing bandage slippage on a limb. High-quality materials give high-quality results. Using inferior products or re-using

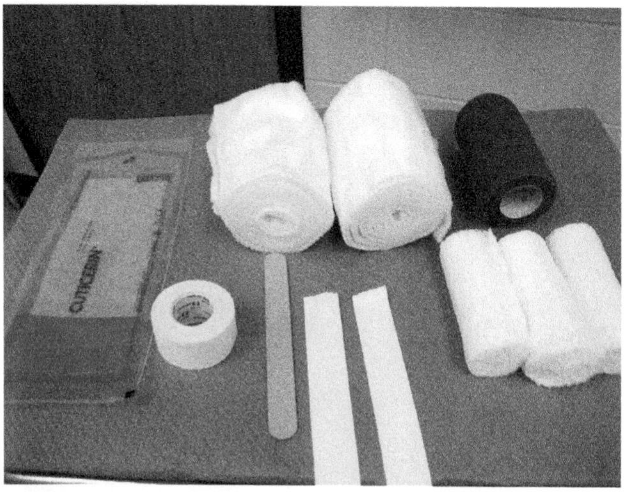

Figure 7.9 Anatomy of a bandage: (L – R) primary wound cover (oil-emulsion gauze), tape stirrups (foreground), and tongue blade to keep stirrups separated, cast padding, elastic gauze (foreground), and protective layer.

materials may save money but cause frustration to the person applying the bandage as the material may tear and fray or not be able to be applied appropriately thus causing patient discomfort. Bandaging is a skill and an art that requires practice. ***A poorly applied bandage may be worse than no bandage at all.***

Bandages applied to the abdomen, chest, and head are all soft-padded bandages. When used on the head, neck, and chest area, care is taken to avoid impeding the ability to breathe and/or eat. Head and ear bandages are kept high enough to avoid eye irritation. If one or both ears may be left exposed, a figure of 8 bandage is applied that aids in keeping the bandage in place. Likewise, chest bandages are often crossed over the front of the chest to keep the bandage from slipping back to the abdomen. Abdominal wraps are difficult to keep in place as they move around and slide backward. A strip of adhesive bandage material or tape applied to the skin serves as an anchor. The rest of the bandage is created with one-half of the width of the anchor strip exposed. After the final layer of material is applied, another strip of adhesive tape is added to include the edge of the bandage and the anchor strip. This anchor tape is left in place for as long as the patient requires the bandage. This avoids excess trauma to the skin from repetitive removal of the adhesive. When no longer needed, the anchor strip is removed with the help of an adhesive remover.

Despite one's best efforts, chest and abdomen bandages are difficult to keep in place. A variety of commercial products are available to provide wound coverage and compression in these areas. They are made of tubular stretch gauze, neoprene, and other materials. Often, they incorporate the legs or allow cutting of holes for legs. Product sizes vary and are custom fitted to individual patients. Some products include Velcro® straps to allow for more customization and others include no leg holes for use following amputation. Wraps are also available with pockets for portable monitoring devices.

Soft Padded

These bandages provide varying degrees of support depending on the amount of padding material. More padding placed under robust compression provides increased stiffness and strong support. Modified Robert Jones (MRJ) or soft-padded bandages provide wound coverage and reduce swelling both preoperatively and postoperatively. They are lightweight with approximately 0.5–2 cm of padding, thus giving only light support and non-rigid stability. However, due to the limited amount of padding, it is easy to apply excess compression thus causing a tourniquet effect on a limb or impeding breathing if applied over a thorax. There are many applications for this bandage for both short- and long-term use. It is the basis for all bandages. During application, the patient may lay in lateral recumbency, with the affected limb up, for orthopedic conditions, or may be standing for other indications. The following section describes the application of a limb bandage; other wraps are similar but without the use of stirrups.

Application of a Limb Bandage (Video 7.1)

1) *Apply tape stirrups to foot* (Figure 7.10): Application of stirrups to the medial and lateral side of the foot is more comfortable for the patient than application to the dorsal and palmer/plantar aspect. It avoids taping the pads together, adhesive material on the pads, and tape trauma to the tender skin over the toes. Location of stirrups may need adjustment to avoid taping over wounds (Video 7.1).

   Stirrups do not need to be long. Extending proximally to the carpus/tarsus and distally to about 10 cm beyond the toes is sufficient. Apply tape under – not over – a dewclaw to avoid compressing the nail into the foot causing a pressure sore. A tongue blade placed between the tape ends that extend beyond the foot keeps them from adhering to each other during bandage application. The tongue depressor is discarded after use.

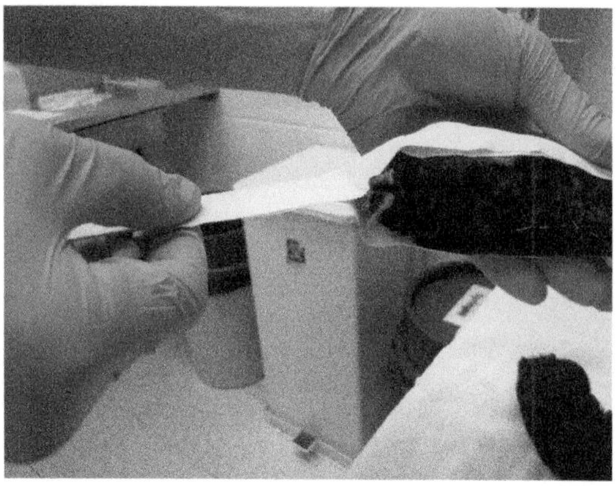

Figure 7.10 Tape stirrups applied to the medial and lateral side of the foot extending to just beyond the carpus or tarsus. A tongue depressor placed between the two tape strips keeps them from sticking together.

2) *Apply primary wound cover* (Figure 7.11): This may be adherent or non-adherent depending upon the patient's condition and needs. (See section on open wound management in Chapter 6 for more information.)

   Care is taken while applying this layer to avoid wound contamination. The use of gloves and not handling the patient side of the primary wound cover decreases the spread of microbes to the lesion. If a wound is located proximally on a limb, delay application of the wound cover until the padding layer reaches its location to keep the wound cover in place.

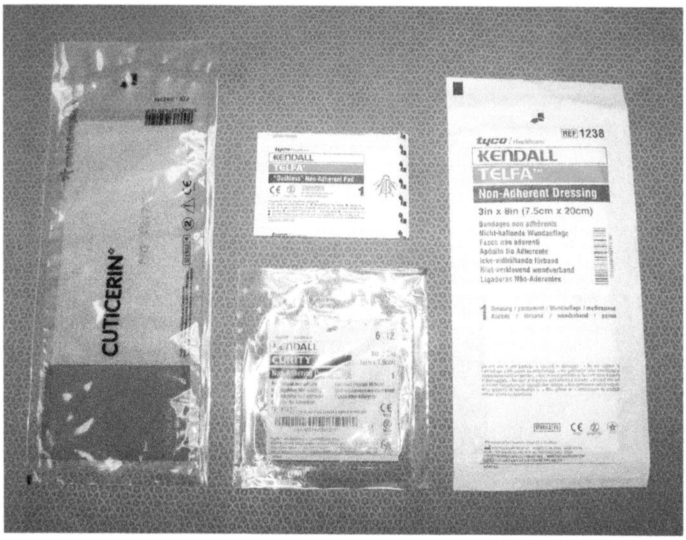

Figure 7.11 Primary wound cover examples: (L-R) oil-emulsion gauze in two sizes and Telfa® pads in two sizes – both items are non-adherent.

3) *Apply padding layer* (Figure 7.12): This layer provides wound protection and absorbs drainage. The thickness varies depending on the patient's needs. For a soft-padded bandage, moderate density is achieved with cast padding. This product is available in a wide variety of materials and widths. The patient's size determines the width of the bandage material. For example, do not use 6″ wide cast padding on a 2-kg patient and reversely while 2″ cast padding can be used on a 60-kg patient; it will take much time and material to cover its leg.

Limb bandages begin at the toes to maintain pressure throughout the leg and to avoid a tourniquet effect. Starting distally also allows fluid to move away from the toes/limb and into the body. Always keep the roll of cast padding near the limb – unroll the material on the leg not in the air. Maintain pressure by unfurling off the "back" of the roll. Note: In small animal practice, there is no preference for wrapping clockwise or counterclockwise. However, after determining a direction – continue in the same direction to avoid loosening the underlying layers.

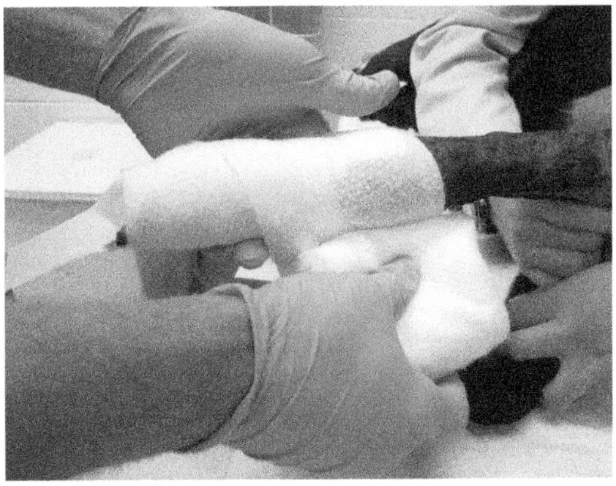

Figure 7.12 Begin by applying the padding layer of a soft-padded bandage. The roll stays next to the limb to control placement, and the cast padding is unfurled off the "back" of the roll to control pressure.

Begin by covering the foot twice with cast padding to secure the material to itself. Unless indicated by the patient's condition (e.g. toe injury), the two center toes of the foot should remain exposed to monitor the foot for rotation, temperature change, swelling, redness, odor, and discharge. After securing the cast padding to the foot, continue wrapping the leg by overlapping the cast padding by about one-half of its width. Placing the material at an angle to the limb avoids creating a horizontal band and tourniquet effect. At the proximal end of the bandage, also wrap the limb twice to secure the cast padding at the top. Continue wrapping the leg moving proximally and distally until the desired amount of cast padding is applied. To maintain the angle of the material, a tuck or tear may be required. The use of even and constant pressure during the application of the cast padding, and avoiding bunching, circumvents bandage sores. The cast padding is applied in even layers to maintain uniform pressure on the limb.

4) *Apply compressive layer* (Figure 7.13): Compression adds some support to the limb by stiffening the padding layer. It also reduces wound swelling by moving fluid away from the limb into the rest of the body. The material of choice for this layer is stretch gauze. It comes in a variety of materials and widths. Veterinary technicians benefit from sampling different products for durability, stretch, and consistency to determine a personal preference. As with cast padding, the patient's size determines the width of the material to be applied

   Stretch gauze is applied over the cast padding beginning at the toes. A small edge of cast padding extends beyond the gauze at both the distal and proximal ends to keep the gauze from cutting into the skin. Cover the foot twice to adhere the gauze to itself. Continue proximally up the limb as with the cast padding while maintaining the gauze at an angle to the limb. Keep the roll of material directly next to the padding and unfurl along the limb, not in the air, to maintain even pressure. To increase/maintain compression, use the hand not holding the roll of gauze to compress the cast padding while bringing the gauze over the hand. For maximum compression over a large quantity of padding, the padding may be compacted from both directions.

   As the stretch gauze is applied, lumps will appear in the bandage. Continue to apply layers of gauze overlapping one-half of the width of the material, moving distally to proximally, until the bandage is smooth and free of bulges. This may require several layers. Even pressure throughout the bandage is imperative to avoid pressure sores and a tourniquet effect – special attention is given to the toes to assure the bandage is as tight over the toes as through its entirety. The bandage should have a uniform firmness.

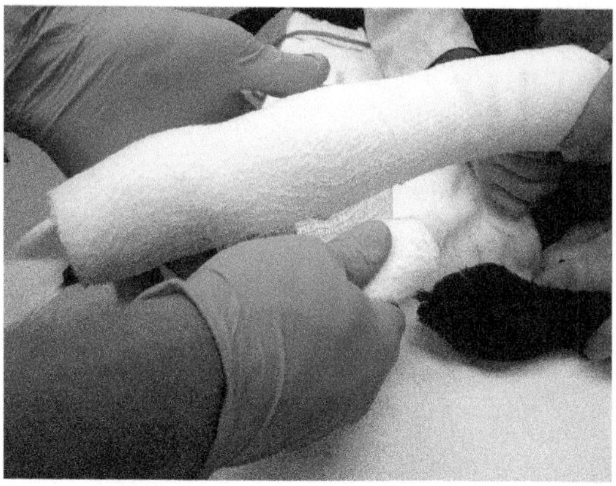

Figure 7.13 The compressive layer is placed over the padding layer to apply pressure to decrease edema and provide stability to the bandage.

5) *Attach tape stirrups to the gauze layer*: The tongue depressor is removed from the ends of the tape stirrups that have been extending distal to the toes. The tape is twisted 180° to place the adhesive surface on the stretch gauze. If needed, the tape is gently pulled proximally to assure exposure of the two center toes.
6) *Apply protective layer*: The protective layer keeps the bandage clean and possibly a bit dry if exposed to a minimal amount of moisture. It is not meant to provide support or compression. Materials used for the protective layer include adhesive-backed elastic tape, white adhesive tape, and self-adhering elastic tape. These products are available in a wide range of widths, colors, and materials. Personal preference has some bearing on choice although each product has its own advantages and disadvantages.
   - Adhesive-backed elastic tape (sizes 1″, 2″, 3″, and 4″ width)
     - *Advantages*: Durable, adheres very well to underlying gauze and skin
     - *Disadvantages*: Scissors are required to cut tape, material must be cut to create smooth curves and edges, adhesive causes skin irritation, easy to over-tighten, and expensive
   - White adhesive tape (sizes 0.5″, 1″, 2″, and 3″ width)
     - *Advantages*: Durable, adheres well to underlying gauze and less so to skin, tears without scissors, available in waterproof style, difficult to put on too tight, and inexpensive
     - *Disadvantages*: Stiff and difficult to conform; strong adhesive makes it difficult to handle and remove from roll
   - Self-adhering tape (sizes 2″, 3″, 4″, and 5″ width)
     - *Advantages*: Easily conforms to body shape, variety of colors, does not adhere to skin, may tear without scissors, and easy to decorate
     - *Disadvantages*: Not waterproof, easy to over-tighten, moderate expense, and prone to wear on bottom of foot

Apply the protective layer in the same manner as the cast padding and stretch gauze. Begin distally at the toes, going around the toes twice to secure the bandage material. Leave a small

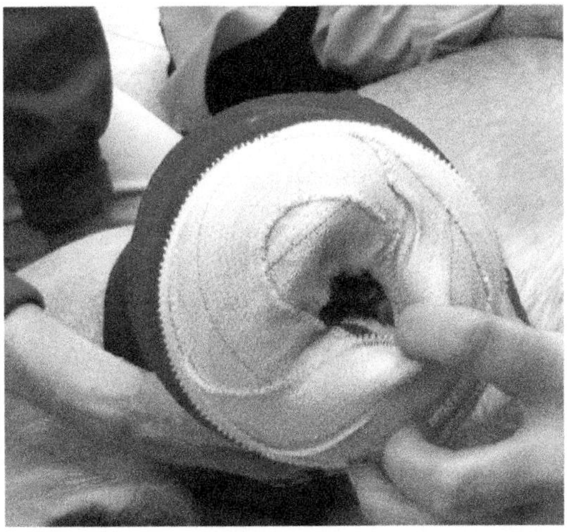

Figure 7.14 The protective layer of self-adhering or adhesive-backed bandaging tape keeps the bandage clean. Bandaging tape applied over the edge of the padding prevents the patient from pulling on the cast padding and may provide better friction for walking.
Source: Courtesy of Jason Bleedorn.

amount of cast padding exposed at the distal and proximal ends of the bandage to avoid the protective layer cutting into the skin. Some patients tend to pull at the cast padding, therefore covering the entire edge of the bandage may alleviate this problem (Figure 7.14). Additionally, bringing the edge of the protective layer over all bandage material and tucking in the edges assuring no direct contact with the skin may keep a patient from bothering the bandage. Elastic bandaging tapes can cut into the skin if applied incorrectly.

After covering the distal end of the bandage, continue proximally on the limb by overlapping the material by one-half of its width and proceeding at an angle to the leg. Cuts or tucks in the material may be needed to go around curves. This material is *not* applied under tension as it provides protection only, not compression. One layer is usually sufficient. On rare occasions, adhesive elastic tape is applied at the proximal end of the bandage to keep it in place. This may occur if the injury is very proximal on the limb and a splint is not desired to keep the bandage from slipping down. However, most properly applied bandages do *not* need this extra adhesion and the adhesive tape causes skin irritation.

The most important parts of the bandage (primary wound cover, padding, and compression) are not what the owners observe. However, the client may perceive the quality of the wrap by its external looks. Assuring the protective layer is smooth, wrinkle-free, and clean provides the client with confidence. Adding decorative elements to the bandage creates an extra personal touch (Figure 7.15a, b).

Robert Jones

The Robert Jones (RJ) bandage is bulky and cumbersome. Its size provides bending, and some rotational, stability to a fracture. The RJ also provides much compression to decrease swelling and apply pressure to a wound. It is used only for injuries distal to the elbows or stifles to provide stabilization of the joint above and below a fracture site. If applied to a femur or humerus injury, the proximal end of the bandage may rest at the fracture site, creating a very heavy fulcrum and causing greater injury to the patient. This bandage takes much time to apply and sedation of the patient may be required. The RJ is meant for short-term use.

The basic elements are the same as the padded or MRJ bandage except for the quantity of materials required. The other difference is to use roll cotton instead of cast padding as the padding layer.

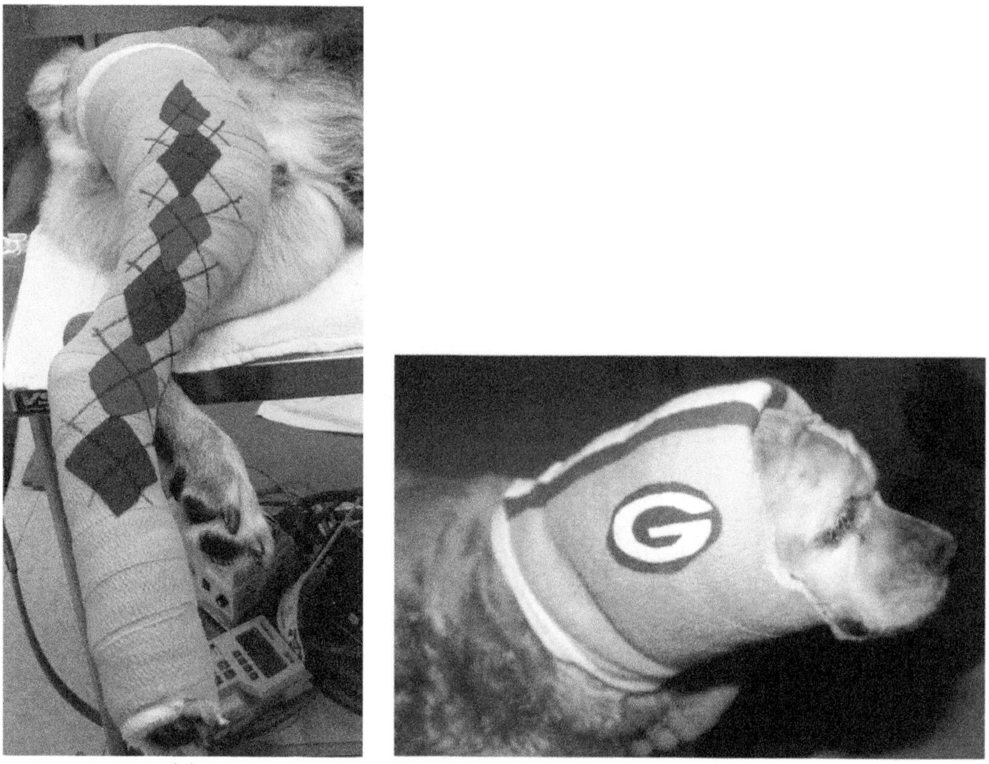

(a) (b)

Figure 7.15 (a) Bandage decoration is fun and entertaining for the client, and (b) showing home team spirit on a bandage.

The stirrups and primary wound cover are applied as described under "padded/MRJ" bandage. As a full-size roll of cotton is unrolled, it is torn in half (width) and re-rolled creating two narrower rolls of cotton. This allows for easier handling and maneuvering around curves of the leg. The entire leg is wrapped, beginning distally at the toes with the two center toes exposed, while overlapping the cotton by one-half of its width. One or two layers of cotton may be needed as well as more rolls of cotton to create the required 4–8 cm of padding. The bandage is extremely bulky at this point.

Stretch gauze is applied in the same manner as for an MRJ – beginning at the toes. Due to the large quantity of cotton to be covered, using as wide a gauze as can be comfortably handled cuts down on the amount of time required to complete the compression. Alternate the gauze roll between the hands and use the opposite hand to compress the cotton. Many layers of gauze are needed to compact the cotton to one-half of its original size. Care is taken to provide even pressure throughout the bandage. When finished, the bandage should "thump like a watermelon." It is difficult, but possible, to apply too much pressure and compression to a Robert Jones bandage.

After compression, the stirrups are attached to the gauze, and the protective layer is applied as with the MRJ bandage. Since this bandage takes an incredible amount of time and materials to complete, it is not meant for a wound requiring frequent attention. Again, it is only meant for temporary fracture stabilization.

Splints

Purposes

Splints have several uses in orthopedic surgery for temporary, supplemental, and primary support. Soft tissue surgical patients may need splints to provide wound stabilization and after skin grafting to avoid tension on the wound/graft. The three main types of splints are as follows.

1) Limb splint = the most commonly applied splint.
   a) *Definitive* stabilization of fractures: young animals, minimally displaced, and distal to elbow or stifle
   b) *Temporary* stabilization of other fractures, luxations, and subluxations distal to elbow or stifle
   c) *Supplemental* post-op support of above conditions
   d) Must be well padded as previously described
   e) Easy to over-compress due to moderate amount of padding
2) Spica splint = Less common, requires much practice to apply properly.
   a) Bandage extends from toes proximal to midline of torso
   b) Includes scapula or hip
   c) *Only* appropriate external coaptation for humeral or femoral fractures (stabilizes the joints above and below the fracture)
   d) *Temporary* or *supplemental* stabilization of fractures
   e) *Definitive* fixation of greenstick fractures of humerus or femur in very young patients
   f) Heavy sedation is needed for application
   g) Lengthy application time
   h) Difficult to use in pelvic limb of male dogs to avoid incorporating the prepuce into the bandage and urine soiling
   i) Cage confinement may be a better alternative if application is only for temporary support prior to internal fracture fixation of humerus or femur

Splint Materials

Clinic-created splints are a soft padded bandage with the addition of a rigid material to provide immobilization. Rigid materials include fiberglass casting tape, thermoplastics, aluminum rods, as well as pre-formed plastic and metal splints. Each of the materials has its own advantages and disadvantages. Newspaper rolls *do not* provide enough support or length to support a fracture (Figure 7.16). The patient shown in Figure 7.16 suffered from bilateral radius and ulna fractures.

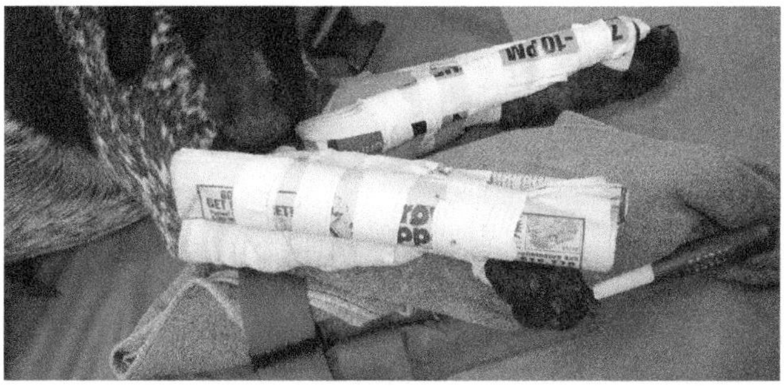

Figure 7.16 Newspaper splints for bilateral radius and ulna fracture provide NO STABILITY for these fractures.

The newspaper splints, shown in the image, are not rigid and do not stabilize the joint proximal and distal to the fracture sites.

1) Fiberglass (2″, 3″, 4″, and 5″ width)
   a) *Advantages*: Easily moldable and cuttable prior to curing, only water is needed to cure quickly (may be set up without water in a humid environment), and easy to use.
   b) *Disadvantages*: Gloves needed to handle, leaves remnants on tables, power tools are needed to cut after curing, may be expensive, and cannot be reformed after cured.
2) Thermoplastics (sheets and rolls, low and high temperatures)
   a) *Advantages*: Easily moldable and cuttable after heating, wide range of sizes and thicknesses available, lightweight, no gloves needed, does not stick to surfaces, easy to use, and can be reformed with re-heating
   b) *Disadvantages*: Hot water and heating source are needed to soften, difficult to cut prior to heating, and may be expensive
3) Aluminum rods (1/8″, 3/16″, 1/4″ 5/16″, and 3/8″ diameters)
   a) *Advantages*: Smaller sizes easily bendable and inexpensive
   b) *Disadvantages*: Not moldable, larger diameters require device to bend, large diameter is required for rigid stability in large patient, and challenging to keep in place
4) Pre-formed plastic or metal (variety of shapes and sizes)
   a) *Advantages*: Rigid fixation if fits properly, no adjustments required, and easy to use
   b) *Disadvantages*: Not moldable or bendable to conform to patient, requires correct size for patient, difficult to immobilize joint proximal and distal to fracture, often misused (e.g. spoon splints used for radius/ulna fractures do not immobilize the fracture), and expensive

Long- term splints, for months or years of treatment, may be custom created from a variety of resources. They often include a neoprene-type material, Velcro® straps for adjustment, and may include a piece of thermoplastic for extra rigidity (Figure 7.17). Specific measurements, taken in-clinic, provide the manufacturer with the appropriate dimensions for splint creation. Each company has its own measuring policy that must be followed precisely to provide optimum fit and patient comfort.

Splint Application

All clinic-created splints begin with a soft-padded bandage as previously described. Prior to application of the protective layer, the splint is applied over the compressive layer. To provide maximum support, splint material must extend the full length of the bandage with a small (1/4″–1/2″) ridge of bandage material extending beyond the splint. This keeps sharp edges of the splint material from cutting into the skin. If using casting tape for splint material, after measuring the required length, the remainder of the roll can be unrolled on the patient or placed on a *covered* countertop – cage papers work well to cover the work area. (Fiberglass leaves semi-permanent remnants on uncovered tabletops.) Rounding the edges of fiberglass and thermoplastics aids in patient comfort. It is easiest to cut these materials prior to curing. Fiberglass, especially, is very sharp with very pointy end threads, when hardened.

- The splint is applied smoothly over the compressive layer, shaping moldable and bendable splint material into the desired position.
- Pre-formed splints must fit the patient perfectly. If this does not occur, the limb may be in the wrong position, not be properly supported, and the patient may develop bandage sores.
- Care is taken when applying a moldable splint to avoid indentations in the material. These may occur from inadvertently pushing on the splint material with the fingers or by creating a crease. Dents in the splint can cause a pressure sore on the patient's skin.

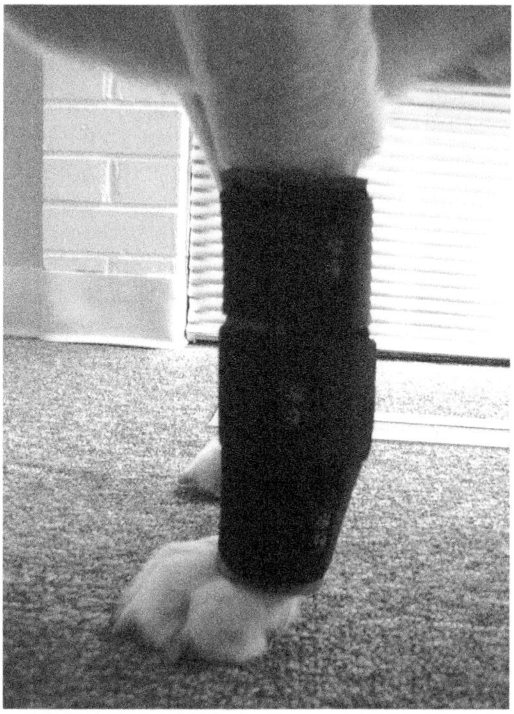

Figure 7.17 Commercially available carpal support, for long-term use, is comfortable, washable, and easily removed. *Source:* Courtesy of DogLeggs Therapeutic and Rehabilitative Products.

- After application of the splint material, it is held in place with an additional layer of stretch gauze or with a protective layer.
- Keeping one's thumbs upright when applying the final bandage layer(s) over the uncured splint material will avoid inadvertent indentations in the splint.
- Stirrups are moved into place over the stretch gauze after splint application but prior to adding the protective layer.
- If fiberglass or thermoplastics are used, the patient is kept immobilized until the product cures. This time varies with the individual material and manufacturer. Follow the instructions on the package insert.

Splints applied to toe fractures provide a challenge. They must extend beyond the toes to provide stability. The patient walks on the splint not on its toes. In order to protect the footpads from cuts and abrasions from the distal edge of the splint material, the toes are often completely covered with bandage material. Unfortunately, this eliminates the ability to assess the toes for swelling, odor, temperature change, and drainage. Stirrups may be added to provide some protection against slipping. They are applied as with a soft-padded bandage, except kept separated with a tongue depressor on each distal end of the stirrup. "Spoon" splints, for toe and carpus fractures, may be manufactured with fiberglass or thermoplastics and are available pre-made. Care is taken for appropriate fitting of the splint with padding added to its distal end to protect the foot.

Spica Splints

Spica splints create a special challenge because their application encircles the chest or abdomen. Their primary use is for patients that require stabilization of a humerus or femur fracture. Due to the length of time and manipulation needed to apply this bandage, the patient is generally under sedation. A spica splint is much better tolerated on the forelimb than rear limb. Therefore, this description is for a spica splint of the front leg.

1) The bandage begins with stirrups and incorporates the same materials as any other limb bandage. The cast padding is applied in a medial-to-lateral (counterclockwise) direction going proximally up the leg (Figure 7.18).
2) As the axilla is reached, the roll goes over the back, around the chest, then around the neck and back down the leg creating a half of a figure of eight or "spica" pattern (Figures 7.19 and 7.20). (The name Spica derives from Latin *spica virginis* "Virgo's ear of grain" [usually wheat][1] – the bandage material forms the same pattern as a wheat grain.) The cast padding applied over the back is spread out to provide padding to extend beyond the edges of the eventually applied splint material. (An assistant is needed to lift the patient as the chest encircling layers are applied.) Cast padding is added until desired thickness is achieved. Stretch gauze is applied over the cast padding, again, moving in a medial-to-lateral pattern. As compression is applied, care is taken to not impede chest movements or compress the neck. However, in order to do its job, the wrap must be snug. One finger should fit between the first layer of the wrap and the chest. After the patient is awake and standing, tightness is re-checked, as this may be difficult to assess in a sedate, laterally recumbent patient.

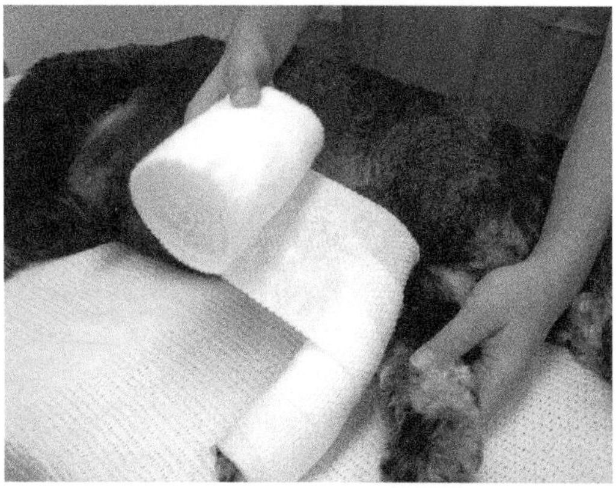

Figure 7.18 Begin a forelimb spica splint by wrapping counterclockwise or from medial to lateral on the limb. A spica splint is the only method of temporarily stabilizing a fracture of the humerus or femur. It may also be used as supplemental support following internal fracture fixation of either of these bones.

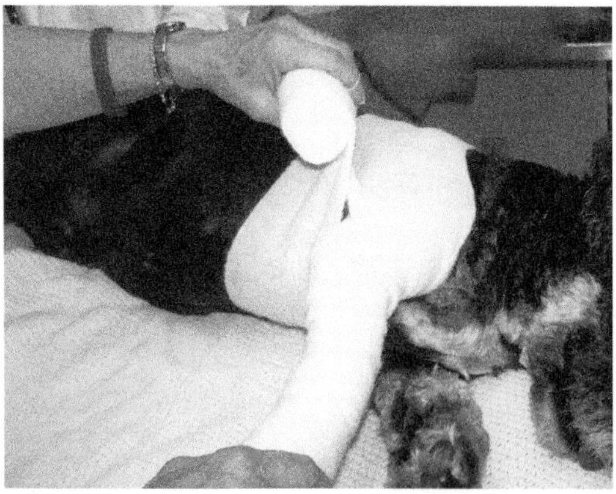

Figure 7.19 Spica splint: After reaching the most proximal aspect of the limb, wrap the bandage material over the back and around the chest, bringing the bandage up behind the caudal side of the limb.

1 http://en.wikipedia.org/wiki/Spica.

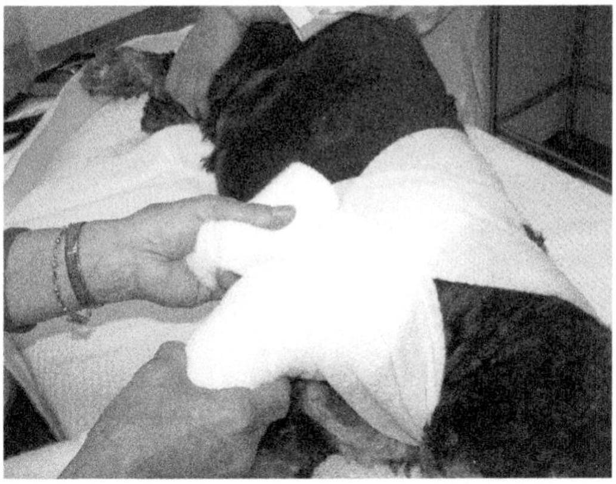

Figure 7.20 Spica splint: Bring the bandage material over the back and around the neck creating a "V" or spica pattern. Continue to add cast padding in this pattern until desired thickness is achieved. Secure the cast padding with stretch gauze placed in the same pattern.

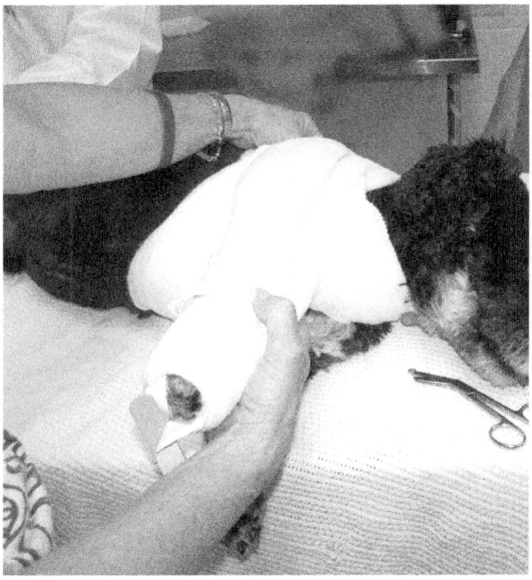

Figure 7.21 Spica splint: Apply splint material to the lateral aspect of the limb, extending to the middle of the back.

3) After application of the compressive layer, the splint material is added. Fiberglass casting tape is the best material to use although splint rods may be employed if sufficiently bendable. The cast material extends from the distal end of the bandage to the midline of the back (Figure 7.21). One or more rolls of cast material may be needed to provide the desired rigidity. Speed is essential when combining two rolls of casting tape into one unit so the first roll does not begin to cure prior to the second roll's application. As with a regular splint, the edges are rounded to avoid points on the corners.
4) Additional stretch gauze or the final protective layer is added to keep the splint in place. Care is taken to avoid indentations in the splint and compression of the chest (Figure 7.22).

Spica splints take much time and materials to apply. They are not meant for daily changes unless necessary for the patient's condition. They take much practice to perfect the technique of application.

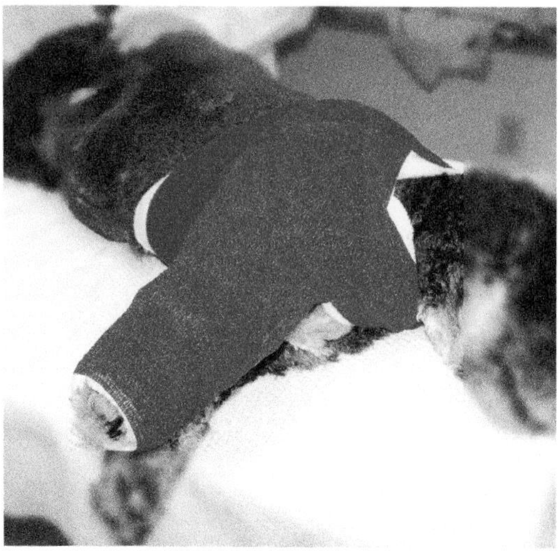

Figure 7.22 Spica splint: Apply stretch gauze to maintain positioning of the splint. Cover with a protective layer in the same placement pattern as the other bandage material.

Casts

The purpose of a cast is to provide fracture stabilization or joint immobilization. They are generally meant for long-term use and therefore must be comfortable for the patient and not cause skin lesions. Casts are initially applied while the patient is anesthetized or heavily sedated. They completely encircle the limb with a rigid material. It may seem counterintuitive but casts actually have less padding than a soft-padded bandage or a splint. While padding is needed to avoid skin irritation, it is the close conformity and proximity of the cast to the limb that provides support. Casts may be used in patients requiring *supplemental* support following arthrodesis or ligament repair. In limited applications, casts may provide *definitive* stabilization for fractures meeting all of the following requirements.

- Minimally displaced
- Non-articular
- Stable
- Transverse or incomplete greenstick
- Distal to elbow or stifle

Cast Application

1) The first layer of a cast is stockinette. This is sized to fit snugly to the leg and to extend a few centimeters beyond the cast in both directions. Cast application follows as outlined under soft padded bandage, except only one to two layers of cast padding are used. The compressive layer is minimal since there is little material to compress.
2) Following label directions, fiberglass-casting tape is applied over the compressive layer. Gloves are worn to keep the fiberglass from adhering to one's hands. The roll is unwound as with other materials, with extreme care taken to avoid any imprints in the cast material. (Indentations in the cast material translate to indentations into the skin causing lesions.) An assistant is needed to stabilize the limb during application. The assistant also wears gloves and only supports the limb with the flat part of the hands, not the fingers.
3) After the initial layers of casting tape are applied to the foot, the assistant pulls up the distal end of the stockinette to create a "rolled-edge" to the cast. After reaching the proximal end of the

cast, the stockinette is similarly pulled down to create the same rounded edge. Casting tape then covers the stockinette up to the rolled edge.

4) Time is essential to apply all layers of the cast before any parts begin to cure thus making the cast a cohesive unit. The cast must cure prior to the patient walking on it.

After application and curing, the cast can be cut on the lateral and medial sides to create two pieces – like a clamshell (Figure 7.23). This is a bi-valve cast that can be removed, as necessary, if skin wounds need attending. The two halves are kept together with adhesive tape.

A cast saw and spreader is required to cut a cast either for bi-valving or for final removal (Figure 7.24). The oscillating blade of a cast saw limits the chance of cutting the patient's underlying skin and is used in an "up and down" not sideways motion. When planning for a bi-valve cast, thin plastic applied over the stretch gauze, prior to application of the cast, keeps the cast material from adhering to the compressive layer. Remove the plastic prior to re-application of the cast.

For very long-term use, casts may be custom-made by an orthotic specialist. Created from thermoplastics, they are well-padded and kept in place with straps and buckles (Figure 7.25). A strained but not severed calcaneus tendon is an example of the use of this cast. It takes many months to heal. The orthotic device is adjusted over time to allow the patient increased mobility and movement in the hock joint (Figure 7.26).

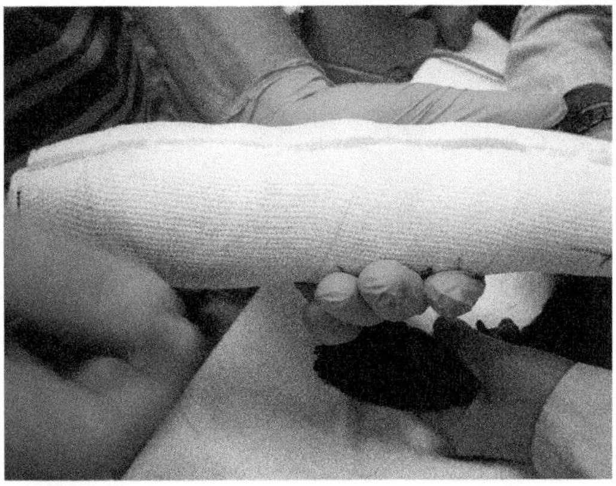

Figure 7.23 Cutting a cast in half (bi-valve) allows for wound care and easy replacement without the need to re-create the cast.

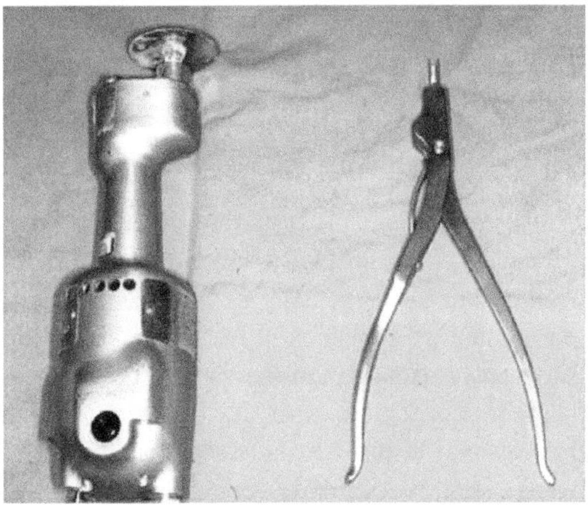

Figure 7.24 The oscillating blade cast saw cuts a cast for removal or bi-valving. The cast spreader opens up the two halves of the cast.

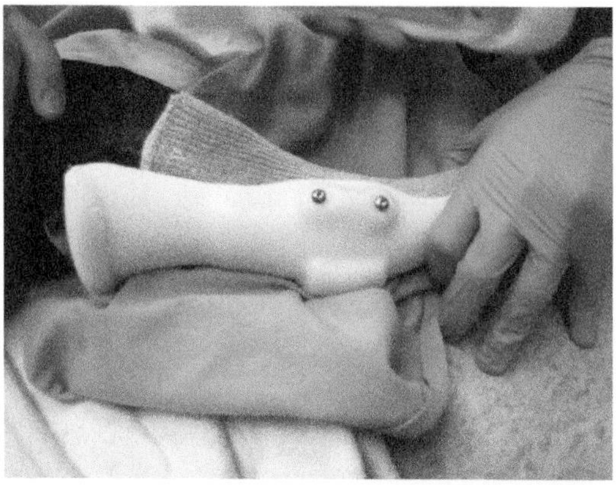

Figure 7.25 Patients requiring a long-term cast or splint benefit from fitting with a custom-made orthotic device. This patient's calcaneal tendon laceration was repaired, however, the repair failed while waiting for the orthotic to be created.

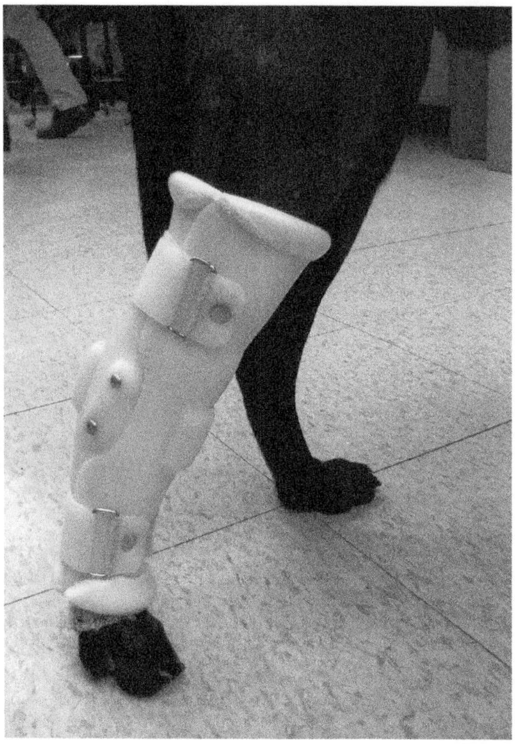

Figure 7.26 Patient seen in Figure 7.25 with the orthotic in place. Patient is able to stand normally and walks well.

External Coaptation Complications and Care

Bandages, splints, and casts require vigilant care to avoid wrap-induced trauma to the patient. Caregivers, in the hospital and at home, must check bandages daily. The skin adjacent to each edge of the bandage is especially susceptible to rubbing and prone to irritation. This varies from minimal redness to abrasions to full-thickness wounds. Catching wounds early and correcting their cause prevents patient suffering and the potential for additional surgery. Bandages are checked daily for odor. This is especially important for limb wraps exposed to moisture and dirt. A smelly bandage may be just wet and need changing or may be a sign of infection. Either way, the bandage needs to be investigated and replaced.

When possible, toes are left exposed to allow monitoring of swelling and temperature change. Both of these condions may be indicative of a bandage being too tight and needing replacement. Clients are advised to compare the temperature of the toes, either hotter or colder, to the toes of the opposite limb. Too cold may mean decreased circulation to the feet and too hot may be another sign of infection.

Any drainage at the edges or soaking through (strike-through) the wrap is a cause for concern. Blood, purulent material, bandage sores, or normal wound drainage can all ooze into and through a bandage. Drainage at the foot of a limb wrap can also indicate wounds or necrosis of the feet from over-tightness of the wrap or the patient chewing on the bandage.

External coaptation must be checked for slipping. For limb bandages, caregivers can monitor the distal location of the bandage in relation to the toes. If the toes were initially exposed and become covered, it means the bandage has moved distally. When a bandage slips, it does not provide the patient with the desired stability. Bandages thus improperly located lead to skin trauma and are potentially harmful to the patient's underlying condition. For example, if a cast slips distally, its proximal end may be directly at the fracture site creating a fulcrum allowing the fracture to bend.

All wraps must be comfortable for the patient. If the dog or cat tries to chew or bite at a bandage, the source of irritation should be investigated, which often includes removing a bandage to search for wounds. Patients with limb bandages that were walking well and then suddenly develop lameness may indicate a problem with the wrap. Clients are also advised to monitor their pet's attitude for changes suggestive of a problem.

Casts, splints, and bandages must be kept clean and dry. If soiled, they must be changed to provide patient comfort and avoid contamination of any underlying surgical or traumatic wounds. When going outside, limb wraps must be protected from the elements. Plastic bags serve this purpose but are often thin, so are checked after each use for holes and tears. They are only attached to the bandage with adhesive tape. While a rubber band will keep the bag in place, the rubber band may slip beyond the edge of the bandage and become a tourniquet on the limb. Used, dry intravenous fluid (IV) bags are great for covering smaller bandages. The port end of the bag is cut off creating a thick plastic pocket. Slits are cut into the bag for lacing of roll gauze or umbilical tape. It is easily tied onto the foot. Commercially available bandage covers come in a variety of sizes, materials, and durability (Figure 7.27). They are longer and cover more of the bandage than plastic or IV bags. Their attached straps keep them in place.

All bandage covers must be removed when the patient is indoors to avoid condensation and heat build-up within the wrap as well as to allow the bandage to "breath."

Some patients, despite the comfort of a bandage, will still chew the bandage or "have fun" pulling out the cast padding. Ingesting bandage material may cause gastrointestinal upset. Removed cast padding leads to loss of integrity of the bandage, cast, or splint and decreases its intended purpose. An E-Collar or other protective device should be used to prevent destruction of the bandage.

The client needs to check the bandage, cast, or splint at least daily. Weekly clinic re-checks are often needed for bandage replacement and professional monitoring. The patient's condition determines bandage change intervals and the required length of time the wrap needs to stay in place. Casts may be downgraded, over time, to splints and soft padded wraps prior to allowing the patient full use of a limb.

Becoming proficient in the application of bandages, casts, and splints takes much time and practice. It is an art to be able to gauge the required pressure, compression, tension, and requirements of the wrap. Practicing on rubber models, staff-owned pets, and patients is a valuable learning experience. Veterinary technicians with bandaging skills become a treasured resource for veterinary surgeons.

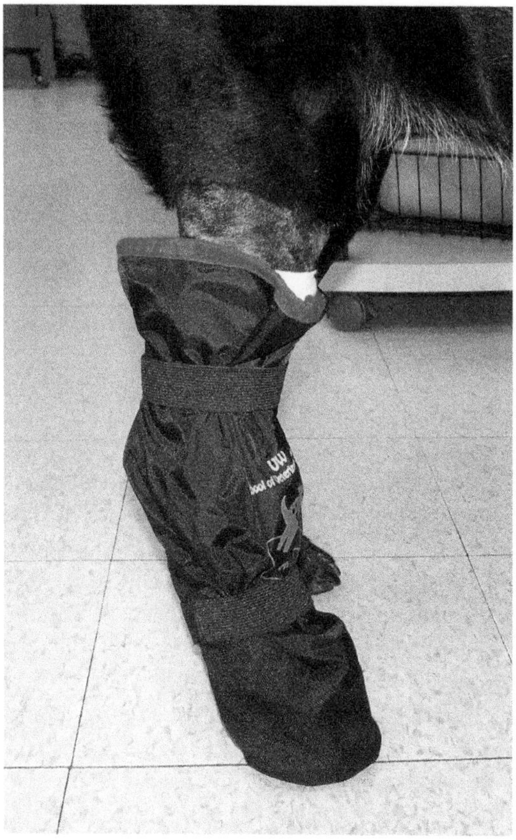

Figure 7.27 Many types of materials are useful for protecting bandages from the environment. Commercially available products are durable and kept in place with Velcro straps. *Source:* With permission of Medivet Products.

External Skeletal Fixation (ESF) Devices

Veterinarians apply ESF or fixation devices. Technicians assist the surgeons in their application and postoperative care. External Skeletal Fixation is employed for comminuted fracture repair, angular limb deformity correction, joint stabilization, tendon laceration immobilization, and a variety of other injuries. The structure includes pins or wires inserted through the bone and held in place with an external device. These include bars, clamps, rings or partial rings, and tubing filled with methyl methacrylate. Clamps and other structures do not contact the skin, thus preventing irritation. The entrances of the pins and wires are cleaned at least daily with dilute chlorhexidine solution or saline to remove any crustiness. If oozing is present, the adjacent skin is cleaned to decrease scalding.

Sterilized foam rubber sponges inserted between the bars and the skin provide postoperative compression to decrease swelling. Initially, a bandage is placed over the entire device to keep the sponges in place. With time, this wrap can be decreased in size, as less compression is needed. Stockinette, stretch tube gauze, or a stocking with the foot removed is often the only protection needed for long-term use. This also allows the client easy access to the insertion sites for cleaning.

All sharp ends of the pins are covered to avoid injury to the patient, client, or staff. Commercially available pin covers or "sharps" covers used for surgical instruments work well (Figure 7.28). Covering all sharp edges and protecting the bars helps to keep the bars from catching on objects and avoids scratches from the pointed ends of the pins (Figure 7.29).

During re-check exams, the ESF clamps and screws are tightened, as needed. Veterinary technicians may remove ESF devices. It is important to review post-application radiographs prior to ESF

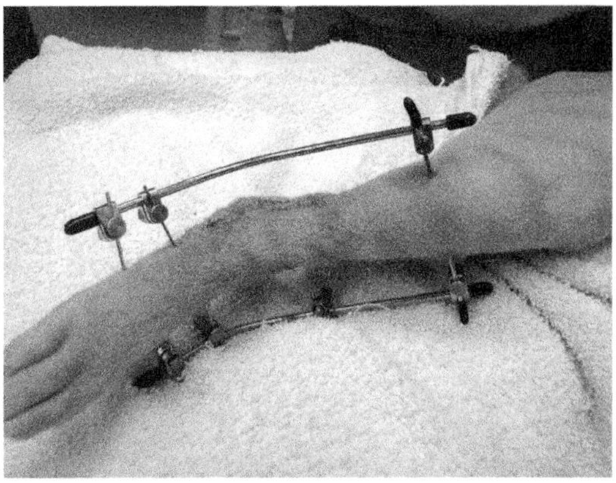

Figure 7.28 Surgical instrument "sharps" covers are perfect for covering sharp ends of external skeletal fixator pins.

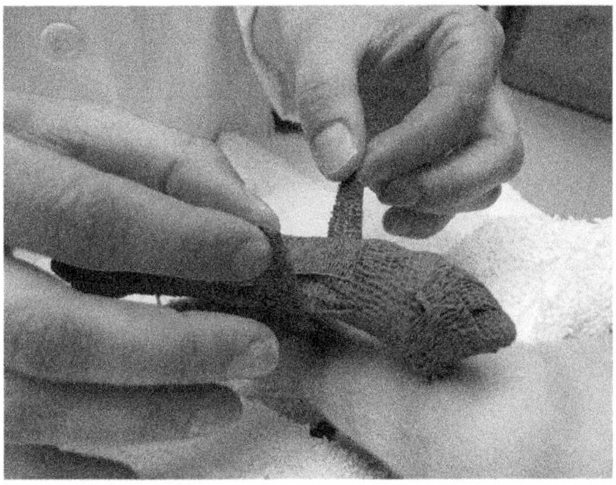

Figure 7.29 Covering the fixator bars with self-adhesive bandaging tape keeps them from being caught on other objects and avoids scratches.

removal. Radiographs provide important information regarding the fixator such as if pins are threaded, completely through both cortices of the bone, their location, and if they have special removal requirements. The external components of the devices (clamps and bars) may be cleaned, sterilized, and re-used for another patient.

Slings

Slings maintain a limb in a specific angle and prevent weight bearing. An Ehmer sling on the hind limb provides abduction and inward rotation of the hip. Its most common use is following closed reduction of a coxofemoral luxation. Various techniques are used for application, including adhesive tape with or without elastic gauze. The adhesive tape alone, however, is very irritating to the skin. Ehmer slings are often difficult to keep in place as they can slide off the butt. The commercially available DogLeggs Ehmer sling provides long-lasting comfort for the patient (Figure 7.30). Keeping a variety of sling sizes in the clinic allows for immediate postoperative use.

A Velpeau sling keeps the forelimb in flexion and prevents weight bearing. It is primarily used after various shoulder surgeries where movement needs to be restricted – such as luxation, minimally displaced scapular fractures, and severe shoulder instability. The sling is created with stretch gauze.

1) Wrap the gauze around the toes (Figure 7.31).
2) Flex the carpus and elbow while maintaining the shoulder in a neutral position.
3) Wrap the gauze around the chest behind the opposite forelimb while encompassing the carpus within the gauze (Figure 7.32).

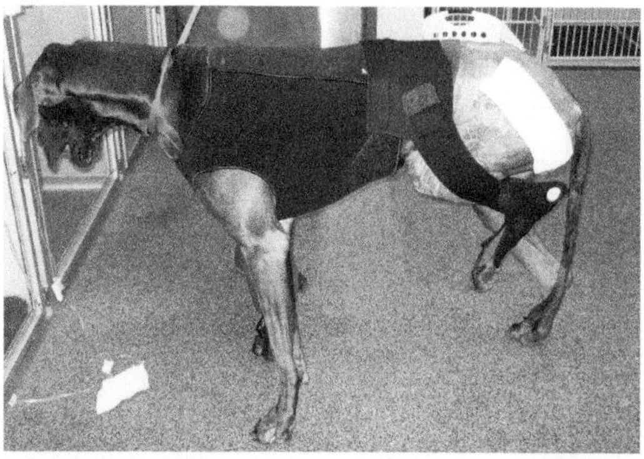

Figure 7.30 Commercially available Ehmer slings maintain the proper position of the rear limb following hip luxation surgery.
Source: Courtesy of DogLeggs Therapeutic and Rehabilitative Products.

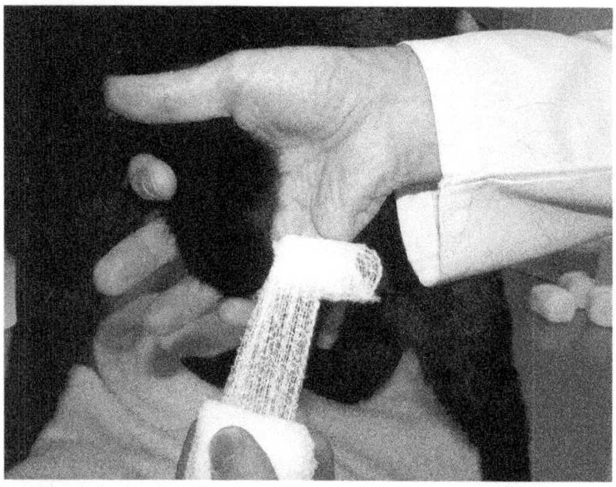

Figure 7.31 Velpeau sling Step 1: wrap stretch gauze several times around the front foot.

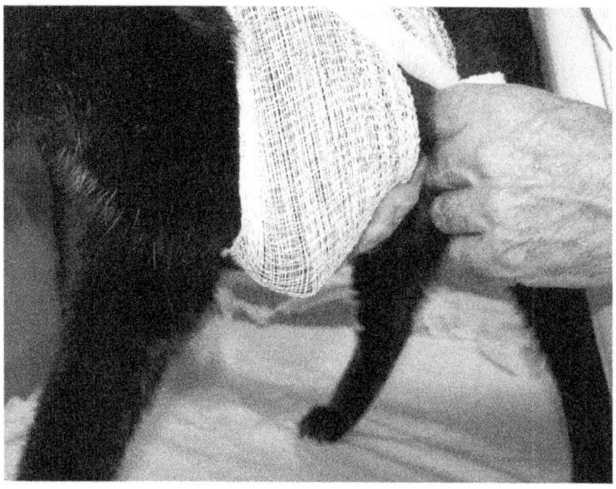

Figure 7.32 Velpeau sling Step 2: While maintaining flexion of the carpus and elbow, create a figure of eight wrap to keep the limb close to the body.

4) Apply multiple layers of gauze as needed to maintain the position of limb.
5) Apply the protective layer (Figure 7.33).

Commercially available Velpeau slings are, also, available (Figure 7.34).

Patients tolerate slings well but they must be monitored weekly for skin irritation and wounds inflicted by the bandage. After two weeks, joint contracture may occur and further use of the sling may be contraindicated [11]. Physical rehabilitation of these patients helps to return them to normal function.

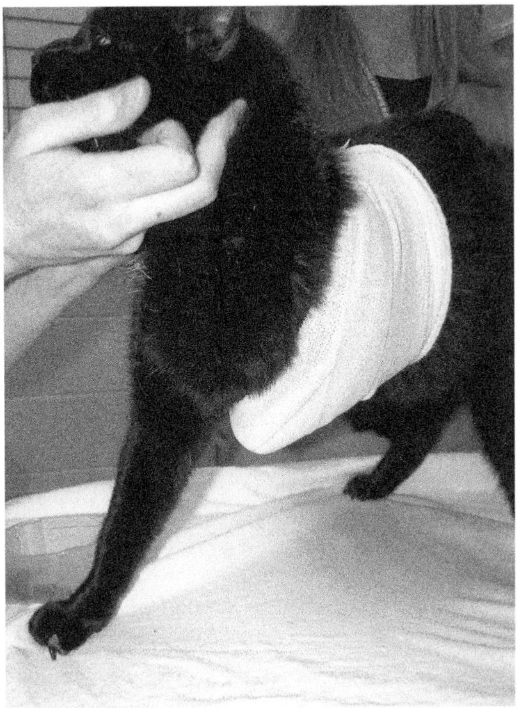

Figure 7.33 Velpeau sling Step 3: Completed Velpeau sling on a Domestic Shorthair cat.

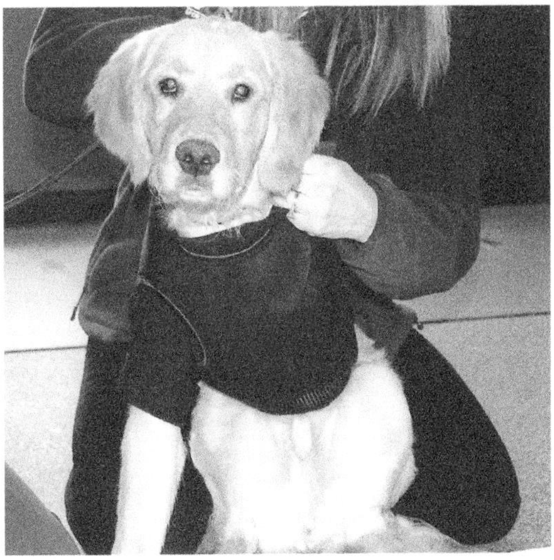

Figure 7.34 Commercially available Velpeau sling used for more long-term use and for patients who areable to get out of a traditional style of sling. *Source:* Courtesy of DogLeggs Therapeutic and Rehabilitative Products.

References

1 McKelvey, D. & Hollingshead, K.W. (2003) *Veterinary Anesthesia and Analgesia*, 3rd edn. Mosby, St. Louis, MO, pp. 249–250.

2 Posner, L.P., Gleed, R.D., Erb, H.N. *et al.* (2007) Post-anesthetic hyperthermia in cats. *Veterinary Anaesthesia and Analgesia*, 34, 40–47.

3 Niedfeldt, R.L. & Robertson, S.A. (2006) Postanesthetic hyperthermia in cats: a retrospective comparison between hydromorphone and buprenorphine. *Veterinary Anaesthesia and Analgesia*, 33, 381–389.
4 Hartman, G. & Shaffran, N. (2006) The postoperative patient. In: Busch, S.J. (ed), *Small Animal Surgical Nursing Skills and Concepts*. Elsevier-Mosby, St. Louis, MO, pp. 295–297.
5 Carney, H.C., Little, S., Brownlee-Tomasso, D. *et al.* (2012) AAFP and ISFM feline-friendly nursing care guidelines. *Journal of Feline Medicine and Surgery*, 14, 337.
6 Fossum, T.W. (2007) *Small Animal Surgery*, 3rd edn. Mosby-Elsevier, St. Louis, MO, pp. 90–110.
7 Piermattei, D.L., Flo, G. & DeCamp, C.E. (eds) (2006) *Handbook of Small Animal Orthopedics and Fracture Repair*, 4th edn. WB Saunders Co., Philadelphia, pp. 49–68.
8 Bohling, M.W. (2012) Burns. In: Tobias, K.M. & Johnston, S.A. (eds), *Veterinary Surgery – Small Animal*. Volume *II*. Elsevier, St. Louis, MO, pp. 1291–1301.
9 Unis, M.D., Roush, J.K., Bilicki, K.L. *et al.* (2010) Effect of bandaging on post-operative swelling after tibial plateau leveling osteotomy. *Veterinary and Comparative Orthopaedics and Traumatology* (impact factor: 0.81), 23(4), 240–244. doi:10.3415/VCOT-09-04-0046.
10 Welch, J.A., Boudrieau, R.J., Dejardin, L.M. *et al.* (1997) The intraosseous blood supply of the canine radius: implications for healing of distal fractures in small dogs. *Veterinary Surgery*, 26, 57–61.
11 Canapp, S.O., Campana, D.M. and Fair, L.M. (2012) Orthopedic Coaptation devices and small-animal prosthetics. In: Veterinary Surgery – Small Animal, *Volume I* (eds. K.M. Tobias & S.A. Johnston), Elsevier, St. Louis, MO. pp. 628–637.

8

Aftercare and Home Care

Gerianne Holzman[1] *and Sandra Engelmeyer*[2]

[1] *University of Wisconsin, School of Veterinary Medicine, Emerita, Madison, WI, USA*
[2] *Blue Pearl Veterinary Partners, Golden Valley, MN, USA*

Instructing and preparing clients for home care is essential for patient healing and return to well-being. This includes verbal and written discharge instructions as well as hands-on demonstrations of wound care, medications, and rehabilitation. Patient care, however, does not end when the animal walks out of the door. Following up with clients within a few days of discharge provides an opportunity to monitor the patient's condition, answer clients' questions, assure compliance, and allay concerns.

Client Instructions

Clients must receive home care instructions to provide their pets with an optimal healing experience. Communication is essential to patient care. Verbal directions are important, but as with preparing for surgery, visual aids are helpful along with written instructions. Engaged clients retain and understand more information. While clients are anxious to be reunited with their pets, talking to them without the distraction of their animal in the room is beneficial. Bringing a client to a quiet area such as an exam room eliminates other disruptions and provides a private setting for a conversation. While providing oral instructions, it is beneficial to emphasize important points in the written instructions. Using a highlighting marker to stress certain aspects of the discharge underscores their importance for the client. When providing instructions for medications, asking the client to repeat the dosing schedule assures their understanding. It is important to provide information on when the next dose of medication is due after the patient is discharged.

Written Instructions

Many studies, in human medicine, compare the appropriate reading grade level for discharge instruction comprehension and the actual reading level created [1]. Studies indicate that the appropriate level of instruction should be at the level of sixth-grade reading [2]. While using medical terms is common knowledge for veterinary professionals, the general public may not understand them. Defining terms provides client with education and understanding. For example,

Surgical Patient Care for Veterinary Technicians and Nurses, Second Edition.
Edited by Gerianne Holzman and Teri Raffel Kleist.

Companion website: www.wiley.com/go/holzman/patient

using the term "medial patella luxation or MPL" in a sentence is clear to the veterinarian and technician; however, a client may not recognize these words. Explaining this in layperson terms states this condition to be "the kneecap dislocates or moves to the inside of the knee." The use of acronyms, "MPL" in the above example, is also confusing and in need of explanation. Discharge instructions must be clear, concise, and free of errors. Creating a defined discharge instruction format for all clinic personnel provides consistency. Electronic records provide easy access to discharge templates. When using any pre-filled form, assure all pertinent information is correct for the individual patient. Include the following information:

- Patient and client names
- Client's contact information
- Caregivers: veterinarian and technician
- Clinic/hospital/emergency contact information
- Diagnosis – medical and layperson terms
- Procedure – medical and layperson terms
- Medication(s)
  - Name of drug (brand and generic)
  - Dose (size in milligrams and quantity per dose)
  - Route of administration (oral, transdermal, injection, topical, etc.)
  - Frequency (how often to give)
  - Quantity dispensed
  - Special precautions (give with food, do not mix with other medications, etc.)
  - *Example*: *Rimadyl® (Carprofen) 25 mg, give one tablet by mouth – with food, twice daily for three days (6 tablets)*
- Duration of medications – as needed, use all medications, etc.
- Feeding instructions – usual diet or special needs and when to start feeding
- Exercise – normal or restricted
- Tests and results – laboratory tests, imaging, etc.
- General instructions for wound care, bandages, rehabilitation, etc.
- Follow-up – call, appointment, suture removal, bandage change, etc.

Using a larger font size (14 pt.) aids in readability. Break down the instructions into short sentences, paragraphs, and bullet points for clarification. Providing extra space allows the client to make notes. Printing on a special color paper may help the client to find the discharge instructions when needed [3]. A separate chart with a medication schedule that the client can post and view at home can assist with medication compliance (Figure 8.1).

Cookie Zimmerman, Medication Schedule (Example)

Medication	Dose	Frequency	Schedule	Date	Date	Date	Date	Date	Date	Date
Rimadyl (Carprofen) – for pain and infla.m.mation	50 mg (1/2 tablet) by mouth with food	2 times per day	6 a.m. and 6 p.m.							
Cephalexin – an antibiotic	500 mg (1 capsule by mouth wi th food)	2 times per day	6 a.m. and 6 p.m.							
Tramadol – for pain	100 mg (2 tablets) by mouth with food	2 – 3 times per day	6 a.m., 2 p.m. 10 p.m.							
Trazadone – for anxiety	100 mg (1 tablet) by mouth with food	2 – 3 times per day if needed	6 a.m., 2 p.m. 10 p.m.							

Figure 8.1 Example of a medication chart to send home with clients to keep track of medications.

While electronically sending discharge instructions to clients after a patient has gone home may be convenient, it eliminates the personal touch of going over every step with the client to assure their understanding. Surgical patients, by definition, may need more client attention than other patients if for nothing more than monitoring the incision site. They often require additional care as outlined later in this chapter. Clients must understand their responsibilities to attend to their pet's special postoperative needs.

Hands-on Demonstrations

Not all clients are proficient in, or knowledgeable about, medicating their pets. Providing a demonstration is important for client compliance. Asking the clients to also perform the task helps them to perfect their technique. Empty gel caps for oral medication, and saline-filled syringes are great teaching aids. Demonstration for drains and feeding tubes can be performed on "dummy" models. The clients can also utilize the models for practice. Figure 8.2 shows a demonstration model of a closed-suction drain that clients may use for practice.

When bandaging is required at home, it is imperative to explain all steps and materials to the client as well as have them practice. Figure 8.3 shows a patient requiring slight compression on a neck incision. Using stretch stockinette as a "hood and shirt" allows the client to replace the gauze covering the wound.

Providing photos, videos, and/or online learning tools help clients who are visual learners. Anatomical models, electronic images, and books are additional aids to enhance client learning and understanding. Offer clients images of scoping procedures and radiographs. Explaining the images to clients enhances their experience and understanding of the procedure. Reviewing charges with the client gives them a perception of all aspects of the surgery and its related costs.

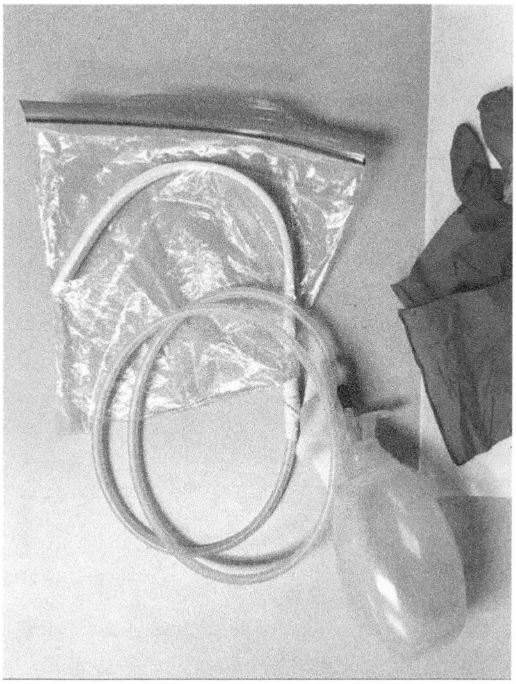

Figure 8.2 Ziploc® bag used as a model to demonstrate to clients how a closed suction drain works and is emptied.

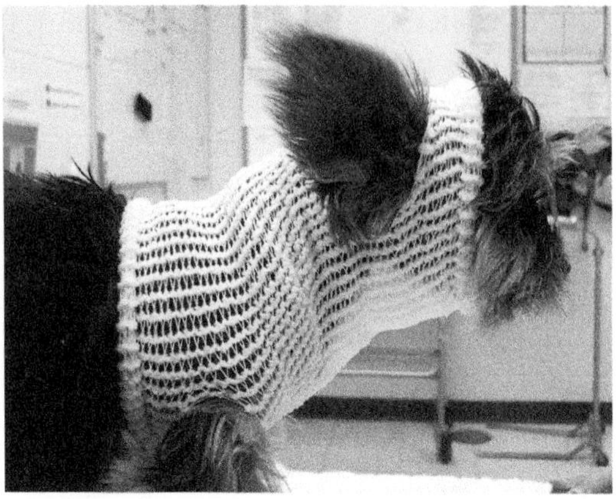

Figure 8.3 Patients may go home with a stockinette bandage, like this Yorkshire Terrier following neck surgery. The bandage, under the stockinette, requires monitoring and changing by the client.

Through all stages of the discharge process, encourage and provide the client with opportunities to ask questions.

Feeding Instructions

Patients may require special diets following their procedure. Short- or long-term needs are explained to the client. This information includes details of how to handle situations immediately after going home when food may need to be restricted to avoid vomiting due to anesthesia or pain medication-induced nausea. Patients are returned to their normal diet as soon as possible to avoid gastrointestinal upset. Some animals benefit from moistening dry kibble to be more palatable. Crushing kibble prior to soaking it in warm water hastens its water uptake. Patients reluctant to eat need coaxing with special foods such as canned pet food, baby food, boiled hamburger or chicken, and water-based tuna. High-fat content food should be avoided to circumvent gastrointestinal issues.

Long-term needs may include diet changes to comply with a specific medical condition, e.g. liver and kidney disease, degenerative joint disease as well as obesity. Pet obesity has been on the rise in the United States. Recent studies indicate veterinary professionals classify 50% of dogs and cats as overweight.[1]

In the same study, about 45% of pet owners felt their dog or cat was obese. This is higher than previous studies when clients did not recognize their pets as being overweight or that pet obesity is a disease. Providing clients with information on weight-related conditions is imperative. These include kidney disease, breathing difficulties, hypertension, osteoarthritis, and type 2 diabetes. Showing and providing a body condition score and chart gives clients a visual aid in determining their pet's current and optimal fitness (Figures 8.4 and 8.5).

Clients need instruction on measuring food intake, determining calorie content, and finding healthy treat alternatives such as raw vegetables. Advice is given on adverse foods not to be given as treats including products containing the artificial sweetener Xylitol, grapes and raisins, chocolate, avocados, garlic, onions, and macadamia nuts.[2]

1 https://petobesityprevention.org/2021.
2 https://www.aspca.org/pet-care/animal-poison-control/people-foods-avoid-feeding-your-pets.

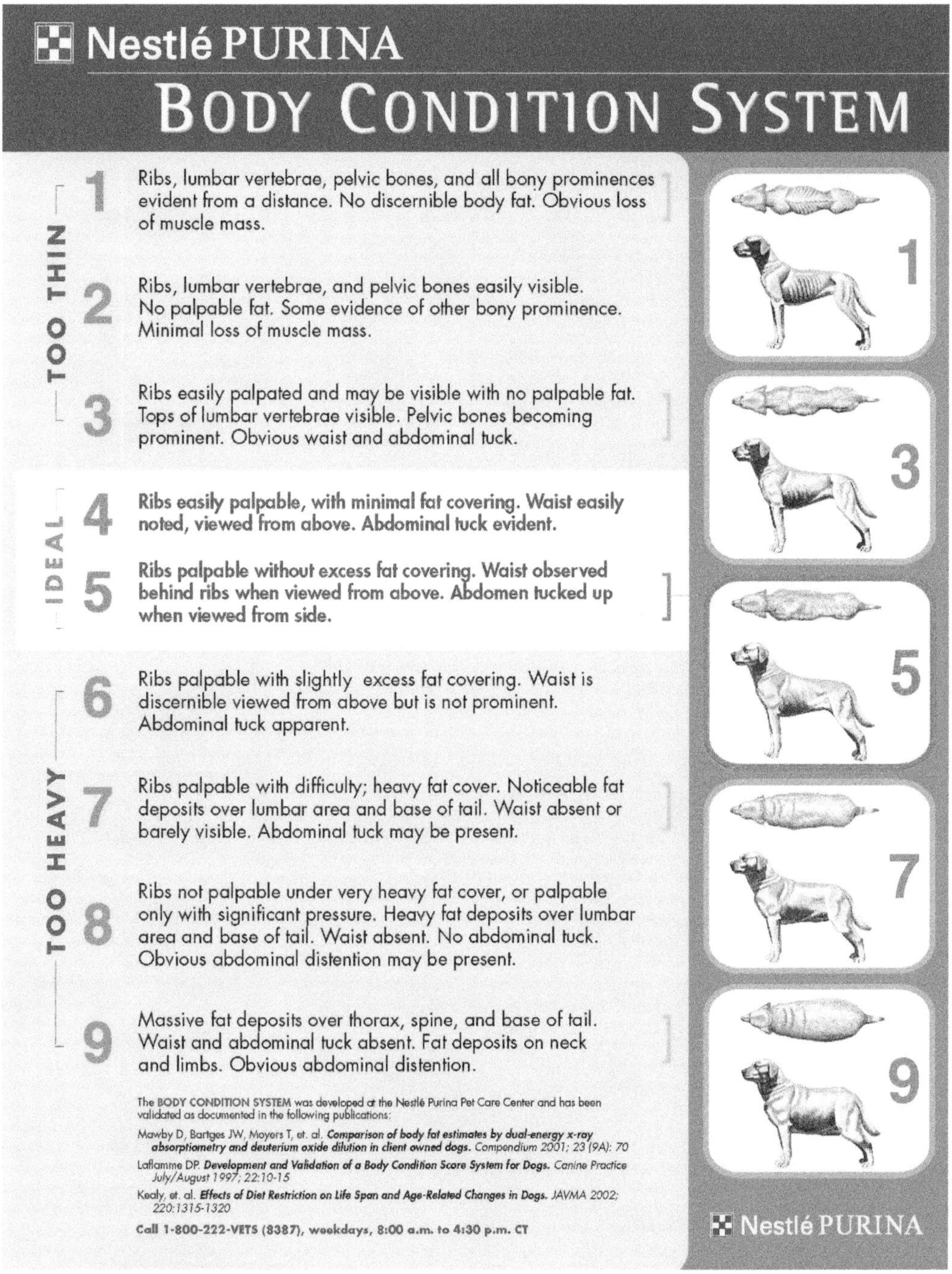

Figure 8.4 Canine body condition system scoring chart. *Source:* Courtesy of Nestle-Purina Petcare Company.

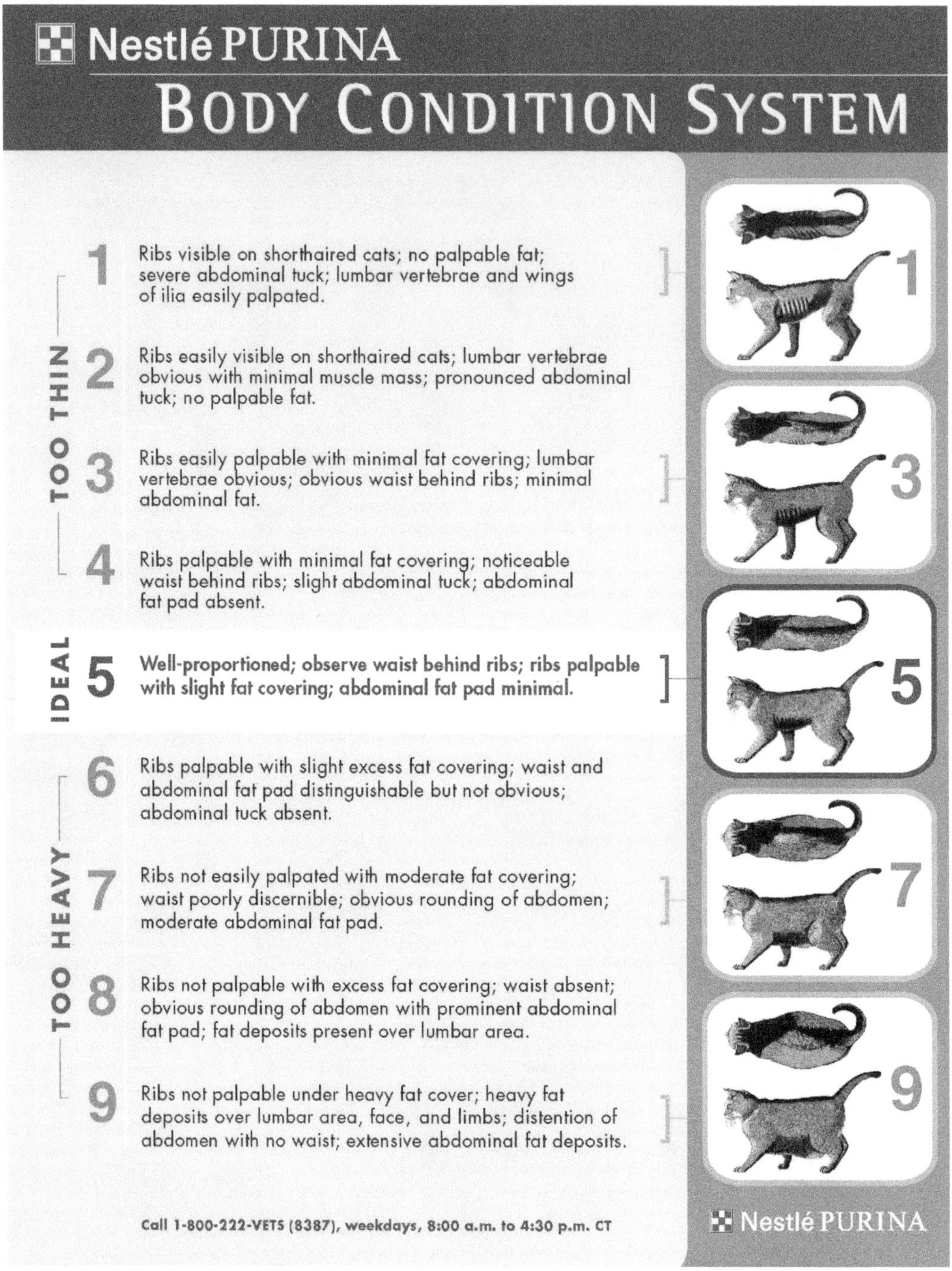

Figure 8.5 Feline body condition system scoring chart. *Source:* Courtesy of Nestle-Purina Petcare Company.

Elimination

The stress of hospitalization, alone, may cause gastrointestinal upset. Clients are warned to watch for vomiting, anorexia, constipation, and diarrhea and to contact the veterinarian or technician if these occur. This is especially true for patients prescribed narcotics and non-steroidal anti-inflammatory drugs (NSAIDs). Patients fasted and deprived of food in the perioperative period and receiving narcotics are less likely to produce bowel movements on a regular basis for a short period after going home [4]. This is generally not a medical concern. However, providing clients with this information allays their concerns. Patients that are unable to urinate **do** require special attention. Often following spinal surgery, patients cannot voluntarily urinate. Carefully explaining the need to monitor urination and demonstrating bladder expression is essential in these patients. When clients are unable to empty their pet's bladder, it may be advisable to continue hospitalization for expression or catheterization. Alternatively, repeat visits to the clinic may be required. Non-steroidal anti-inflammatory medications may cause vomiting and diarrhea. Clients are warned to contact the clinic if these occur, as it is imperative to stop the NSAID before the gastrointestinal condition worsens.

Exercise

Following any surgery, the patient is rested to provide an opportunity for the wound to heal. The extent of these restrictions depends upon the patient's individual condition. All patients are kept from running, jumping, and playing in the immediate postoperative period. This includes playing with other pets in the household. Exercise restriction continues, at least, until the incision is well healed and sutures or staples are removed. Clients are advised that the outside of the skin may quickly look healed but deeper levels of tissue need additional time to heal completely. Walking dogs on short (5 ft or less) leashes for elimination purposes, with no off-leash exercise, aid in recovery by lessening stress put on healing tissues. Emphasizing the length of time and frequency of walks as well as the length of the leash improves client compliance. To avoid rambunctiousness, when unattended, the patient is restricted to a crate or small, unfurnished (e.g. bath or laundry) room during the client's absence. Cats should be kept indoors with limited activity. Active cats can be confined to a large dog kennel with a litter pan and water to prevent jumping and running indoors.

Patients undergoing orthopedic procedures need more extensive exercise restrictions. This includes additional time after suture removal and may be as long as 10 weeks or more. Along with leash walking, support with a sling or towel keeps the patient from falling and aids in the use of stairs. Use of the repaired leg is often encouraged; thus, the sling is not meant to hold the patient off the ground. Patients going home with an Ehmer or Velpeau sling are the exception to encouragement of limb use.

Slowly returning patients to normal activity advances as their condition dictates. This includes incrementally increasing leash walks by 5 to 10 minute intervals every few days or weekly. Comparing an injured pet to an injured athlete gives the client a point of reference for increasing activity. For example, a runner with an anterior cruciate ligament (ACL) tear would not immediately run a marathon but would gradually work up to that point. Similarly, a Labrador Retriever recovering from a similar cranial cruciate ligament (CCL) injury does not immediately resume field trial work.

Support Devices

Patients recovering from orthopedic and neurologic surgery or those with neurologic deficits benefit from supportive devices to assist their mobility. Towels provide support as do a variety of commercially available support devices (Figure 8.6). Patients may need help to rise off the ground, walk, use stairs, etc. Clients are advised on how much support to provide. For example, a patient

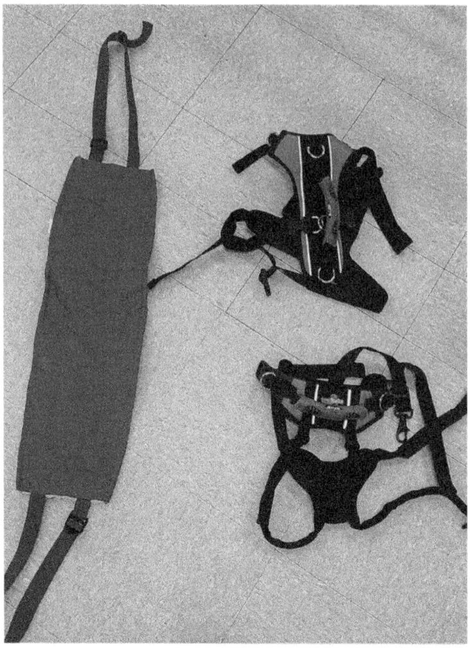

Figure 8.6 Slings and harnesses come in a wide variety of styles for multiple uses.

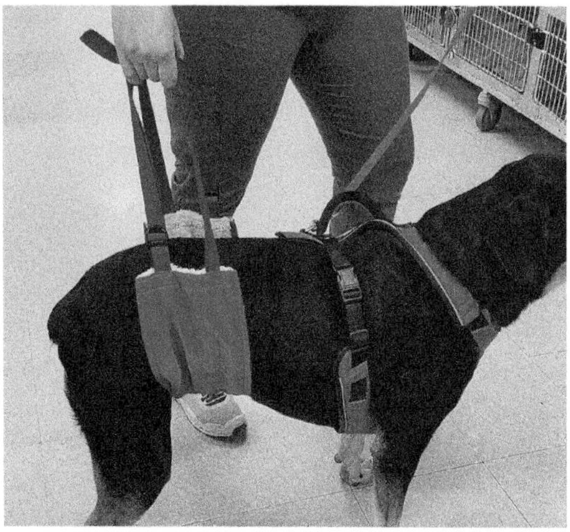

Figure 8.7 Slings provide support while allowing patients to bear some weight on their limbs.

recovering from a tibial plateau leveling osteotomy is encouraged to use the affected limb and gain strength. A support sling or harness in this circumstance is meant to keep the patient from falling while allowing the animal to bear some weight on the leg (Figure 8.7). A patient who has undergone a hemilaminectomy or has paraparesis may not have immediate use of the rear limbs and will need complete assistive support to walk around (Figures 8.8 and 8.9).

Physical Rehabilitation

Orthopedic and neurologic patients require rehabilitation to return to normal or near-normal conditions. While it begins in the hospital, it is often the client who provides the majority of this care. Careful client instructions and demonstrations are essential to provide the patient with appropriate therapy. Large referral practices may offer rehabilitation services by a certified canine rehabilitation therapist (CCRT) or a veterinary technician specialist (Physical Rehabilitation). A CCRT/VTS (Physical Rehabilitation) is specialist in therapy and rehab. Veterinary technicians may also gain the title of certified canine rehabilitation assistant (CCRA). (In many areas, "Physical Therapy (PT)" is a protected term in that one cannot state they are providing PT if they are not a physical therapist and often only applies to treating humans.) In addition to immediate postoperative treatment, long-term therapy is beneficial for patients suffering from osteoarthritis and for conservative management of orthopedic and neurologic conditions. Providing strength and conditioning for working dogs helps healthy patients to maintain fitness (Figure 8.10). The goal of physical rehabilitation is to aid in recovery, improve function, and promote well-being.

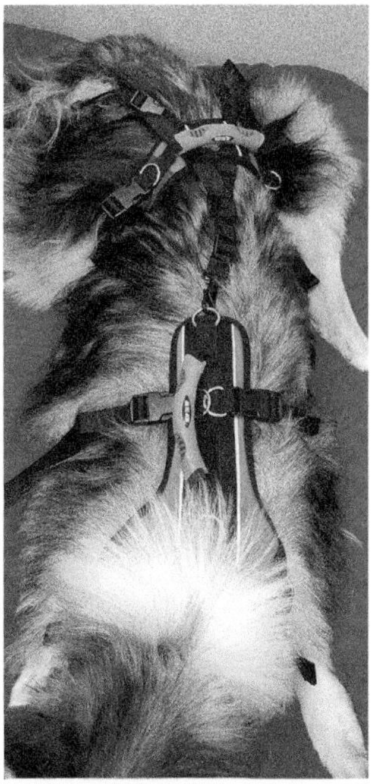

Figure 8.8 Non-ambulatory patient fitted for a full body harness.

An individual plan is developed for each patient to provide for its optimal rehabilitation needs. Timing of rehab depends upon the patient's condition. Following some joint surgeries (e.g. arthroscopy, osteochondritis dissecans, femoral head and neck ostectomy, and extra-capsular stabilization of a cranial cruciate rupture), patients are strongly encouraged to immediately begin use of their limbs. Patients undergoing other surgeries (e.g. fracture repairs, osteotomies for cranial cruciate rupture, and intervertebral disc decompression) may benefit from more moderate therapy. Instituting the incorrect treatment at the wrong time may lead to poor outcomes [5]. Pre-rehabilitation measurements of the affected joint's range of motion and the circumference of its accompanying muscles provide a starting point for gauging effectiveness of treatment. The use of a goniometer and a tape measure is employed for these measurements. Knowledge of the normal range of motion of joints aids in determining a long-term goal for therapy (Table 8.1). Subsequently, after recovery, similar readings are taken for comparison. However, in the end, the goal is to have a comfortable, happy, and ambulatory patient. Physical rehabilitation is an excellent way for clients to be intimately involved with their pet's recovery.

Figure 8.9 The harness is used to lift non-ambulatory patients and help them to move around.

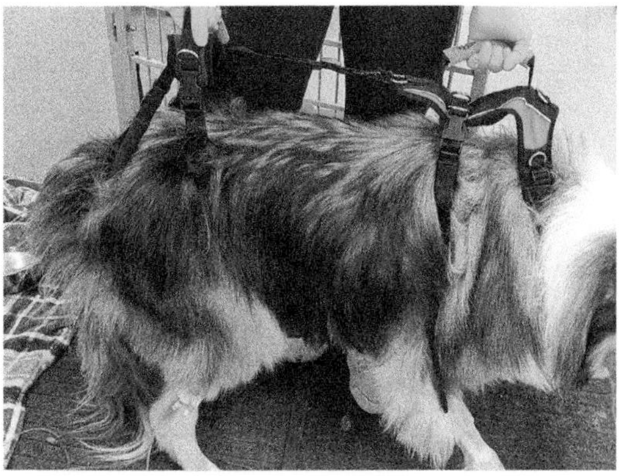

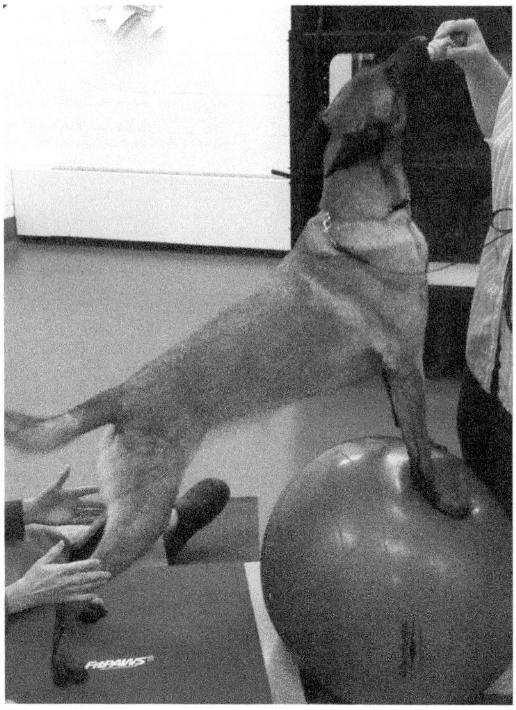

Figure 8.10 Patient receives strength and balance training while on a ball. *Source:* Courtesy of Courtney Arnoldy.

Table 8.1 Normal range of motion – flexion and extension.

Joint	Dog (degrees)	Cat (degrees)
Shoulder		
Flexion	60–70	60–70
Extension	65–75	90
Elbow		
Flexion	70–75	50–60
Extension	70–75	80–90
Carpus		
Flexion	155–160	130–140
Extension	20–30	30–40
Hip		
Flexion	70–80	50–60
Extension	80–90	100–110
Stifle		
Flexion	65–75	50–60
Extension	65–75	90
Tarsus		
Flexion	65–75	50–60
Extension	90–110	90–110

Source: Adapted from Newton [6].

Cryotherapy

Cryotherapy is one of the first stages of rehabilitation and is used in the acute stage of healing. Ice packing is done at specific intervals in the immediate postoperative period. It minimizes inflammation and provides pain relief. Cold applied to the skin causes vasoconstriction and decreases nerve conduction velocity. Muscles may cool by 1–4 °C (33–39 °F) and the skin by 12–13 °C (53–55 °F) [7]. The effects of cryotherapy may last for 15–30 minutes. Bags of crushed ice, frozen peas or corn kernels, and commercially available freezer gel packs are great sources of cooling. To avoid incision contamination and keep the skin from getting too cold, a washcloth or paper towel is placed between the ice pack and the skin. Towels may be used but should not be too thick to impede the flow of cold to the skin. Incisions must be protected from cross-patient contamination in the hospital. The source of cold therapy is cleaned with a disinfecting solution between patients. Cryotherapy is applied for 10–15 minutes up to every 4 hours depending on the client's schedule. This continues for the first 72 hours following surgery. Patients with cold sensitivity are monitored closely for distress.

Heat

Heat is used for long-term therapy beginning on days 3–4 of the postoperative period. It is not used when acute inflammation is present as it may increase hemorrhage and edema. Heat is not applied to active infections, tumors, or pregnant uteruses. Heat therapy creates vasodilation and muscle relaxation and improves stretching ability. Hot packing provides superficial heating. (Deep heating may be achieved by a certified therapist with the use of therapeutic ultrasound.) Prior to the application of a hot pack, the skin and incision are protected as with cryotherapy. Heat is applied with warmed towels or commercially available gel packs. This continues for 10–15 minutes, again up to every 4 hours. The patient must be monitored closely for redness and skin irritation. Clients monitor the temperature of the pack by application to their own skin. If it is too hot for them, it is too hot for their pet. **Heating pads are never used for heat therapy as they become too hot and provide a focal point for potential burns.**

Massage

Massage soothes the patient and may provide a bonding experience for the client. It improves the flow of the lymphatic system, and in patients with distal edema, aids in moving fluid from the extremities to the rest of the body. Massage also softens adhesions and relieves muscle contracture. Following hyperthermia treatment, massage prepares patients for exercises and stretching. Massage treatment always begins distally and works proximally to move fluid into the body. Beginning with soft strokes, the massage intensity increases to provide pressure to the muscles. The sessions proceed for 5–15 minutes as the patient tolerates.

Passive Range of Motion

The passive range of motion (PROM) exercises involve moving a joint through its full motion. It increases joint flexibility while providing extension to the surrounding muscles, tendons, and ligaments. Passive range of motion improves nutritional support of the synovium and increases blood flow. PROM is beneficial to maintain mobility and avoid joint contracture. However, to improve strength and reduce muscle atrophy, active range of motion is a better option. This includes the patient walking on its own with assistance, underwater treadmills, swimming, and other therapeutic exercises as described later in this chapter. To perform PROM, the limb is grasped distal to the joint of interest. The limb is supported proximal to the joint with the other hand. With the leg maintained in an even plane, the joint is slowly flexed and extended (Figures 8.11 and 8.12).

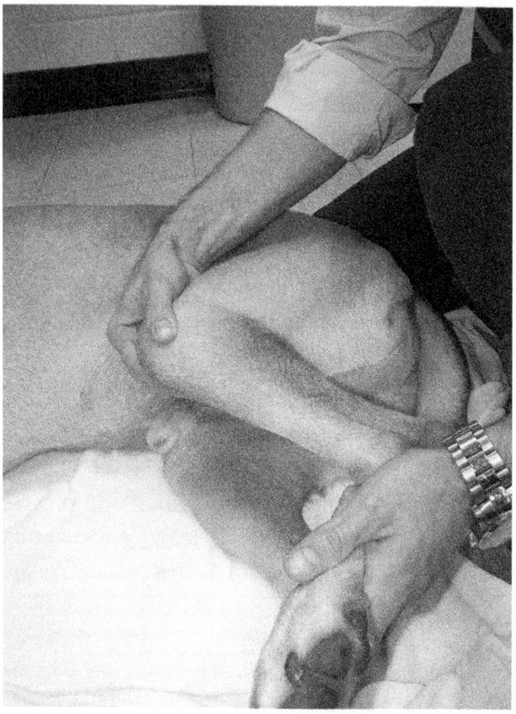

Figure 8.11 Passive range of motion: stifle flexion.

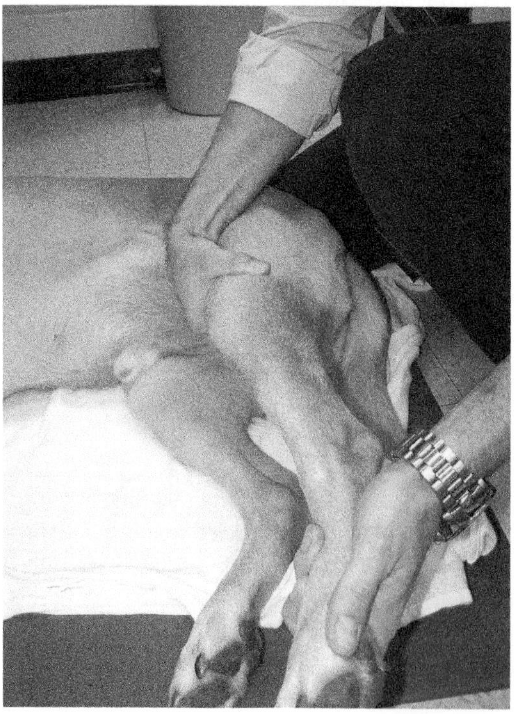

Figure 8.12 Passive range of motion: stifle extension.

Initially, it may not be possible to reach a full range of motion – the patient's comfort dictates the extent of movement. As each motion (flexion or extension) is reached, it is held for 15–30 seconds. Twenty repetitions performed three to four times daily are sufficient. Each individual joint of the affected limb is taken through a PROM. "Bicycling" movements by grasping the foot and imitating a walking movement *do not* provide full range of motion to all of the joints.

Therapeutic Exercises

Therapeutic exercises may be performed by a certified therapist and can be incorporated into home care. Exercise improves a patient's attitude, range of motion, muscle strength, and limb use. As with all rehabilitation methods, therapeutic exercise is individualized for the patient. As the patient improves, exercise is increased in repetitions, duration, and intensity. Simply standing with assistance improves patient balance, muscle tone, and patient attitude. Initially, the patient is helped to stand on an even, stable, non-slippery surface. Sufficient time is allowed between standing exercises to allow the patient to rest. As the patient's condition improves, standing time is increased, while support is decreased. Therapeutic round and peanut-shaped balls assist standing and balancing exercises.

Sit-to-stand and down-to-stand exercises improve muscle strength of the quadriceps, semimembranosus, semitendinosus, as well as the biceps and triceps. Range of motion and joint mobility are improved. If a patient is unable to stand or rise on its own, the patient is assisted with sling support. When performing this exercise, the patient is encouraged to sit/stand symmetrically without tilting to either side. As with all training, the use of treats rewards and encourages the behavior. Begin this exercise slowly (1–5 repetitions) twice daily until the animal is able to sit/stand squarely. As the patient tolerates, more repetitions are added.

Veterinary hospitals with rehabilitation facilities may offer clients in-house rehabilitation with the use of an underwater treadmill. While manufacturers differ slightly, underwater treadmills use a holding tank and filtration system that warms and chlorinates the water for recirculation during the patient's session. (The water is changed between patients.) A leak-proof, clear-sided chamber encloses the treadmill. Depending on the particular product, adjustments are available for speed and incline. The chamber is filled with water to the appropriate level for the patient. The water is deep enough to provide buoyancy and still keeps the patient's feet on the treadmill – generally to the height of the sternum (Figure 8.13).

The water buoyancy causes a reduction in gravity that provides for a lower-impact exercise. The reduced stress on joints allows for ease of movement, longer strides, and extended range of motion. Walking against the flow of water aids in muscle strengthening while the warmth of the water relaxes muscles and eases pain. Over time, the level of the water may be lowered to provide more impact.

Underwater therapy does not begin until all incisions are healed. Patients are always attended when on a treadmill; small or non-ambulatory animals are assisted by a therapist in the water with the patient. Flotation devices provide extra safety for all patients. The exercise begins slowly in very short sessions of one to two minutes, gradually increasing by five-minute intervals as the patient tolerates. The patient is monitored very closely for signs of fatigue and the exercise stopped immediately when this is noticed. Clients with land treadmills in their homes, with time and patience, may be able to teach their pets to use these devices between sessions on the underwater treadmill.

Swimming is a great exercise for rehabilitation, active range of motion, strengthening, and coordination. This low-impact activity improves muscle mass and stamina. (All incisions and skin lesions must be completely healed prior to beginning any water therapy.) Swimming occurs in an underwater treadmill (without the treadmill portion in use), pool, lake, or other body of water.

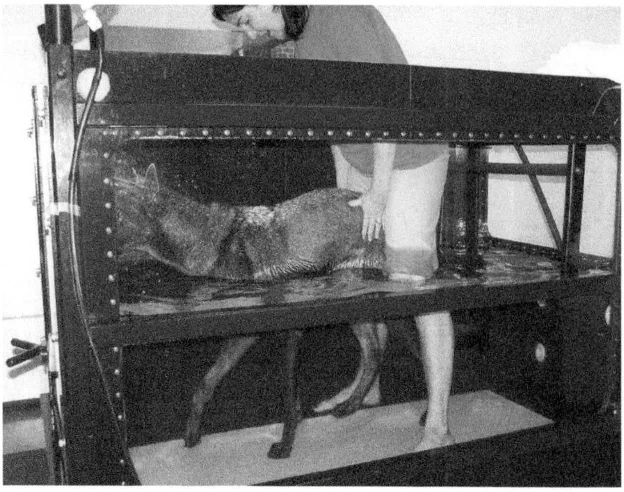

Figure 8.13 An underwater treadmill provides active range of motion to all four limbs while the water lessens the impact of the exercise. *Source:* Courtesy of Courtney Arnoldy.

Most four-legged dogs swim primarily with their front legs. However, patients missing one forelimb swim well with their back legs providing extra strengthening exercises for their remaining legs. Dogs not used to being in water, must slowly be acclimated to it, and some patients will never accept swimming. Flotation devices provide safety and allow the patient to rest. The animal is accompanied in the water or within very close proximity. During rehab, dogs are encouraged to walk into the water and not to jump from a dock or pier to minimize impact on their joints. As with the underwater treadmill, patients are monitored closely for fatigue.

Another exercise, requiring more impact, includes controlled walks at a slow pace. When forced to move at a leisurely pace, pets are more likely to use all of their limbs. When trotting or running quickly, animals have more momentum to allow walking on three legs and carrying the injured leg. (Watching an amputee's walk demonstrates this phenomenon well. Three or even two-legged veterinary patients move better at a faster speed and are more easily fatigued at a slower pace.) Walking provides an active range of motion exercise to increase joint mobility as well as muscle strengthening. Additionally, walking over and around obstacles provides more thoughtful movement as the patient navigates the obstruction. Stair climbing and walking on an incline or decline strengthen muscles and force flexion of the joints. Impact activities are not instituted until the patient is sufficiently healed from surgery. For less ambulatory patients, sling support is beneficial.

Clients are advised to gradually introduce the exercises and slowly increase their duration. Varying rehabilitation techniques provide more stimulation for the patient, less boredom for the client, and different joints are put through their range of motion while different muscles are strengthened.

Follow-Up

Clients are often stressed and nervous when caring for their recuperating pets. They may not want "to bother" the veterinarian or veterinary technician with a call. They may not understand or remember some of the instructions provided at discharge. Patient follow-up is important to monitor progress, answer client questions, and assure compliance with discharge instructions (Figure 8.14).

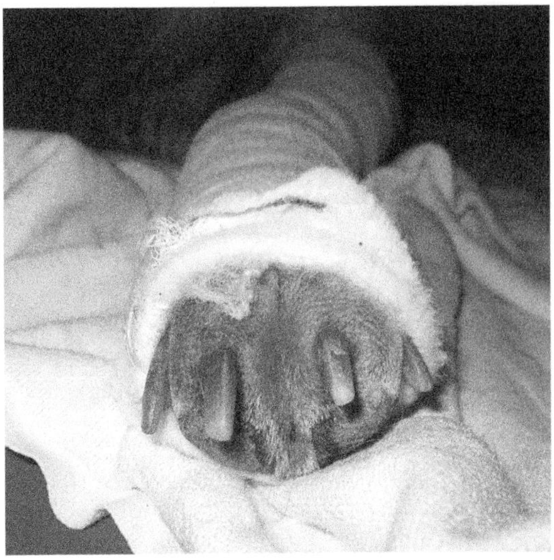

Figure 8.14 Postoperative swelling of toes from bandage tightness. Following bandage application, clients monitor toes daily for problems. *Source:* Photo courtesy of Susan Schaefer.

Contacting a client within 24–72 hours of surgery [8] conveys the veterinary staff's concern for the patient's welfare. Minor problems caught early can avoid major complications. Client correspondence provides an opportunity to confirm dosing schedules, create rehabilitation plans, and discuss wound care. Clients are quizzed on the appearance of an incision and its surrounding skin – is it red, warm, swollen, or is there any drainage – clear, bloody, or purulent? (Figure 8.15)

Clients are also asked about the condition of any bandages that were placed. Is the animal bothering the bandage? Clients may need additional instructions for wound and bandage care. If there is a problem, a return visit to the clinic/hospital is in order (Figure 8.16).

Monitoring a patient's eating and elimination is especially important when many medications are prescribed. Antibiotics, non-steroidal anti-inflammatories, and narcotics may all cause nausea, anorexia, and/or abnormal urination or defecation. Diarrhea may be present from some treatments and advising clients to monitor for blood in the stool is imperative. They must call if bloody stools or melena are evident to prevent serious complications. Providing dietary suggestions, such as a bland diet of boiled hamburger or chicken and rice in the event of vomiting and diarrhea, helps clients to provide nourishment for their pets. If a fentanyl patch or adhesive bandage has been placed, clients may need advice on their removal. It is helpful to send patients home with odor-free adhesive remover packets for use with patches and possibly bandages.

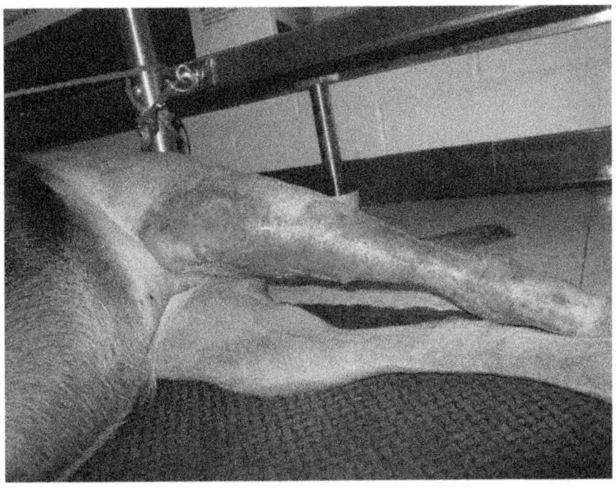

Figure 8.15 Observing the skin, every day, for redness, bruising, drainage, and irritation prevents severe problems. *Source:* Photo courtesy of Jason Bleedorn.

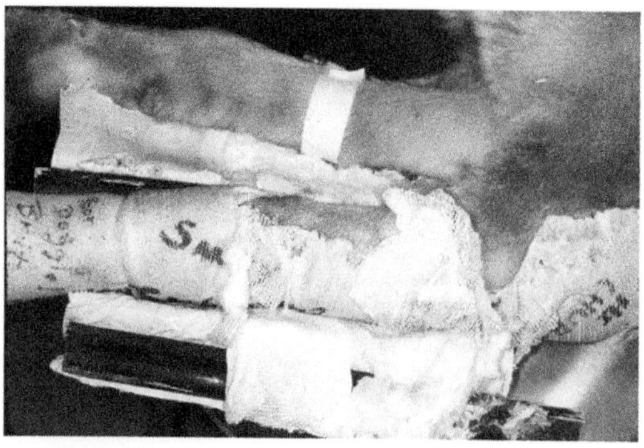

Figure 8.16 Without protection, patients chew bandages and casts. A chewed cast may indicate an underlying problem and needs to be investigated. *Source:* Photo courtesy of Susan Schaefer.

Follow-up communication provides an opportunity for scheduling suture/staple removal along with re-check exams and client updates. It also gives the client an opportunity to discuss any new symptoms that may have arisen after the patient went home. Clients are always encouraged to call with other questions and are provided with emergency contact information. Experienced veterinary technicians may answer most of a client's questions; however, they must never hesitate to seek the advice of the attending surgeon. Keeping all members of the surgical team informed and updated provides the best patient care. Veterinary technicians and nurses perform an integral role in excellent patient care from the client's first phone call, through hospital care and surgery, and postoperatively until the patient is well. Healthy and happy patients and content clients are the goals of all animal care.

References

1 Bukata, R. (2012) With discharge instructions, less is more. *Emergency physicians monthly* 01/2012.

2 Somes, J. (2003) *Reading levels of ED patients compared to level of discharge instructions.* Emergency Nurses Association Virginia Henderson International Nursing Library, Indianapolis, IN.

3 Day, D. 5 Ways to Help Patients Recall Their Post-Visit Discharge Instructions. *The Care Transitions Journal,* Sirona Health, South Portland, ME June 2012 see web: http://www.caretransitions.com/health_call_center_blog/bid/57106/5-Ways-to-Help-Patients-Recall-Their-Post-Visit-Discharge-Instructions [accessed on June 20 2012].

4 Papich, M.G. (2007) *Saunders Handbook of Veterinary Drugs,* 3rd edn. Saunders Elsevier, St. Louis, MO.

5 Arnoldy, C. (2010) Rehabilitation for dogs with cranial cruciate ligament rupture. (ed. P. Muir), Advances in the Cranial Cruciate Ligament. pp. 249–253 Wiley-Blackwell, Ames, IA.

6 Newton, C.D. (1985) Normal joint range of motion in the dog and cat – Appendix B. In: Newton, C.D. & Nunamaker, D.M. (eds), *Textbook of Small Animal Orthopedics.* JB Lippincott, Philadelphia, PA.

7 Knap, K., Johnson A.L., Schulz K. (2007) Fundamentals of physical rehabilitation. (ed. T. W. Fossum), Small Animal Surgery Textbook, 3 pp. 111–129. Mosby Elsevier. St. Louis, MO.

8 SironaHealth (2012) *7 Steps to Successful Post Discharge Follow Up Care – Using Inbound and Outbound Calling Programs.* SironaHealth, South Portland, ME. e-book.

Glossary

Abrading Removal of the superficial layer of the skin
Abrasion Skin wound less than full skin thickness
Acetabulum "Socket" part of the hip joint
Adhesions Fibrous bands of scar tissue that form between internal organs and tissues, joining them together abnormally
Aerosolized Converted from liquid or solid state to a gaseous state
Alopecia Lack of hair
Ambulation Ability to walk
Analgesic Medication or treatment that reduces pain without inducing unconsciousness
Anesthetic Medication administered to reduce the perception of pain; it may (or may not) produce unconsciousness
Anomalous Deviation from normal
Antibiotic Medication to kill or inhibit the growth of bacteria
Anti-inflammatory Generally a drug that reduces inflammation
Anti-microbial Agent that kills or suppresses growth of microorganisms
Appose Bringing edges of a wound together
Arrhythmia An abnormal heart rhythm
Arthrocentesis Joint tap, obtaining synovial fluid via a syringe and needle inserted into the joint
Arthrodesis Fusion of two or more bones of a joint
Arthrogram Radiographic demonstration of the joints employing contrast media
Arthroplasty Surgery to restore function of a joint
Arthroscopy Internal visualization of a joint through a camera and employing instruments through ports to perform intra-articular surgery or for diagnosis
Aseptically Perform a technique without introducing microorganisms into the area or field
Atrophy Wasting away or a decrease in the size of an organ or body part such as muscle from lack of use
Aural Of the ear
Austenite A solid solution of ferric carbide or carbon in iron
Autogenous Originating from the host, self-generating
Avascular Without blood flow or blood supply
Avulsion Tearing away

Surgical Patient Care for Veterinary Technicians and Nurses, Second Edition.
Edited by Gerianne Holzman and Teri Raffel Kleist.

Companion website: www.wiley.com/go/holzman/patient

Biceps tenosynovitis Inflammation of the biceps brachii tendon and its synovial sheath
Bipolar (cautery) Electric current passes only through the tissues between two electrodes
Box lock Joint or point of union of two sides of a ring handled instrument
Bradycardia Slow heart rate

Calculi Plural of calculus; abnormal concretions (stones) formed of minerals in the kidneys, urinary bladder, or gallbladder; calcified plaque on the teeth
Cancellous Bone having a lattice-like or spongy structure
Cardiovascular Of the heart and blood vessels
Cavitation Action of an ultrasound to produce small bubbles that then burst when they contact an item, to clean the item
Celiotomy Surgical incision into the abdominal cavity
Cerclage To encircle a bone with wire to aid in the repair of a fracture
Cesarean section (C-section) Incision into the uterus (hysterotomy) to remove fetuses, may be performed with an ovariohysterectomy
Cholecystectomy Surgery to remove the gall bladder
Circumferential Encircling, peripheral
Coaptation Fitting together two parts, e.g., two ends of a fracture or edges of a wound
Cortex Outer layer of a long bone
Cortical Pertaining to the outer layer of a bone
Cryotherapy Cold treatment to reduce inflammation and pain, e.g., ice packing
Cystic Relating to the urinary bladder, gall bladder, or a cyst
Cystocentesis Obtaining a urine sample using a syringe and needle through the abdominal wall
Cystogram Radiographic demonstration of the bladder employing contrast media
Cystotomy Surgical incision into the urinary bladder
Cytotoxic Causing a toxic effect on cells

Debridement Surgical removal of dead, devitalized, or contaminated tissue and/or foreign material
Deciduous Primary teeth or first set of teeth
Decompression To release or remove pressure
Decubital ulcer Skin wound caused by compression
Degloving Loss of skin and underlying tissue
Dehiscence Rupture or break open (surgical wound)
Developmental Occurring during growth
Diaphysis Shaft of a long bone
Disinfectant Product that kills many, but not all, microorganisms present on an inanimate object
Dissection To cut apart or separate
Distal Away from the center or point of attachment
Distended Swollen, expanded
Distichiasis Eyelash that grows from an abnormal location or abnormal direction
Dominant Strongest or most commonly used
Dosimeter Instrument used to measure and indicate the amount of radiation absorbed over a certain period of time

Echocardiogram Image produced from ultrasonic waves examining the structures and function of the heart
Ectropion Eyelid turning out and away from the eye
Edema Swelling of organs, skin, or other body parts due to fluid accumulation
Efficacy How efficient or well something performs
Effusion Fluid escaping from blood or lymphatic vessels into tissue or spaces
Emaciated Extremely thin, usually related to disease or lack of food
Endothelin Proteins that constrict blood vessels and raise blood pressure
Enterogram Radiographic demonstration of the intestines employing contrast media
Entropion Eyelid turning inward and toward the eye
Enucleation Removal of an eye
Erythema Redness
Esophagram Radiographic demonstration of the esophagus employing contrast media
Everting Edges of the wound turning outward
Exteriorization To remove or bring out of a body cavity
Extrahepatic Outside of the liver
Extravasation Accumulation of fluid outside of the joint
Extruded Protruded out from the original position

Fenestrated Solid sheet of material that has a window of material purposefully removed
Fissure Crack, tear, or groove in a body part
Fragmented medial coronoid process Portion of the medial coronoid process of the ulna separates from parent bone

Gastric dilatation volvulus (GDV or bloat) Stomach is twisted causing enlargement (may have simple dilatation without volvulus [twisting])
Gastro-intestinal (GI) Relating to the stomach and intestines
Granulation Small, fleshy protuberances on the surface of a healing wound

Hematocrit Percentage by volume of red blood cells in a sample of blood after centrifugation
Hematoma A lump or swelling filled with blood that is not flowing
Hemilaminectomy Unilateral decompression of the spinal cord via removal of a portion of a vertebral body to relieve pressure; provides access for removal of extruded intervertebral disc material
Hemoglobin Iron-containing substance in red blood cells that transports oxygen from the lungs to the rest of the body
Hemostasis Control of blood loss
Hip dysplasia Genetic disorder where the hip is malformed and the head of the femur does not sit properly in the acetabulum
Hyperextension Extending beyond the normal range of motion of a joint
Hyperflexion Flexing beyond the normal range of motion of a joint
Hypertension Elevated blood pressure
Hyperthermia Higher than normal body temperature
Hyperthyroid Overactive thyroid gland
Hypoextension Extending less than the normal range of motion of a joint
Hypoflexion Flexing less than the normal range of motion of a joint

Hypotension Low blood pressure
Hypothermia Lower than normal body temperature
Hypothyroid Underactive thyroid gland

Ileus Mechanical or functional bowel obstruction
Infestation Large number of parasites causing damage
Inflammation Protective tissue response to injury
Insufflation Infusing gas into a body cavity to aid in visualization, e.g., during laparoscopy
Insufflator Machine used to perform insufflation
Integrity Whole or undivided
Integument Outer covering of the body: skin, hair, etc.
Intrahepatic Inside the liver
Intraoperative Time during surgery
Inverting Edges of the wound turning inward

Laceration Wound with sharp edges
Laminar air flow System of circulating filtered air in parallel-flowing planes
Laparoscopy Examination of the abdominal cavity using an endoscope
Larynx Opening at the proximal trachea to control breathing and prevent food from entering the trachea
Lavage Act of washing or rinsing with fluid
Ligation Use of suture to tie around a vessel or tissue mass to achieve hemostasis or closure
Lobectomy Surgical resection of lobe of an organ, e.g., lung or liver
Locomotion Ability to move
Longevity Length of time something survives
Luxation Dislocation of an anatomical part, e.g., hip or patella

Martensitic Formed in stainless steel by rapid quenching, consisting of a supersaturated solid solution of carbon in iron
Mastectomy Surgical removal of mammary tissue
Memory Ability of suture to return to its packaged form
Menace (reflex) Poking finger toward eye to test vision; normal response is closing of the eye
Modulation Synapse of the neurons in the nucleus caudalis in the medulla of the brain
Monofilament Single strand of suture
Monopolar (cautery) Electric current passes from the active electrode to the lesions, through the body, and exits via a return electrode
Multifilament Multiple strands of suture braided together to form a single strand
Musculoskeletal Muscles and bones

Neoplasia Tumor, new tissue
Nephrectomy Surgical removal of a kidney
Neuromuscular Condition affecting the nerves and the muscles
Nociception An unpleasant sensation that may be associated with actual or potential tissue damage and that may have physical and emotional components
Nystagmus Rapid, involuntary eye movements

Obtunded Mentally dull
Occlude To prevent the passage of

Onychectomy Declaw, removal of the third phalanx of each digit
Orchiectomy (neuter/castration) Sterilizing a male dog to prevent breeding
Orthotic Orthopedic appliance used to support a body part
Ossification Formation of bone from fibrous tissue
Ostectomy Removing all or part of a bone
Osteoarthritis Degenerative joint disease; joint inflammation characterized by cartilage degeneration
Osteochondritis dissecans (OCD) Incomplete endochondral ossification causes cartilage to remain; fissure in this cartilage creates a flap that may loosen causing a "joint mouse"
Osteotomy Cutting a bone
Ovariohysterectomy (OHE, neuter, spay) Sterilizing a female dog to prevent breeding

Palmar Underside of the front foot
Palpation Feeling parts of the body to determine normal or abnormal conditions
Parameters Measurable factors
Patent Ductus Arteriosus (PDA) Persistent opening between two main heart vessels
Pathogen Disease-causing microorganism
Penetrating Poke through or into
Perineal urethrostomy – feline (PU) Penile amputation to alleviate chronic urethral obstruction not relievable by other means
Perineum Area of the body including the rectum and urogenital openings
Perioperative Period of time surrounding surgery including preoperative, intraoperative, and postoperative
Persistent right aortic arch (PRAA) Vascular ring anomaly
Pharynx Funnel-shaped structure in the back of the oral cavity including the larynx, esophagus, tonsils, etc.
Pheromones Chemical secreted by an animal that affects behavior of the members of the same species
Pinna External part of the ear
Pitting Creation of small dents or "pits" on a surface, e.g., pitting edema
Plantar Underside of the rear foot
Plaque Biofilm on the teeth containing bacteria and glycoproteins
Platelet Disc-shaped cell fragment in blood that aids in clotting
Pliability Ease of suture workability
Polydipsia Increased thirst
Polyuria Increased urination
Portography Radiography of the portal vein with contrast
Portosystemic shunt (PSS) Blood vessels bypass the liver and drain from the stomach, intestines, spleen, and pancreas directly into the circulatory system, thus partially eliminating the liver's filtering properties; may be intrahepatic or extrahepatic
Postoperative Time after surgery
Povidone Iodine infused into the product
Preoperative Time preceding surgery
Proprioception Awareness of one's movement based on sensations
Proximal Nearer the center of the body or attachment
Puncture Penetrating injury
Pyoderma Skin infection

Ratchet Toothed tabs that interdigitate and lock as on a ring handled instrument
Rehabilitation (rehab.) Treatment of physical conditions to restore normal function
Renal Of the kidneys
Residual effect Duration of efficacy after application

Seroma Local accumulation of serum within a tissue or organ
Serrated Cutting edge of a scissors that has small teeth for grasping and then cutting tissue
Sphincter Circular muscle constricting an orifice
Splenectomy Surgical removal of the spleen
Stabilization Secure to eliminate movement
Stenotic nares Nostrils with very narrow openings
Sterilization Act of removing or killing microorganisms; unable to reproduce
Supplemental In addition to the regular amount
Synovial fluid Joint fluid

Tachycardia Fast heart rate
Tensile strength Amount of tension that can be withstood before suture breaks
Thoracotomy Surgical incision into the chest wall between two ribs or through the sternum
Thrombin Protein in blood that aids in clotting by converting fibrinogen to fibrin
Tranquilizer Sedative
Transduction Conversion of the unpleasant sensation into electrical impulses by a free afferent nerve ending
Transmission Transports electrical impulses along nerve fibers to the nucleus caudalis of the brain
Transverse Horizontal plane of a surface; crossing from side to side
Tympanic membrane Eardrum

Ultrasound Sound waves greater than 20,000 Hz/s
Ununited anconeal process Anconeal process does not attach to proximal ulna
Urinalysis Laboratory analysis of urine to aid in the diagnosis of a medical condition
Urogenital Relating to the urinary and genital organs and their functions

Valgus Outward turning of a bone
Varus Inward turning of a bone
Viability Ability of an item or organism to live or survive
Visualization Ability to see a structure

Xiphoid Caudal end of the sternum

Index

a

abdomen
  clipping guidelines 52
  exam 14, 198
  instrumentation, retractors 105–106
  intestinal forceps 106
  patient preparation 52
  surgical procedures 52, 196–212
abdominal procedures 52, 106, 154
abdominocentesis 25
absorbable sutures
  monofilament 178–179, 219, 220
  multifilament 179
absorbable *vs.* nonabsorbable sutures 176–177
Adson forceps 100
alanine aminotransferase (ALT) 18, 19
alkaline phosphatase (Alk Phos) 18
allergies 1, 3, 10
alligator forceps 104, 110, 168
allis tissue forceps 105, 106
ALT *see* alanine aminotransferase
analgesics
  anti-inflammatory drugs 3, 38
  CRI 42
  cyclooxygenase (COX) 41
  DEA 42
  narcotic drug 294, 324–325
  NSAIDs 41, 42, 325
  University of Wisconsin Pain Scale 39
  “wind-up” 38
anal sacculectomy
  patient prep 57
  positioning 263
  surgical procedure 262–263
anesthesia recovery 289–290
antibiotics
  injectable broad-spectrum 37
  ovariohysterectomy/castration 37
Army-Navy retractor 103
arrhythmia 3, 14, 218
arthrocentesis
  IMPA 25
  synovial fluid 25–28
arthrogram 37
arthroscopy
  instrumentation 120–122, 222
  procedure specific duties 173
aseptic technique
  monitoring 193
  rules of aseptic technique 193
  source of surgical wound infection 273
aspartate aminotransferase (AST) 18–19
assistant “running” suture 181
AST *see* aspartate aminotransferase (AST)
attitude
  calming fears 7
  sedative agents 8
aural
  instruments
  patient preparation 57

Surgical Patient Care for Veterinary Technicians and Nurses, Second Edition.
Edited by Gerianne Holzman and Teri Raffel Kleist.

Companion website: www.wiley.com/go/holzman/patient

aural (*cont'd*)
  positioning
  surgical procedures 57
autoclave
  loading 145–146
  maintenance 146
  sterilization 143–146

b

Babcock intestinal forceps 106
Backhaus penetrating towel clamps 63, 97
bacterial contamination 273
Balfour retractor 105, 123, 173, 198, 199, 203, 208
bandage
  application 299–303
  scissors 95, 96
  tie-over 276–278
battery-operated orthopedic equipment 113
BCS *see* body condition score
biceps tendon conditions 12
blood urea nitrogen (BUN) 17, 19
body condition score (BCS)
  charts 5
  dogs and cats 6
  obese pug (BCS) 6
  thin pug (BCS) 6
bone cutters 113
bone graft site 159
bone holding forceps 159
bone plates 114, 117–120, 232, 248, 249, 251, 252
bone screws 113, 114, 117–120, 236, 249, 251, 252
boxes/hiding spots 293

c

cage height 293–294
canine body condition 323
canine rehabilitation therapist (CCRT) 327
cardiovascular system
  cardiac pathology 15
  femoral pulse 15
  sinus arrhythmia 14
  surgical conditions 256
cast
  application 310–311
  purpose 310
cautery *see* electrosurgery
CCL *see* cranial cruciate ligament
certified canine rehabilitation assistant (CCRA) 327
chemical burns 282, 287
chisels 111, 114
chlorhexidine 52, 59–61, 72, 74, 78, 127, 158, 314
chloroxylenol (PCMX) 74
circulating nurse/technician
  opening packs 188–192
  room set-up 187–188
circulating water blankets 69–70
cleaning solutions
  accelerated hydrogen peroxide 50
  potassium peroxymonosulfate 50
  quaternary ammonium compounds 50
  sodium hypochlorite 49
client compliance
  elimination 324–325
  exercise 325
  feeding 322–325
  hands-on demonstrations 321–322
  support devices 325–326
  written instructions 319–321
clipping
  description 51
  proper angle 51
  technician and surgeon, communication 51
colony forming units (CFU) 274
complete blood count (CBC)
  anticoagulant 18
  definition 18
  reference values 18
compressive layer 298, 301, 302, 306, 309, 310
computed tomography (CT) 28, 31–33, 212, 214, 217, 225, 227, 228, 230, 232, 233, 236, 238, 239, 245, 254, 255, 257, 258, 263
constant rate infusion (CRI) 42
contamination 21, 25, 27, 45, 46, 51, 58, 90, 113, 137, 150, 151, 162, 189, 190, 198, 204, 269, 272–274, 278, 279, 284, 290, 291, 293, 300, 313, 329
continuous suture patterns
  assistant "running" suture 180, 181
  simple continuous 180–181
convection warming systems 70

cranial cruciate ligament (CCL) rupture
  diagnosis 249
  radiographs 249
  "sit test" 9
  surgeries 250
creatinine kinase (CK) 20
CRI *see* constant rate infusion
Crile hemostatic forceps 99
Crile-Wood needle holder 102
cryotherapy 217, 233, 234, 236, 286, 329
cutting suture
  external 185
  internal 184–185
cyclooxygenase (COX) 41
cystic calculi 1, 2, 36
cystocentesis 21–24, 223
cystogram 36
cytology 27, 28, 217, 264

d

DCP *see* dynamic compression plate
Debakey thumb tissue forceps 101, 107
declaw bandage 241, 242
decubital ulcer 269
Derf needle holder 102
double pelvic osteotomy (DPO) 247
Dowling spay retractor 104
Doyen intestinal forceps 106
drills 113, 115, 117, 119, 123, 124, 171, 173, 227, 228, 230, 232, 233, 236, 238, 239, 244, 246, 250, 251, 253, 255, 256
dynamic compression plate (DCP) 117, 118

e

elbow dysplasia 222
electrical burns 287
electrolytes 18, 20, 197, 198, 200, 211, 278
electrosurgery 48, 49, 123, 159, 164, 167–170, 187, 188, 194, 198, 199, 201, 203, 208, 210, 212, 214, 218–221, 227, 228, 230, 233, 234, 236, 244–247, 249–251, 253, 254, 256, 258, 259, 262–264
enterogram 37
esophagram
ethylene oxide sterilization (ETO)
  description 147
  indicators 148, 149
event-related shelf life 150
exercises
  lower impact 331
  sit-to-stand and down-to-stand 331
  swimming 330
  underwater treadmill 330
external coaptation
  care and complications 312–313
  concepts 295–296
  considerations 297–298
  types of support 296–297
external skeletal fixation (ESF) devices 238, 295–298, 314–315

f

feeding instructions
  adverse foods 322
  canine body condition 323
  feline body condition 324
  gastrointestinal upset 322
  medical condition 322
feline body condition 324
femoral head and neck excision (FHNE)
final paint solutions, patient prep 60–61, 63, 72, 158
fine needle aspirates (FNA) 24, 27–28, 33, 217
Finochetto retractor 106
first intention healing 274
foam rubber pads 291
follow-up 320, 332–334
Ford interlocking continuous pattern 181
foreign bodies
  gastric 197–198
  intestinal 198
fractures
  casts 297, 298, 310
  clipping guidelines 55
  external coaptation 296
  external skeletal fixation (ESF) 296, 314
  internal fixation implants 110, 114
  patient preparation
  slings 315
  splints 297, 305–307
  surgeries 55, 57
fragmented coronoid process (FCP) 233–234
Frasier laminectomy retractor 124
Freer periosteal elevator

frostbite
- causes 286
- treatment 286–287

g

Gelpi retractor 108, 109, 250, 262
gloving
- assisted 89, 90
- closed 83–86
- double 90–91
- open 86–89
- removing contaminated gloves 90

glucometer 17
gowning 78, 80–83
grooved director 104

h

hammock beds 292
hand-held retractors
- Army-Navy 103
- description 102
- Senn 103

healing chronology, wound 270
heated surgery tables 69
heat therapy 329
hemostasis
- clamp securing 168
- energy source
  - monopolar 167
  - bipolar 167
- non-energy source 167, 169

hemostatic forceps
- description 98
- Kelly 99
- mosquito 98–99
- Rochester-Carmalt 99
- Rochester-Ochsner 99
- Rochester-Pean 99

hip dysplasia
- clinical signs and causes 243
- surgeries 243

Hohmann retractors 109, 238, 247, 249
home care, verbal instructions 319
honey 278, 279
horizontal mattress 182–184
hot air warming systems 71
Hug-U-Vac® positioning device 68

i

imaging
- computed tomography 31–33
- contrast studies 36–37
- magnetic resonance imaging 32–33
- personal protection 29
- radiographs 30–31
- ultrasound 33–36

immune-mediated polyarthritis (IMPA) 25
inflammation 10, 24, 41, 184, 249, 262, 270, 271, 273, 283, 329
instrumentation, surgical
- alligator forceps 104, 110
- allis tissue forceps 105, 106
- description 92
- Dowling spay retractor 104
- groove director 104
- hand-held retractors, *see* hand-held retractors
- hemostatic forceps, *see* hemostatic forceps
- lubrication 129–130
- maintenance 130–131
- manual cleaning 127
- manufacturing 92–94
- needle holders, *see* needle holders
- needle rack 104, 105
- pack
  - preparation 131–136
  - wrapping and instrument packaging 136–141
  - scalpel handles and blades 97–98, 164
  - scissors, *see* scissors
  - Snook spay hook 104
  - thumb tissue forceps, *see* thumb tissue forceps
  - towel clamps, *see* towel clamps
  - ultrasonic cleaning 127–129

instrument table 132, 154, 163–165, 171, 172, 190, 191
interlocking nails 114, 117, 230
internal fixation implants
- bone plates 117–120
- bone screws, *see* bone screws
- description 114
- interlocking nails 117
- orthopedic wire 115
- pin/bolt cutters 116
- wire twisters 115–116

interrupted suture patterns
  cruciate 183
  horizontal mattress 182–183
  simple interrupted 182
  vertical mattress 184–185
intestinal foreign body 198

j
Jacob's chuck 113
Jones towel clamps 97
juvenile pubic symphysiodesis (JPS) 245, 246

k
Kelly hemostatic forceps 99
knot tying (sutures) 182, 184

l
laparoscopic instruments 122–123, 207, 225
lavaging 163, 165–166
Lembert, Cushing, and Connell patterns 182
limb splint 305
locomotion assessment
  "bunny hops" 8
  grades 9
  lameness/gait abnormalities 8, 9
  "sit test" 9
Lorna (Edna) non-penetrating towel clamps 97
Lyme disease 10
lymphatic system 329
lymph nodes 10, 223, 264

m
malleable retractor 106, 201, 210, 212
Mallet 111, 137, 234, 245, 249, 253
manual cleaning 127, 129
Mathieu needle holder 94, 102, 103
Mayo dissecting scissors 95
Mayo-Hegar needle holder 102
medical history
  allergies 3
  current and prior medications 3
  diet 2–3
  mnemonic device 4
  parasites 2
  patient's lifestyle 3
  vaccinations 2
medications, current and prior
  stomach ulceration 3
  "wash-out" period 3
Metzenbaum dissecting scissors 95
Meyerding retractors 109
minimally invasive
  laparoscopy 223–224
  thoracoscopy 224–226
Modified Robert Jones (MRJ) 299, 303, 304
monofilament *vs.* multifilament sutures 177–178
mosquito hemostatic forceps 98–99
muscle atrophy 9, 329
musculoskeletal examination
  Achilles tendon 12
  biceps flexion test 12
  carpal hyperextension 11
  patella luxation 12, 14
  ROM 11, 13
  ulna 11

n
narcotic drugs 42
natural *vs.* synthetic sutures 43
needle holders
  Crile-Wood 102
  Derf 102, 211
  description 101
  Mathieu 94, 102, 103
  Mayo-Hegar 101, 102
  Olsen-Hegar 101, 102, 211
negative pressure wound therapy (NPWT)
  advantages 281
  disadvantages 281
  foam/gauze 281
  non-healing wound 281
  shear injury 280
nervous system
  brain and mental status 15
  conscious proprioception (CP) deficits
    hemi-standing/walking 16
  orthopedic or neurologic 15, 16
neurologic
  exam
  instrumentation 123–126
  patient prep 55
  positioning 154
  surgical procedures 55–56

non-absorbable suture
monofilament 179
multifilament 179–180
non-orthopedic draping
communication 160
contamination risk 162
fingers, folds 159–161
proposed incision site 160, 161
towel 159–162
non-steroidal anti-inflammatory drugs (NSAIDs) 41, 42, 325
nutritional support 284, 294, 329

o

OCD *see* osteochondritis dissecans
oil emulsion gauze 279, 298, 300
Olsen-Hegar needle holder 101, 102, 211
onychectomy, declaw 240
open wound
clipping 58
irrigation 227, 275
management 300
opening packs
glove pack 189–191
peel pack 191, 192
wrapped pack 188–190, 192
operating scissors 94, 95, 184
ophthalmic procedures
instruments 124–126
patient preparation 56
positioning
surgical procedures 215–216
oral pharynx 10
orthopedic
draping 162–163
implants
IM pins 115, 239, 255
plates 114, 239, 255
screws 239, 255
wire 95, 115, 256, 260
instruments 108–120
surgical procedures
clipping 54–55
forelimb 55
hindlimb 55
patient preparation 54–55, 63–65
orthopedic procedures 54, 55, 65, 91, 120, 159, 162, 195, 325
oscillating blade cast saw 311
osteochondritis dissecans (OCD)
arthrogram 37
distal humerus
cause 234
clinical signs 234
flap 234, 235
postoperative care 236
removal 235
proximal humerus 232–233
osteotomes 111, 137, 234, 245, 249, 253
oxidizing agents

p

passive range of motion (PROM)
muscle atrophy 329
proper technique
stifle extension and flexion 330
patella luxation 12, 14, 253, 320
clipping 55
patent ductus arteriosus (PDA)
after ligation 257
caudal lung lobe abscess 256
chest tube 256
Finochietto retractor 256
hemorrhaging 257
internal stapler 256
before ligation 256
oxygen cage 256
post lung lobectomy 256
patient draping
bone graft site 159
non-orthopedic 159–162
orthopedic 162–163
patient follow-up
chew bandages and casts 334
diarrhea 333
fentanyl patch/adhesive bandage 333
postoperative swelling 333
skin observing 333
patient positioning 66, 154
dorsal recumbency 66, 154, 155, 157, 197–199, 201–204, 206, 208, 210, 214–216, 218, 220, 224, 225, 227, 233, 234, 236, 238, 246, 249–253, 256, 259, 261, 264

instrument table 154
leg 25, 26, 64, 66–68, 155, 239, 261
leg tie with a half hitch on a limb 67
ophthalmic procedures 68, 155
patients in lateral recumbency 68, 206, 212, 214, 217, 224, 230, 233, 236, 239–241, 244–246, 249, 254–256, 258, 259
prep process 66
rubber rollers 66, 155
sandbags/vacuum aids 66, 68, 155, 156
on surgery table 66, 68, 155, 156
specific procedures 155
surgery table "V" 66, 155
thoracic positioner, dorsal recumbency 66
ventral recumbency 66, 158, 262, 263
patient preparation
abdominal procedures, *see* abdominal procedures
aural surgeries 57
clipping, *see* clipping
head and mouth procedures 57
neurologic procedures 55–56
open wound clipping 58
ophthalmic procedures 56
orthopedic procedures, *see* orthopedic procedures
perineal procedures, *see* perineal procedures
thoracic procedures, *see* thoracic procedures
patient prep patterns
orthopedic prep 63–65
perianal/perineal procedures 65–66
target pattern 62–63
patient skin preparation
description 59
surgical scrub products, *see* surgical scrub products
patient sterile prep 71–73
patient warming
alternative warming devices 71
circulating water blankets 69–70
convection warming systems 70
heated surgery tables 69
normal body thermoregulatory systems 69
solid warming pads 70
PCMX *see* povidone-iodine, chlorhexidine, and chloroxylenol (PCMX)
pelvis
fractures 230
hip dysplasia, *see* hip dysplasia
radiography 243, 245
surgical procedures 243–249
perforated mats 291–292
perineal procedures
patient preparation 57
surgical procedures 57–58
periosteal elevators 110, 123, 214, 227, 228, 230, 249, 252
persistent right aortic arch (PRAA) 224, 256–258
personnel preparation
attire 73–74
gloving, *see* gloving
gowning, *see* gowning
hand rub 74, 78
hand scrub 74, 78
hands and arms, drying 78–80
stress mats
pheromones 294
physical exam parameters 5
physical rehabilitation
goniometer and tape measure 327
orthopedic and neurologic 326, 327
osteoarthritis 327
physical therapy (PT) 327
range of motion 327
strength and balance training 328
pin/bolt cutters 116
plasma sterilization 147–148
pneumatic drill 123, 227
portosystemic shunt (PSS)
ameroid constrictor 203
cause and clinical signs 203
definition 203
instruments and postoperative care 203
surgical procedure 203
potassium peroxymonosulfate (Trifectant®) 50
Potts Smith scissors 107
povidone-iodine 52, 53, 59–61, 74
primary support 297, 305
primary wound cover 298, 300, 303, 304
pyoderma 10, 40

q

quaternary ammoniums compounds 50
quiet, alert, and responsive (QAR) 7

r

radiation exposure 29, 30
radiography
  abdomen 30, 31
  avian/reptile 31
  extremities 31
  OCD
    phosphor crystals
    spine/skull 31
    technique chart 30, 31
    thorax 30, 31
    x-ray photons 30
range of motion (ROM) 11–13, 67, 236, 239, 243, 246, 297, 327–329, 331, 332
rat toothed thumb tissue forceps 100
redness and skin irritation 329
reproductive
  Cesarean section
    gravid uterus 204
    postoperative care 204
    resuscitation of newborn 205
  orchiectomy 204–206
  ovariohysterectomy 206–207
respiratory system 14, 218–222
retractors
  abdominal
    Balfour 105
    malleable (Not found)
  orthopedic
    Gelpi self-retaining 108
    Hohmann 109
    Meyerding 109
    Weitlaner self-retaining 109
  thoracic
    Finochetto 106
    malleable 106
right-angle mixter forceps 107
rinsing agents, patient prep 60
Robert Jones (RJ) bandage 298, 303–304
Rochester-Carmalt hemostatic forceps 99
Rochester Ochsner hemostatic forceps 99
Rochester Pean hemostatic forceps 99
Roeder towel clamps 97
ROM *see* range of motion
ronguers 110, 113, 123, 227, 228, 236, 245, 253
Russian thumb tissue forceps 101

s

Satinsky/Cooley clamp 107–108
scalpel handles and blades 97–98, 164
Schroeder-Thomas splint (Not found)
scissors
  bandage 95, 96
  description 94
  Mayo dissecting 95
  Metzenbaum dissecting 95
  operating 94–95, 184
  ophthalmic 95, 96
  orthopedic 95
  suture removal 92, 96
second intention healing 274, 285
self-adhering tape 302
Senn double-ended, hand-held retractor 103
serum chemistry panel
  bilirubin 20
  calcium 19
  cholesterol 20
  creatinine 20
  glucose 20
  magnesium 20
  metabolic panel 18
  phosphorus 20
  protein 20
  reference values 19
  triglycerides 20
serum glutamic oxaloacetic transaminase (SGOT) 18
serum glutamic pyruvic transaminase (SGPT)
single-and double-action ronguers 110, 228
skin staples 185–186
slings 227, 228, 247, 249, 253, 290, 295, 315–317, 325, 326, 331, 332
snook spay hook 104
sodium hypochlorite 49
soft-padded bandages 236, 297, 299–301, 305–307, 310
solid warming pads 70
splints
  aluminum rods 306
  application 306–307
  pre-formed plastic/metal 306

purposes 305
spica 307–310
sponge/instrument count 171–173
staple remover 96
stenotic nares 10, 221–222
sterile patient prep 71, 157–158
sterilization process
autoclave 148
biological indicators 149–150
chemical indicators 148–149
EtO 147
glutaraldehyde 142
physical/chemical 142
physical monitors 148
plasma 147–148
steam 143–147
stifle
CCL rupture 12, 249–252
patella luxation 12, 14, 253
stomach ulceration 3
stress mats 91
stretch gauze 280, 299, 301, 302, 304, 307–311, 315, 316
subcutaneous ureteral bypass (SUB), *see* urinary surgical procedures
suction 21, 48, 49, 58, 127, 168–170, 187, 194, 197–199, 201, 203, 204, 208, 210, 212, 218, 220, 221, 224, 225, 227, 228, 230, 233, 234, 236, 242, 244–247, 249–254, 256, 262, 281, 321
supplemental support 296–297, 308, 310
surgical scrub products
chlorhexidine 59
for patient prep 59–60
povidone-iodine 59–60
surgical attire
beard covers 46
Bouffant hat 46
scrub suits 46
masks 47
shoe covers 46
surgeon's cap 46
surgical hood 46, 47
surgical instruments-passing to the surgeon
ring-handled 164–165
scalpel handle and blade 164
thumb tissue forceps 165
surgical site infection (SSI) 10, 47, 60, 273
surgical suite cleaning
in between cases 48
before the first case of the day 48
solutions, *see* cleaning solutions
terminal cleaning, end of day 49
surgical suite preparation 45
suture materials
characteristics 174–176
classification 176–178
sizing 176
suture removal scissors 92, 96
synovial fluid 25–28

t

tape stirrups 63, 298–300, 302
TA® reusable stapler 186
target prep pattern 62–63
Telfa® pads 279, 300
temperature, pulse, respiration (TPR) 5
anesthetic protocol 5
feline and canine 5
therapeutic exercises, *see* exercises
thermal burns
division 282
hyperthermia 282
treatment 283–284
third intention healing 274
thoracic
clipping guidelines 52, 54
exam 219, 221
instruments
retractors 106
scissors 106
vascular clamps 107
patient preparation 52–54
surgical procedures 256–262
thoracic procedures 51, 52, 54, 159
thyroidectomy
patient preparation
positioning 218
postoperative care 218
thumb tissue forceps
Adson 100
Debakey 101
description 99
rat tooth 100
Russian 101
tibial crest osteotomy 252

tibial plateau leveling osteotomy (TPLO)
  implants 251
  instrument set 251
  physical rehabilitation 251
  surgical procedure 251
tibial tuberosity transposition (TTT) 253
Tightrope® 250
total ear canal ablation (TECA) 212–214
total hip arthroplasty (THA)
  assistant's role 247
  instruments and template set 246–247
  postoperative care 247
  surgical procedure 246–247
total hip replacement (THR), *see* total hip arthroplasty
towel clamps
  Backhaus penetrating 97
  description 97
  Jones 97
  Lorna (Edna) non-penetrating 97
  Roeder 97
traffic, operating room 47
Trifectant® 50
triple pelvic osteotomy (TPO) 247–249

u

Ultrasonic cleaning
  process 129
  solution 128
ultrasound
  mechanical/electronic transducers 34
  shaving 33
  sound waves 33, 34
  transducer 33–35
United States Nuclear Regulatory Commission (USNRC) 29, 30
ununited anconeal process 11, 236
upper respiratory system
  elongated soft palate 218–220
  laryngeal paralysis 220–221
  stenotic nares 221–222
urethral blockage
urinalysis
  bladder infection 24
  catheters 21, 22, 24
  cystocentesis 21–24
  tests 24
urinary bladder care 294–295
urinary surgical procedures 208–212
urinary system
  calculi, *see* cystic calculi
  exam
  surgical procedures 208–212
  urolith 209
U.S. Army retractor 103

v

Vac-Pac® positioning device 68
vacuum-assisted closure (VAC) 280–282, 286
vacuum positioning aids 68, 155
vascular clamps
  Mixter 107
  Satinsky/Cooley 107
VCP *see* veterinary cuttable plates
ventral bulla osteotomy (VBO)
  patient prep 57
  positioning 214
  surgical procedure 57, 214, 215
veterinary burn card 284
veterinary cuttable plates (VCP) 118
V-troughs 29

w

Weitlaner self-retaining 109, 123
wire twisters 101, 115–116, 256
Wobbler syndrome 227
wound care 232, 239, 274–287, 296, 298, 311, 319, 320, 333
wound management
  care 274–282
  delays, healing 272–273
  inflammation 270
  maturation 272
  proliferation 270
  tie-over bandage 276–278
  types 269
  wet-dry bandage 277
  wet gauze 276
  wound cleaners 275
wrapping packs 138–141

x

X-rays *see* radiography